# PATIENT EDUCATION IN REHABILITATION

Olga Dreeben, PhD, MPT, PT
Associate Professor
Physical Therapy
University *of* North Texas
Health Science Center *at Fort Worth*

**JONES AND BARTLETT PUBLISHERS**
*Sudbury, Massachusetts*
BOSTON    TORONTO    LONDON    SINGAPORE

*World Headquarters*
Jones and Bartlett Publishers
40 Tall Pine Drive
Sudbury, MA 01776
978-443-5000
info@jbpub.com
www.jbpub.com

Jones and Bartlett Publishers
Canada
6339 Ormindale Way
Mississauga, Ontario L5V 1J2
Canada

Jones and Bartlett Publishers
International
Barb House, Barb Mews
London W6 7PA
United Kingdom

Jones and Bartlett's books and products are available through most bookstores and online booksellers. To contact Jones and Bartlett Publishers directly, call 800-832-0034, fax 978-443-8000, or visit our website www.jbpub.com.

Substantial discounts on bulk quantities of Jones and Bartlett's publications are available to corporations, professional associations, and other qualified organizations. For details and specific discount information, contact the special sales department at Jones and Bartlett via the above contact information or send an email to specialsales@jbpub.com.

This publication is designed to provide accurate and authoritative information in regard to the Subject Matter covered. It is sold with the understanding that the publisher is not engaged in rendering legal, accounting, or other professional service. If legal advice or other expert assistance is required, the service of a competent professional person should be sought.

**Production Credits**
Publisher: David Cella
Associate Editor: Maro Gartside
Production Manager: Julie Champagne Bolduc
Production Assistant: Jessica Steele Newfell
Senior Marketing Manager: Barb Bartoszek
Manufacturing and Inventory Control Supervisor: Amy Bacus
Composition: Publishers' Design and Production Services, Inc.
Cover Design: Kristin E. Parker
Cover Image: © Photos.com
Printing and Binding: Malloy, Inc.
Cover Printing: Malloy, Inc.

**Library of Congress Cataloging-in-Publication Data**
Dreeben, Olga.
 Patient education in rehabilitation / Olga Dreeben.
   p. ; cm.
 Includes bibliographical references and index.
 ISBN 978-0-7637-5544-7 (pbk. : alk. paper)
 1. Medical rehabilitation. 2. Patient education. I. Title.
 [DNLM: 1. Patient Education as Topic—methods. 2. Communication. 3. Health Promotion.
4. Occupational Therapy—methods. 5. Physical Therapy Modalities. W 85 D771p 2010]
 RM930.D74 2010
 615.8'515—dc22

2009001184

6048

Printed in the United States of America
13 12 11 10 09   10 9 8 7 6 5 4 3 2 1

*This book is dedicated to my mother, Ana.*

*As a health care provider, she treated her patients with skill, empathy, and compassion.*

*Those whom she touched will always remember her with love.*

# CONTENTS

# PREFACE

Rehabilitation interventions have evolved from simple treatments to restore basic function lost in injuries and diseases to the contemporary evidence-based professions of physical and occupational therapy. Both disciplines are dynamic professions founded on theoretic and scientific knowledge as well as logical applications to restore, maintain, and promote optimal physical function. In addition to the anatomy and physiology of the human body, advanced expertise is required in relation to the applied physics of human motion, the sequence of human development and behavior, the electrochemical aspects and function of nerves and muscles, the pathology of disorders, and many other complex concepts that concern rehabilitative care. Unquestionably, the proficiency needed in physical and occupational therapy expanded exponentially in the 20th century and will continue its further development in the 21st century. Professional education in physical therapy is presently at the graduate level with a doctoral terminal degree, and the same may be expected in the discipline of occupational therapy in the near future.

In addition to the increase in educational training for the rehabilitation practitioner, it has become widely recognized that patients must be actively involved in their own restorative process. The patient-centered approach to medical diagnostics and interventions has been given greater prominence with resultant successful outcomes. The need for more patient involvement in preventative health measures and promotion of optimal function is equally important. Recognition of these aspects of health care has increased the requirement for the health care practitioner to act as an educator as well as an expert clinician. It is the purpose of this text to explore various teaching and learning theories and models of instruction as well as communication, ethical, legal, and cultural variables involved in patients' education.

This book is organized into five sections that include 19 chapters. Section I, *Basic Concepts of Patient Education*, describes the significance of teaching and learning in health care and physical and occupational therapy as well as the historical development of patient education. This section also contains a definition of patient education for rehabilitation and an exploration of predictors that contribute to effective patient instruction. Section I is divided into five chapters: Chapter 1, "Significance of Patient Education for Health Care and Rehabilitation"; Chapter 2, "Historical Outlook of Patient Education in American Health Care"; Chapter 3, "Historical Outlook of Patient Education in Physical and Occupational Rehabilitation"; Chapter 4, "Patient Education in the Context of Physical and Occupational Rehabilitation"; and Chapter 5, "Predictors of Effectual Patient Education."

Section II of this book, *Patient Education Variables: Adherence, Communication, and Behavioral Modifications*, discusses adherence approaches and specific communication strategies for patient education. Appropriate communication methods and behavioral modification techniques are suggested. Section II is divided into three chapters: Chapter 6, "Patient Education and Adherence Variables"; Chapter 7, "Patient Education and Communication Variables"; and Chapter 8, "Patient Education and Behavioral Modification Variables."

Section III of this text, *Teaching and Learning Theories: Applications to Patient Education*, includes basic learning theories and their significance in patient education. Applications of educational strategies to the individual's stages of cognitive and psychosocial development are presented in this section. Section III is divided into four chapters: Chapter 9, "Main Teaching and Learning Theories and Patient Education"; Chapter 10, "Additional Teaching and Learning Theories and Patient Education"; Chapter 11, "Adult Learning and Patient Education"; and Chapter 12, "Cognitive/Psychosocial Stages of Development and Patient Education."

Section IV, *Ethical, Legal, and Cultural Variables in Patient Education*, emphasizes the major ethical, legal, and cultural aspects of patient education. Section IV is divided into four chapters: Chapter 13, "The Role and Significance of Ethical Systems for Health Care"; Chapter 14, "Morality and Values in Patient Education"; Chapter 15, "Ethical and Legal Aspects of Patient Education"; and Chapter 16, "Cultural Factors in Patient Education."

The final section of this book, Section V, is *Selected Topics in Patient Education: Examples in Rehabilitation*. This section describes specific learning approaches in motor learning and examples of instructional design applied to wellness and preventative care. Section V is divided into three chapters: Chapter 17, "Teaching and Learning Strategies for Motor Performances"; Chapter 18, "Patient Education for Older Adults Related to Exercises/Activities and Internet Utilization"; and Chapter 19, "Teaching and Learning Considerations for Wellness, Health Promotion, and Disease Prevention."

It is the author's hope that this text will help to expand the role of physical and occupational therapists and assistants as patient educators in achieving successful rehabilitative outcomes. The aim of *Patient Education in Rehabilitation* is to encourage therapists to become more aware of how they teach and how they might teach more effectively. Many of the teaching and learning concepts depicted here can be readily implemented while others may require some planning and modification. Nevertheless, each topic was chosen to stimulate the therapist's thinking about patient education and interrelated variables. This text also may be used as a reference in conjunction with material regarding patient evaluation, the planning of care, and interventions. The objective is to enable clinicians to assess and improve their teaching and learning skills by developing and applying various instructional strategies and approaches described in this book, ultimately to benefit the patients.

# REVIEWER RECOGNITION

Thank you to the reviewers of this text. Your voices, criticism, and support have truly made this a better text:

**Suzanne Robben Brown, MPH, PT**
Director, School of Physical Therapy
Touro University–Nevada
Henderson, NV

**Heather Hayes, DPT, NCS**
Assistant Professor (Clinical)
Rehabilitation and Wellness Clinic
Department of Physical Therapy
University of Utah
Salt Lake City, UT

**James Johnson, MD**
Professor
Canyon College
Carmichael, CA

**Michael T. Lebec, PT, PhD**
Assistant Professor
Department of Physical Therapy and Athletic Training
Northern Arizona University
Flagstaff, AZ

**Everett B. Lohman, III, DSc, PT, OCS**
Assistant Dean of Graduate Academic Affairs–SAHP
Orthopedic Track Coordinator, Entry-Level PT Programs
Director of Post-Professional PT Programs
Professor
Department of Physical Therapy, School of Allied Health Professions
Loma Linda University
Loma Linda, CA

**Nelson Marquez, PT, EdD**
Program Director
Physical Therapist Assistant Program
Polk Community College
Winter Haven, FL

**Tsega A. Mehreteab, PT, MS, DPT**
Clinical Professor of Physical Therapy
Department of Physical Therapy
New York University
New York, NY

**Marilyn E. Miller, PhD, PT, GCS**
Faculty, University of St. Augustine for Health Sciences
San Diego, CA

**Ann Greenan Naumann, PT, OCS, MS**
Physical Therapist
Fletcher Allen Health Care
Burlington, VT

# BASIC CONCEPTS OF PATIENT EDUCATION

Section I of this book, "Basic Concepts of Patient Education," describes the importance of teaching and learning in health care and physical and occupational therapy rehabilitation as well as the historical development of patient teaching and learning. Section I concludes by defining patient education within the context of rehabilitation and providing an in-depth exploration of predictors that contribute to effective patient instruction.

Section I is divided into the following five chapters:

Chapter 1: Significance of Patient Education for Health Care and Rehabilitation

Chapter 2: Historical Outlook of Patient Education in American Health Care

Chapter 3: Historical Outlook of Patient Education in Physical and Occupational Rehabilitation

Chapter 4: Patient Education in the Context of Physical and Occupational Rehabilitation

Chapter 5: Predictors of Effectual Patient Education

# SIGNIFICANCE OF PATIENT EDUCATION FOR HEALTH CARE AND REHABILITATION

## Objectives

After completing Chapter 1, the reader will be able to:

- Identify the significance of patient education in health care.
- Discuss the importance of patient education in physical and occupational rehabilitation.
- Compare and contrast the impact of patient education in health care and in rehabilitation.
- Understand the importance of patient education as related to health care and rehabilitation practices.
- Identify the general significance and benefits of patient education and health education.

## The Significance of Patient Education in Health Care

In contemporary health care, patient education is a patient's right and a health care provider's responsibility. U.S. governmental efforts regarding health and patient education are illustrated in the *Healthy People 2000* and *Healthy People 2010* initiatives. These initiatives have encouraged the United States as a whole to participate in health promotion and disease prevention through exercising, appreciating better health and fitness, avoiding workplace injuries, immunizing children against disease, and participating in preventive screening programs. The upcoming *Healthy People 2020* expands the goals for health promotion and patient or client teaching and learning by incorporating specific health objectives for various races and ethnicities. It also includes a larger, contemporary definition of the concept of health equality in relation to health risks caused by various genetic differences and predispositions to diseases or disorders.

## PATIENT EDUCATION VERSUS HEALTH EDUCATION

Patient education is a significant component of modern health care.[1] Patient education can be divided into two large categories—clinical patient education (or clinical teaching and learning) and health education. Clinical patient education is a planned, systematic, sequential, and logical process of teaching and learning provided to patients and clients in all clinical settings.[2] It is also a continuous teaching and learning process involving the health care provider and the patient or client (and/or the patient's family). The goals of clinical teaching and learning are based on the patient's assessment, evaluation, diagnosis, prognosis, and individual needs and requirements related to interventions.

Health education is also a teaching and learning process similar to patient education. However, it concentrates mostly on wellness, prevention, and health promotion. Additionally, health education can be provided to individuals, groups, and communities. The basic focus of health education is to change and improve societal health behaviors. In regard to both contemporary clinical patient education and health education, patients and clients are taking a more informed and active role in health care–related decisions. This new approach to health can be attributed to a variety of factors, including educational materials distributed by health care providers, the abundance of medical information found on the Internet, and clinicians' increased involvement in patient education. Furthermore, all health care providers have been learning new risk assessment techniques in the context of current health promotion and prevention. The illness-based thinking process has been changing to a risk-based one that involves the patient as a collaborator and partner of care, sharing responsibilities with the clinician.[1] The degree to which risky behaviors are reduced depends mostly on the patient's understanding of the significance of the risk and the importance of change. In this context, the primary role of the health care provider is that of patient educator and supporter, to better help patients progress and effect the needed life modification.

## THE PATIENT-CENTERED CARE MODEL

Health professionals are increasingly encouraged to involve patients in treatment decisions, recognizing patients as experts with a unique knowledge of their own health and their preferences for treatments, health states, and outcomes. Increased patient involvement in health care represents an important part of quality improvement of all health care organizations.[3] Patients' participation in health care assessments has been largely associated with better health outcomes. As a result, health care providers need to expand their patient-centered care practices. Modern health care has been evolving away from a disease-centered model toward a patient-centered model. The patient-centered approach demonstrates the highest quality of care, offering the most effective interventions, including education, for an individual patient.[4] In addition, care that is truly patient-centered considers patients' cultural traditions, personal preferences and values, family situations, and lifestyles. The patient and his or her family are an integral part of the health care team, actively collaborating with health care providers in making clinical decisions.[4] Consequently, patient clinical teaching and learning is essential in this context because it increases patients' responsibility for important aspects of their self-care, monitoring, and continuum of care. Patient-centered care also assures coordinated and efficient teaching and learning between health care professionals and providers involved in each patient's treatment.[4]

## THE BENEFITS OF PATIENT EDUCATION IN HEALTH CARE

Health care institutions are recognizing the benefits of patient education in improving patients' safety and adherence to interventions as well as patients' satisfaction. In contemporary health delivery, patient education has the potential to counter the rise in health care costs by reducing expenses and helping patients manage pricey chronic conditions. Adopting patient education programs can help health care providers and organizations produce better outcomes and enhance quality of care. Effective educational materials can help patients understand medical complexities while reducing anxiety and increasing compliance with instructions. Patient educational resources have the ability to change communication into actions and improve health. Furthermore, in modern health care, patient education is supported because it adds value to the management of various diseases and disorders. Specific interventions aimed at increasing the patient's knowledge can improve the treatment outcomes of many acute and chronic illnesses. For example, when they become ill, educated patients remain motivated and adherent with treatment programs.[1] Direct patient involvement in treatment decisions increases motivation, empowerment, adherence, and satisfaction.

Patients should receive education and training specific and appropriate to the care, treatment, and services provided. Patient education content should be personalized to each patient depending on cultural differences and specific needs.[1] Patient education should also be available in appropriate reading levels and be customizable to individuals. Successful patient education is the result of comprehensive, proven solutions that are thoughtfully set up by health care providers and integrated into the patient health care delivery system. Additionally, an efficient patient education program can yield better quality of care in fiscally responsible health care settings.

# The Significance of Patient Education in Physical and Occupational Rehabilitation

In the 21st century, patient education has become an important focus of health care provisions. Teaching and learning are essential concepts to be included in the patient's interventions. From the beginnings of organized rehabilitation services, rehabilitation providers have been using patient education practices to help individuals become actively involved in the goals, outcomes, and selection of interventions. Physical and occupational therapists and assistants, as providers of rehabilitative care, have also been involved in teaching patients. The role of the therapist in patient education has been enlarged to incorporate a variety of learning styles, theories, and educational strategies for patients and clients. Patient and family education is not just telling patients "what to do," but involves a more complex mechanism. This includes adequate selection of teaching and learning strategies to be able to make an impact on patients' outcomes in the clinic and in the continuum of care at home.

The role of physical and occupational therapists and assistants as educators is now becoming more central to their scope of practice than ever before. Therapists have a key role in patient teaching and learning. The focus of contemporary patient education is to help individuals and their families become informed participants to manage their own illnesses and to facilitate their adaptive responses to illness.[2] Additionally, while considering socioeconomic and cultural factors, rehabilitation providers must be able to teach individuals activities and techniques to perform in the clinical setting and at home, and also to facilitate health promotion and prevention measures.

Rapid discharge from acute care facilities is increasingly forcing patients to be more independent in managing their own health. Appropriate teaching and learning methods can increase patients' adherence with therapeutic rehabilitation programs and their independence in the community. Today, entering the second decade of the 21st century, clinical patient education and health education have been greatly enhanced in physical and occupational rehabilitation. Therapists use clinical teaching and learning regularly in their patients' examination, evaluation, plan of care, and interventions. The goal of rehabilitation providers is to help their patients learn about the disorder (disease) affecting them and actively participate in the planning of interventions. The overall scope is to assist their patients' return to participation in activities they need and want to achieve.

In regard to health education, many physical and occupational therapy practices have been increasingly focused on prevention and health promotion. Pre-diabetes and diabetes prevention is just one example of an area where the expanding teaching role of physical and occupational therapists is helping to positively change patients' lifestyles. Obesity (as a risk factor in American health) represents another important education topic for prevention. Rehabilitation professionals use patient teaching to design safe, effective fitness and wellness programs. Strong skills in ergonomics, work conditioning, and work simulation allow physical therapists to collaborate with occupational therapists in coordinating injury prevention programs and functional capacity evaluations in occupational health. Consultation services provided by pediatric occupational therapists promote assessments in technology and wellness, and a greater involvement in mental health interventions for pediatric depression and autism.

Physical and occupational therapists and assistants have been refining their skills not only to teach rehabilitative tasks to their patients, but also to improve the health of the population as a whole. Through health education and advocacy on behalf of their community, these rehabilitation professionals can support patients' individual needs as well as influence the policies and programs that affect the health of their communities. In the second decade of the 21st century, it is projected that the future of health care will go beyond eliminating health disparities to achieving health equity and also increasingly addressing environmental factors that contribute to individual and community health.

## THE BENEFITS OF PATIENT EDUCATION IN PHYSICAL AND OCCUPATIONAL REHABILITATION

Patient teaching concepts are an intrinsic part of interventions in the rehabilitation professions. For decades, physical and occupational therapists and assistants have been teachers of rehabilitative interventional programs and also health educators, promoting primary and secondary prevention. They have been helping their patients acquire a heightened awareness of risk behaviors and assisting and guiding them toward positive health behavioral changes. Today's health and patient education emphasize the patient's personal benefits of eliminating risk behaviors and exploring all viable options for a plan of behavior change. Physical therapists, as movement specialists, are able to identify risk factors that potentially can lead to physical impairments and functional limitations.

In physical and occupational therapy, the major purpose of patient teaching and learning is to increase the patient's competence to manage his or her own health requirements. The goals of patient education are to enhance the patient's self-dependence and the continuity of care in his or her own environment. For almost four decades, the physical therapy profession, as with other health care professions, has greatly increased its emphasis regarding patient education.[2] In the past, although patient instruction was considered an inherent part of physical therapy interventions, many therapists did not have sufficient training and experience to conduct appropriate patient instruction. Also, several decades ago, American health care did not emphasize the active role of the patient in the health care delivery system. Now attitudes have changed. Health care providers have the accountability and patients have the entitlement to appropriate education. Patient participation in treatment goal setting as a patient-centered care approach is recognized and valued by all rehabilitation professionals. Patient education is extended not only to the patient, but also to the patient's family and the community in which the patient lives. Patient education, educational theories, and various teaching and learning techniques have been an intrinsic part of physical and occupational therapy schools' curricula. The role of the physical and occupational therapist as a teacher is evident everywhere, including in rehabilitation research.[2]

In physical and occupational therapy, therapists' frequent clinical contacts with patients allow them to make a unique contribution to the patients' teaching and learning, helping them achieve planned intervention goals. In addition to patient education, therapists use health education to prepare wellness, prevention, and health promotion activities geared toward individuals and communities. Clinical patient education and health education are beneficial to all patients (**Table 1.1**).

| Table 1.1 | **Major Benefits of Clinical Patient Education and Health Education** |
|---|---|
| | Patient education enables patients to assume better responsibility for their own health care, improving patients' ability to manage acute and chronic disorders.[3] |
| | Patient education provides opportunities to choose healthier lifestyles and practice preventive medicine.[3] |
| | Patient education attracts patients to the provider and increases patients' satisfaction with their care, while at the same time decreasing the provider's risk of liability. |
| | Patient education promotes patient-centered care and as a result, patients' active involvement in their plan of care.[4] |
| | Patient education increases adherence to medication and treatment regimens, leading to a more efficient and cost-effective health care delivery system. |
| | Patient education ensures continuity of care and reduces the complications related to illness and incidence of disorder/disease. |
| | Patient education maximizes the individual's independence with home exercise programs and activities that promote independence in activities of daily living as well as continuity of care. |

# HISTORICAL OUTLOOK OF PATIENT EDUCATION IN AMERICAN HEALTH CARE

## Objectives

After completing Chapter 2, the reader will be able to:

- Describe the development of patient education in health care.
- Identify the transition from health education to patient education in the health care system.
- Outline the contributions of various organizations to the development of health and patient education.

## The Beginnings of Patient Education in the American Health Care System

Health and health care services in the United States have changed dramatically over the years. The American health care system has evolved from one symbolized by the country doctor with little, if any, training to one comprised of an incredibly complicated and sophisticated array of providers and institutions. The health care system today bears little resemblance to the health care services available in colonial America. During this time, epidemics of acute infectious diseases such as plague, cholera, typhoid, and smallpox struck entire communities and killed large numbers of the population. Many of these diseases were spread through impure food, contaminated water supplies, inadequate sewage disposal, and the generally poor living conditions of the time. Public health programs such as sanitation, purification of water, quarantine, and hygiene leagues only were established in the late nineteenth century. These programs were effective in drastically reducing the morbidity and mortality caused by epidemics.

## EARLY AMERICAN HEALERS AND PATIENT EDUCATORS

Patient instruction has been a part of health care since the first healer gave the first patient advice about treating his or her ailments.[5] Patient and health education in general have been an intrinsic component of the caring process for centuries. In colonial America, patient education was totally dependent on local resources and local healers. Caring for the sick was based mostly around the home and family, although at that time there was little health care that could be provided at home. Most health care was palliative and long-term while the disease ran its course. In 1658, the first informal American hospital with six beds was opened in a small poorhouse supported by a church in New Amsterdam.[6] This small hospital for the poor and the sick served approximately 1,000 inhabitants of Manhattan and is considered the forerunner of Bellevue Hospital in New York City.[6] However, the first documented American hospital was the Pennsylvania Hospital founded in 1751 by Dr. Thomas Bond and Benjamin Franklin.[6] The Pennsylvania Hospital cared for, and at the same time isolated, residents of Philadelphia who were sick, poor, and afflicted by mental illnesses.[6] Later, in 1798, the passage of a nationwide act for the relief of sick and disabled seamen established a federal network of hospitals for the care of merchant seamen.[6] This hospital network represents the foundation of today's U.S. Public Health Service as well as symbolizes the first official establishment of the American health education system.

## THE FIRST DEVELOPMENT OF ORGANIZED HEALTH CARE

The American health care system started to become organized for the first time around the middle to late 1800s.[6] During that time, community epidemics were still prevalent, with many Americans dying young from acute infections such as influenza and pneumonia. The first institutionalization of health care began around 1850 when the first large hospitals in New York (Bellevue Hospital) and Boston (Massachusetts General Hospital) began to flourish.[6] However, growth in the hospital field was still very slow. Prior to the mid-1800s, health care primarily consisted of an unorganized collection of individual services functioning independently, with little or no relationship to one another.[6] Hospitals were few in number, small in bed size, characterized by high mortality rates, and stigmatized as indigent care institutions whose role was to isolate the sick from the rest of society.[6] The majority of people who became ill were not ready or willing to use the health care facilities of the 1800s. The inadequate sanitary conditions in these facilities were viewed by the public as the last resort to medical care. The hospitals were actually considered a final alternative before death.[6] As a result, much of the care was still provided by members of the patient's family.

In regard to patient education in the 1800s, the health care provider's role was to teach the patient's family how to treat the patient at home and how to protect themselves from the disease, especially when caring for infectious and contagious diseases.[6] At that time, patient education was performed mostly by nurses and doctors. Nurses taught family members how to take care of the sick, proper sanitary precautions, and disease prevention. In addition, nurses who were in contact with the patient and patient's family more often than the doctor commonly were also able to interpret the doctor's instructions to the patient.[7]

## THE SECOND DEVELOPMENT OF ORGANIZED HEALTH CARE

In 1900, the average life expectancy in the United States was 47 years, and the most common causes of death each year were various infectious diseases.[6] During the beginning of the 1900s, the American health care system began to move forward with the introduction of the scientific method into medicine, symbolizing the second phase of development of the health care system.[6] Scientific discoveries and advances played a central role in the growth of medical treatments and surgical practices. Powerful diagnostic tools started to be developed, and new vaccines and antibiotic medications came into use. Medical knowledge increased, as did technological improvements, bringing in new concepts of health care. During this time, the American Medical Association (AMA) sponsored medical schools, trying to improve the quality of medical education and strengthen the licensing requirements of medical doctors. Better medical education, coupled with more effective surgery and treatment practices, permitted better trained physicians and surgeons to increase their intervention in disease processes.[6] As a result, patients' mortality rates decreased. Education programs in sanitation, immunization, and maternal and child health became important components of the U.S. public health system. These programs, taught by nurses, doctors, and other health care providers, created the U.S. health education system. The National League of Nursing Education described that in the 1900s, preventive and educational activities of public health nurses were considered to be the essential elements of public health work.[6] The health education provided in the 1900s became a precursor to modern patient and health education.

## THE THIRD DEVELOPMENT OF ORGANIZED HEALTH CARE

The third phase of development of the American health care system started after the Depression and World War II (WWII). The exceptional scientific accomplishments and the development of the civil rights movement after WWII resulted in profound changes in the country's health care delivery system. Before the war, most American physicians were still general practitioners. By 1960, 85% to 90% of medical graduates were choosing careers in specialty or subspecialty medicine.[6] The egalitarian spirit of post-WWII society originated a new view about health care delivery. Health care became a fundamental right of all citizens, not merely a privilege. This change in attitude was financed by the rise of third-party payers that brought more and more Americans into the health care system.[6] The social and organizational structure of health care concentrated on financing health, forming health insurance plans, and increasing the federal government's involvement in health care delivery services. The need for educating patients as part of organized health was growing.

# *The Introduction of Patient Education in the American Health Care System*

During the third phase of development of the American health care system, infections started to be replaced by disabilities and chronic diseases such as rheumatic fever, tuberculosis, and diabetes as sources of health disorders.[6] The military veteran population increased to 19 million individuals by the 1950s. More than 50,000 WWII veterans had tuberculosis.[6] As a result, the Veterans Administration (VA) hospitals started to offer for the first time *selected patient education* as part of total patient care. The term *patient education* was first documented in literature in the 1950s in relation to the VA hospitals.[7] In addition, public awareness of chronic diseases and disabilities increased. Moreover, the concept of health education expanded from disease prevention to management of chronic diseases and disabilities. For example, the National Tuberculosis Association started to teach patients and their families about the disease and its treatment as part of its public health service.[7] Many programs teaching the public about specific chronic diseases such as this became available. These programs were supported and funded by the federal government. Health education and patient education concepts were used interchangeably. Nevertheless, patient education was provided sporadically and on a case-by-case basis. As a separate concept of care, patient education was in its developing stage.

## INDIVIDUALIZED PATIENT EDUCATION

Still in the third phase of American health care development, private medical insurance companies like Blue Cross and Blue Shield began providing health care insurance to millions of middle-class citizens. In 1965, the U.S. government became involved in the financing of health care services with the passage of Titles XVIII and XIX of the Social Security Act, which created the Medicare and Medicaid plans, respectively. These programs were designed to pay for health care services for the medically needy, the aged, and the poor. Also, the concept of patient education evolved to focus on educating the patient to assume increased responsibility for maintaining personal health. Health care providers offered patient instruction for special patient groups who were treated for various diseases and disorders.[7] This instruction was different from health education. Patient education went beyond disease prevention and focused on the patient fully understanding the disease and its treatment. Patients were becoming consumers of health care, having responsibilities and rights at the same time. Toward the end of the 1960s, the American Public Health Association formed a committee that recommended patient education become an organized health care activity.[7] Patient instruction also had to be based on each patient's individual needs. In addition, the committee mentioned that the educational prescription for each patient should be included and remain as part of the patient's record.[7] Historically, this represented the first mention of *individualized patient education* as an organized health care activity.[7]

In 1971, the Department of Health, Education, and Welfare officially introduced the new concept of patient education by describing in its publication *The Need for Patient Education* the requirement for a more specific, individualized form of patient education.[7] This new concept included teaching patients to stay healthy and providing individualized information about diseases and treatments. The publication also recognized the need for a formal approach regarding patient education that would concentrate on a continuous organized program instead of on a sporadic, incidental basis.

# The Beginnings of Structured Patient Education in the American Health Care System

In the 1970s, patient education was officially included as part of organized health care in American hospitals. President Nixon appointed a committee to explore the feasibility of a public and private health education foundation.[7] President Nixon's committee mandated, through the Department of Health, Education, and Welfare, that hospitals offer patient education to patients and families of patients.

## PATIENT EDUCATION INCLUDED IN PATIENT'S BILL OF RIGHTS

President Nixon's committee also recommended that the American Hospital Association (AHA) had the obligation to provide educational programs for patients in hospitals or other health care institutions. These programs were required *to include all health professionals in patient education activities* in order to improve the quality of patient care, provide better utilization of outpatient facilities, and offer shorter lengths of stay and reduced health care costs.[7] Through all these educational programs, patient education during the 1970s started to affect not only the welfare of the patient, but also the health care delivery system.

In 1973, the AHA published the first *Patient's Bill of Rights*, authorizing that patients should receive information in understandable terms that would enable them to make informed decisions about recommended treatments or procedures.[6] Although the initial statement on a patient's rights did not specifically mention patient instruction, health care providers had to be able to explain the most important points of the diagnosis, treatment, and prognosis in terms the patient could understand. Consequently, patient education became the responsibility of the health care professional as well as the *patient's right*. Because patient education was recognized as a patient right and a necessary part of quality patient care, health professionals also were held legally liable for acts of omission or commission in regard to instructing patients and their families.[6] For example, the first legal court ruling to substantiate this patient right was applied in Iowa in 1974.[7] The court ruled that a physician who failed to advise a patient properly could be tried for negligence.

During the 1970s, patient education and health promotion were given increased recognition with the Canadian Lalonde Report of 1974 and the U.S. Surgeon General's *Healthy People* report of 1979.[8,9] Both reports addressed the notion that individuals play an important part in modifying behaviors to sustain or improve their health. To legitimize patient education even more, in 1975 the House of Delegates of the AMA adopted a formal statement that made patient education an "integral part of high quality health care."[7(p.28)] Although the AMA emphasized the role of the physician as the main education provider, other health care professionals such as pharmacists, nurses, dieticians, dentists, and rehabilitation practitioners were also considered responsible for patient instruction.[7]

In 1976, following President Nixon's committee report, the National Consumer Health Information and Health Promotion Act was signed into law by President Ford.[7] Consumer organizations became more alert to the possibility of increasing their right to receive quality products and services, including health care. Because of the consumer movement and the *Patient's Bill of Rights*, patients became more demanding about receiving information on their condition and treatment, and about becoming involved in decisions regarding their care.

## PATIENT EDUCATION INCLUDED IN THE ACCREDITATION MANUAL FOR HOSPITALS

The reinforcement of patient education as a right and expectation of quality health care was specified in the 1976 edition of the *Accreditation Manual for Hospitals* published by the Joint Commission (formerly known as the Joint Commission on Accreditation of Healthcare Organizations).[7] In the manual, patient education was expanded to include outpatient and inpatient services. The patient had the right to be informed of any technical procedure that needed to be performed, including the type of procedure, the reason for the procedure, and the person responsible for performing the procedure.[7] Also, the manual solidified patient education as an entitlement. This required the health care provider to make available to the patient information about the patient's medical problem, the type of problem, the prognosis, and the necessary treatment to be implemented.

The 1980s provided rapid and dramatic changes for the health care industry. Regulatory and competitive pressures, in addition to rising costs and developing technologies, pushed health care providers, payers, and consumers into new behaviors.[6] Providers behaved more defensively and payers behaved more aggressively, while consumers carried the burden of decreased public and private payer willingness to pay for health care services. This led to the business-imposed approach of managed care. For example, health maintenance organizations (HMOs), which were promoted in the 1970s as alternatives to fee-for-service medicine, began to introduce cost savings strategies limiting the utilization of medical services. Nevertheless, the largest benefit of managed care was that it forced the medical profession for the first time to think seriously about costs, encouraging greater attention to patients as consumers.

# National Health Education Programs

The 1980s were the beginning of an era of cost containment and reorganization of the methods of financing and delivering health care. Health care trends concentrated on disease prevention and the promotion of healthful behaviors. These developments brought about much good in regard to the growth of *national health education* programs. As a result of this, and also following the U.S. Surgeon General's *Healthy People* report of 1979, the U.S. Public Health Service issued the *Healthy People 2000: National Health Promotion and Disease Prevention Objectives* report in September 1990.[9,10] The document established specific goals for health promotion, disease prevention, and health protection in 21 critical areas. *Healthy People 2000* also called for the creation of data and surveillance systems to track progress towards the goals and established national health care objectives for a nation-wide patient education initiative.[10] In the U.S. health care industry, this document served as the basis for the development of state and community plans that laid the foundation for a national patient education agenda called *Healthy People 2010*.[10] The same as its predecessors, *Healthy People 2010* was developed through a broad consultation process, built on the best scientific knowledge of the time and designed to measure health programs over time.[10]

## TWENTY-FIRST CENTURY HEALTH EDUCATION PROGRAMS

The *Healthy People 2010* national initiative offers a powerful idea to provide health objectives in a format that enables diverse groups to combine their efforts and work as a team.[10] *Healthy People 2010* can be considered a *contemporary national health education* or patient education road map to better health for all. The Healthy People Consortium consists of more than 400 national membership organizations, all state and territorial health departments, and key national associations of state health officials working to advance health. Individuals, groups, and organizations are encouraged to integrate *Healthy People 2010* into their programs, special events, publications, and meetings.

The U.S. Department of Health and Human Services issued an addition to *Healthy People 2010* called *Communicating Health: Priorities and Strategies for Progress*.[10] This document enhances the two main goals of *Healthy People 2010*: to increase quality and years of healthy life and to eliminate health disparities by adding new action plans to American health care (**Table 2.1**).

The *Healthy People 2010* campaign supports health professionals such as physical and occupational therapists, providing improved, accurate, and understandable information to patients. Also, all rehabilitation providers are asked to encourage their patients to pursue healthier lifestyles and participate in community-based programs.

| Table 2.1 | *Healthy People 2010 New Action Plans*[10] |
|---|---|
| To improve all disease prevention. |
| To increase Internet access for specific populations. |
| To improve health literacy among policy makers and organizational leadership. |
| To increase research and evaluation of health communication activities. |

In the 21st century, patient education and health education are continuously expanding and evolving areas recognized as essential components of modern health care. Patient education and public or health education programs are among the fastest growing components of health care in the United States. Currently, patient education and health education programs are available in almost every health care institution. Although no exact numbers are available, it is assumed that, since 1970, the number of health educators also has greatly increased. More health care professionals, including rehabilitation providers, are completing professional preparation programs as well as participating in training and workshop programs to develop skills in providing effective, high quality clinical patient education and health education. In addition, patients and clients are becoming well-informed health consumers. It is estimated that annually more than 70 million Americans use the Internet to search for medically related Web site information pertaining to their health.

Patient education is growing among health care providers as well as with patients. Patient education invites patients to participate in decision-making aspects of their care using a patient-centered approach to health care. In this Internet age, health care providers are being challenged to take a proactive role in helping their patients find and understand medical information provided on Web sites. Ultimately, the future of patient and health education is for health care providers to build their own digital libraries and Web sites. Clinical patient teaching and learning and health education programs will enhance health care environments, making them safer, more effective, patient-centered, efficient, timely, and equitable organizations.

# HISTORICAL OUTLOOK OF PATIENT EDUCATION IN PHYSICAL AND OCCUPATIONAL REHABILITATION

## Objectives

After completing Chapter 3, the reader will be able to:

- Discuss the beginnings of patient education in rehabilitation professions.
- Describe how the Reconstruction Therapy era affected the development of patient education.
- Distinguish the American Physical Therapy Association's contribution to the progress of patient education.
- Explore the modern trends of patient education and health education in physical and occupational therapy.

## The Beginnings of Patient Education in Physical and Occupational Rehabilitation

Historically, patient education was not associated with rehabilitative interventions at the same heightened level as in nursing care. The reason may be related to the social and political trends that affected the health care industry for several decades. Health care policies requiring the integration of patient education in health care evolved slowly. Only after the middle of the 20th century, in the 1960s, did hospitals create positions for patient education coordinators.[5] During that time, education committees appeared, and projects were developed to provide evidence that patient education was having a positive impact on

American health care. In 1976, the Joint Commission (formerly known as the Joint Commission on Accreditation of Healthcare Organizations) specified that inpatient facilities must have a systematic, multidisciplinary program of patient and family education.[5] Therefore, inpatient facilities also included physical and occupational therapists and assistants in their multidisciplinary approach of patient education.

In the past there was little documented data to help trace the role of patient education in the evolution of rehabilitation in general, and in physical and occupational therapy in particular. Many health care professionals still consider patient education to be entirely part of nursing care. The reason for this assumption is related to the role of nurses who, for decades, educated patients and patients' families in care of the disease, prevention, nutrition, and personal hygiene. A 1937 curriculum guide in nursing emphasized that nurses were essentially teachers.[7] Also, the nurses' professional organizations and their practice acts required, as early as the 1950s, that nursing school curricula should prepare nurses to assume the role of teacher of others.[11] Furthermore, the nursing literature is filled with references about patient education, and much of the research in methodology and outcomes of patient education also has been done by nurses.[11]

Rehabilitation professionals such as physical and occupational therapists and assistants also have been teaching patients. It can safely be assumed that since the beginnings of rehabilitation, physical and occupational therapists have had an important role in preventing physical disabilities by educating and advising patients during their course of treatment. Patient instruction is considered an intrinsic part of the rehabilitation intervention process. When evaluating patient education in rehabilitation facilities, physical therapists have stated that the treatment is incomplete without an element of advice or education.[12] In addition, because physical and occupational therapists spend a large amount of time with patients, patients often seek advice regarding general health-related matters. Informally, through patient instruction, physical therapists as rehabilitation providers had been making a substantial contribution to general health education, including health promotion and impairment prevention.[13]

## HEALTH PROMOTION EDUCATION AT SARGENT SCHOOL OF PHYSICAL TRAINING

From a historical perspective, patient education most likely started during the Reconstruction Therapy era of World War I (WWI). Physical therapy training was initiated in 1881 at the Sargent School of Physical Training in Cambridge, Massachusetts.[14] The students at the Sargent School were professional masseurs and corrective exercise nurses who later became Reconstruction aides during WWI. At the Sargent School, students learned training techniques to strengthen and improve the physical capabilities of all people, including both disabled and healthy individuals. The school founder, Doctor Dudley Allen Sargent, was an innovator in physical conditioning and health promotion. Doctor Sargent also had a novel and deep-seated conviction in the importance of preventive medicine and comprehensive health, preparing the teachers and practitioners of physical and occupational therapy of the 19th and 20th centuries to impart information about disease conditions and prevention.[14]

## PATIENT INSTRUCTION AT REED COLLEGE

The role of patient education in physical therapy also was promoted by Mary McMillan, one of the first educators of physical therapy science and the founder of the modern national physical therapy association, the American Physical Therapy Association (APTA). McMillan can be compared in many ways with Florence Nightingale, the founder of modern nursing. Like Nightingale, McMillan understood the importance of proper conditions in hospitals to improve health care and to teach patients about the need for fresh air, exercise, and personal hygiene. An outline of the early physical therapy curriculum developed by McMillan at Reed College does not specifically mention education.[5] However, it may be assumed that at least some of the 66 hours of remedial exercises or 163 hours of clinical practice may have included the concept of teaching patients.[14] This assumption is supported by evidence that, during WWI, the heavy patient load necessitated that Reconstruction aides teach the injured to self-administer exercises.[5] Furthermore, the curriculum at Reed College included 10 hours of study of the psychological effects of injury and recovery.[14] This incorporated psychosocial forms of patient instruction to foster patients' adjustment and acceptance of changes[14] that occurred with injury. It is reasonable to assume that the Reconstruction aides used patient education for vocational training and to help the WWI soldiers' recovery process. For example, during the 10 hours of psychological studies at Reed College, the students were taught to use "cheerfulness against adversity and mental training to assist the badly wounded soldiers to forget the lost functions and cultivate new ones."[14(p.54)]

# *Organized Patient Education in Physical Therapy*

In the 1950s and 1960s, when physical therapists became autonomous for their educational curriculum, patient education was introduced as a criterion of the APTA's accreditation of educational programs. Physical therapy curricula emphasized courses in administration, education, and professional issues.[5] Later, as accreditation criteria changed from a focus on subject matter hours of instruction to the competencies expected of the graduate, the role of the physical therapist and later the physical therapist assistant as a teacher became better defined.

## PATIENT EDUCATION AS AN ACCREDITATION CRITERION

The first accreditation criterion related to education was developed by the APTA in 1978.[5] It stated that the physical therapy graduate should be able to apply basic educational concepts of learning theories in designing, implementing, and evaluating learning experiences in order to teach patients and families and to design and implement community education in-service programs.[5]

Although patient education was perhaps informally offered in rehabilitation care since its beginnings, because of health care trends in the United States and the APTA's accreditation efforts, for the last four decades, patient education has been formally recognized as part of standard rehabilitation interventions. In contemporary health care, it is essential that patients, clients, and their families are prepared to assume responsibility for self-care management.[15] In physical and occupational rehabilitation, the same as in nursing, the focus of care is on functional outcomes demonstrating the extent to which patients, clients, and their families have learned the knowledge and skills for independent living.

## PATIENT EDUCATION IN ITS EARLY YEARS

In the early years of patient education, patient instruction in all health care fields, including rehabilitation, was equivalent to giving directions or obtaining consent for procedures.[5] The education also consisted of information about medications, exercises, diet, or behaviors that need to be avoided, such as alcohol abuse and smoking cessation. In the 1950s and 1960s, medical information was considered extremely technical and beyond the patient's understanding.[5] Many health care providers genuinely believed that patients did not want to know details about their conditions. Although some health care providers informed their patients about their disorders, the information was very limited. In addition, the patients were considered passive recipients of care and were expected to perform what they were told without asking questions. These patients were considered adherent or nonadherent, depending on how well they followed the provider's instructions.[7,11]

In the 1950s and 1960s, patient education literature concentrated on the evaluation of the efficacy of instruction in the care of patients.[5] The research studies changed many health care providers' attitudes in regard to patient instruction because they showed that patients wanted to learn about their conditions and have control of their health decisions. One of the first articles emphasizing the importance of teaching as a fundamental part of the treatment process appeared in the physical therapy literature in 1958.[5] The article described that physical therapists appreciated patient education but they were not fully committed to the concepts of teaching and learning.[5] The problem was that besides knowing *what* to teach, the therapists had to be able to know *how* to teach the material. The authors of the article also promoted the importance of involving the patient in the learning process and adapting the learning activities to the needs of the patient.[5] The 1958 article's results (of therapists being unsure of teaching and learning concepts) are understandable for their time. Many physical therapy providers of the 1950s were not trained in how to provide teaching and learning. In addition, specific health and patient education topics were taught only as early as the mid-1970s in the physical therapy curricula.

# *Contemporary Patient Education Trends in Physical and Occupational Therapy*

For at least four decades, the Commission on Accreditation in Physical Therapy Education (CAPTE), as part of the APTA, has considerably increased its emphasis on the teaching and learning concepts of the professional physical therapy curriculum.[15] Physical therapy graduates must be able to effectively educate others using culturally appropriate teaching methods that are appropriate to the needs of the learner.[15] Physical therapy education also must be based on students' foundational knowledge and skills in educational theory, health promotion, fitness and wellness programs, health education, and health behavior.[15] Physical therapy educators have been designing learning experiences for their students that go beyond traditional clinical settings to being actively engaged in health education in diverse settings.[16] Physical therapy students have been learning to be involved in patient and health education and also in health promotion not only with their individual patients, but also with the communities in which they live.[16]

## PATIENT EDUCATION DEVELOPMENTS IN PHYSICAL THERAPY EDUCATIONAL PROGRAMS

Currently, all physical therapist education programs devote a large amount of attention to patient education. Some programs do a better job than others by also including and developing patient education procedural skills for physical therapy students.[17] For example, some schools, besides teaching students concepts of teaching and learning, have the students demonstrate patient education during the practical exams, as well as show evidence of these skills in their clinical affiliations. At present, many clinical educators have increased their emphasis on teaching students and giving them feedback in how to modify their level or type of language when talking to patients.[17] Physical therapists and physical therapist assistants are trained to be able to effectively educate others using culturally appropriate teaching methods that are commensurate with the needs of the learner.[18] Also, the physical therapist's plan of care should be patient-centered, including a collaborative problem-solving approach with the patient. Patient instruction may also consider teaching the patient self-management skills, especially for chronic diseases or disorders. This form of education may improve outcomes and also reduce cost.

Clinical educators can offer students actual teaching environments to integrate their patient education school curricula with clinical practice. In the clinical settings, students have opportunities to learn from their clinical instructors and from patients how to effectively model the role of the therapist as a teacher.[19,20] Reciprocal teaching and learning is facilitated by "creating and sustaining therapeutic alliances with patients"[20(p.314)] and accurately understanding their health beliefs. Students' clinical experiences when teaching and learning could be successful or unsuccessful, especially when selecting patient education strategies. Nevertheless, the primary sources for learning about patient education in the clinical practices are patients, clients, caregivers, families, clinical instructors, other health care professionals, and students' continual reflection about their experiences in teaching. The first step for students to be able to learn from their patients is to create therapeutic partnerships with the patients. After that (and using various educational approaches), students can facilitate patient learning by taking into account patients' cultural, social, and economic differences. For every student, the most significant factors for becoming a proficient clinician and teacher are: (1) self-reflection of successes and failures when trying to understand patient's needs; and (2) self-growth and development during clinical experiences.[19,20] Students' reflective journals about teaching and learning with patients can provide deliberate exploration of reasons for challenges in patient education processes.[20]

## PATIENT EDUCATION DEVELOPMENTS IN PHYSICAL THERAPY CONTINUING EDUCATION

More and more therapists, who in the past received little education about teaching and learning concepts, are starting to appreciate continuing education programs about how to teach effectively.[18] Those therapists feel that the role of the teacher in current rehabilitation care is growing quickly, as is evidence-based practice (EBP). EBP is important because it incorporates new ideas and research findings into the professional body of knowledge. The EBP literature found that, in general, all physical therapists approve the use of evidence-based findings in clinical practices.[19] However, there is a difference in the therapists' understanding of the importance of EBP. For example, younger therapists with the highest professional degrees who had been licensed for fewer years were more likely to say that EBP is necessary because it improves patient quality of care and also reimbursement rates.[19] Therapists with baccalaureate degrees as their first professional or highest degree were less likely to understand the terms involved with EBP than those with a postbaccalaureate professional degree or an advanced master's degree or doctorate as their highest degree.

The EBP understanding phenomenon may be the same in regard to patient education. All rehabilitation providers are increasingly recognizing the importance of patient teaching and learning. They know that patient education is an instructional requirement of contemporary health care trends. However, many therapists need to gain more knowledge about multiple methods of transmitting information to their patients. All rehabilitation clinicians must be aware that in order to serve their patients more effectively, they need: (1) to be able to inform each patient about their condition and how to deal with it; (2) to address the patient's understanding; and (3) to ensure that the patient has access to necessary information or materials.[18]

In modern health care, physical therapists whose training included little or no patient education find that continuing education courses can facilitate their use of the patient-centered care model. This model, also called the patient-practitioner collaborative model, can help the clinician to better focus on interventions that are dependent not only on the condition (disorder), but also on the patient's needs and wants.[21] Connecting with the patient in a therapeutic relationship and appreciating the patient's beliefs are essential elements in the establishment of a plan of care for interventions that also incorporates patient-needed teaching and learning strategies.[21] Knowing a patient's belief system helps set priorities and maximize resources.[21] As a result, physical therapy clinicians can achieve effectual health outcomes including patient adherence with interventions and health promotion activities.

## CONTEMPORARY TRENDS OF PATIENT EDUCATION IN PHYSICAL THERAPY

In the current health care environment where efficiency, effectiveness, and cost containment are considered major factors, patient education is an extremely significant function in the rehabilitation process. The focus of physical and occupational rehabilitation is on facilitating patient independence, increasing patients' self-management, and continuing rehabilitation in the patients' own environment. This requires the therapist to have the knowledge, skills, and attitudes to design effective and efficient education programs that will improve the patients' health and quality of life. Teaching is an important and, at the same time, difficult skill. In physical therapy, teaching was described to be similar to research.[20] Comparable to research, teaching requires careful planning, rigorous design, systematic implementation, analysis of results, and communication of outcome.[20] As an introduction to the teaching and learning process, it has been established that effective teaching with students or patients involves several steps that may include the teacher's ability to comprehend the material, deliver the information in an understandable and interesting format, and engage the learner in an active educational process (**Table 3.1**).

In physical and occupational therapy, teaching and learning are two inseparable processes and must work well together. At any given moment, the patient, the therapist as the rehabilitation provider, or the patient's family member can be the learner or the teacher. The teacher's role can also depend on the learner's style of acquiring information. With physical therapy teaching and learning, three events typically must occur (**Table 3.2**). These are related to the teacher's knowledge and experience and his or her ability to use different educational techniques and assist the learner in gaining the necessary knowledge.

Physical therapists of the 21st century, through professional education or continuing education courses, are becoming more familiar with the complex process of patient education. They are starting to better understand patient instruction that requires a variety of inputs and the need to accept the significant role of active listening, teaching, and learning, as well as using evaluation and intervention tools that have a patient-centered approach in physical therapy practice. The APTA's *Guide to Physical Therapist Practice* incorporates patient-related instruction as part of physical therapy procedural interventions in every clinical setting including musculoskeletal, neuromuscular, cardiovascular and pulmonary, and integumentary practices.[22] The guide's position also establishes that physical therapists educate patients, clients, students, facility staff, communities, and organizations and

| Table 3.1 | **Effective Teaching Concepts**[21] |
|---|---|
| The teacher deeply comprehends the information to be taught. |
| The teacher transforms and presents the information in a format that is understandable for students. |
| The teacher engages the student in active collaborative learning experiences. |
| The teacher teaches the student how to learn by using constant inquiry and reflection. This helps the student acquire his or her own knowledge and comprehension. |

Table 3.2

## Events that Facilitate Teaching and Learning[21]

The teacher should (1) understand the topics very deeply; (2) have a passion for the topics; and (3) continually seek new knowledge in order to reflect on new experiences.

The teacher should know his or her students very well in order to be able to effectively impart the information to them (by capturing their curiosity and interest).

The teacher should be acquainted with various educational techniques to facilitate learning for diverse groups of students.

agencies. In addition, therapists provide consultative services to health facilities, colleagues, businesses, and community organizations and agencies.

Rehabilitation professionals' roles are growing to include complex and demanding teaching that goes behind disease pathology, wellness, fitness, and prevention. Issues such as a patient-centered approach to care, patient compliance and motivation, continuity of care, cultural competency, illiteracy, and accurate application of teaching and learning in patient education permeate the current health care delivery system. These issues increase the need for trained physical and occupational therapists and physical and occupational therapist assistants to properly teach others and help them learn in this modern era of health care reform.

## CONTEMPORARY TRENDS OF PATIENT EDUCATION IN OCCUPATIONAL THERAPY

Historically, occupational therapy may have included better organized patient education practices when compared with physical therapy. The reason could be related to the fact that the domain of occupational therapy consists of role function in seven occupational areas where teaching and learning have been closely integrated with rehabilitative interventions. *Occupational Therapy Practice Framework: Domain and Process* describes seven areas of occupational therapy practice consisting of activities of daily living, instrumental activities of daily living, education, work, play, leisure, and social participation.[23] The focus of occupational therapy is on patient engagement in occupation. As a result, occupational therapists are very involved in patient education to actively help facilitate patients' engagement.

Patient teaching and learning are essential in occupational therapy interventions. Patient teaching is used to communicate goals and objectives. In occupational therapy, patient teaching does not commence in the acute phase of illness or injury but later in the convalescent stage, when the patient is returning home.[23] As in physical therapy, patient education consists of several topics that may include description of disorder (etiology and prognosis), provision of interventions (self-care or ways to prevent recurrences), and provision of information to patient and family about community services and resources.[23] For patients with long-term conditions, patient teaching and learning is more complex, involving adherence to taking medications, wearing corrective splints, and following home programs of exercises or activities.

The professional education of occupational therapists, similar to physical therapists, places particular importance on communication and the patient teaching and learning processes.[23] Occupational therapy development in health education also includes prevention programs to maintain the community's health and to help individuals function in the presence of unfamiliar environments.

For the 21st century, occupational therapy's goals are trying to provide innovative and modern interventions that place value on teaching skills and tasks most meaningful to patients and clients. Patients' needs have been changing from simple to more complex skills and tasks. Consequently, patients' teaching goals are shifting from patient education for self-care to patients' active involvement in societal life. Additionally, new areas of practice have been emerging in patient education and health education, teaching compensation techniques for hearing and visual deficits. Educational opportunities for occupational therapists and assistants may also be found in newer specialties of disease prevention and health promotion such as home and business modifications for wellness and life and job coaching.

# PATIENT EDUCATION IN THE CONTEXT OF PHYSICAL AND OCCUPATIONAL REHABILITATION

## Objectives

After completing Chapter 4, the reader will be able to:

- Describe patient education in relation to the nursing profession.
- Explore the definition of patient education in relation to the practice of physical and occupational rehabilitation.
- Value the unique characteristics of patient teaching and learning in rehabilitation.
- Explain the modified ASSURE paradigm for a teaching plan of care.

## Major Considerations When Defining Patient Education

In general, when discussing patient education, a variety of terminology has the same meaning. For example, the terms *patient education* and *patient instruction* are used interchangeably in the nursing field.[11] Also, language such as *educating*, *instructing*, and *teaching* the patient, or *providing information* to the patient also applies to patient education. In *Taber's Cyclopedic Medical Dictionary*, patient education encompasses health information and instruction to help patients learn about general and specific medical topics such as preventive services, healthy lifestyles, proper use of medications, or home care of various injuries and diseases.[24] This seems simple when relating patient education to the multifaceted aspects of modern health care. Contemporary health care policy advocates patient education as an essential aspect of health care delivery. Patient education is recognized as a fundamental tool of treatment and is mandated by health care accrediting agencies and health care payers. In health care, patient education is described as the responsibility of every health care professional and provider, and also as a part of total health care including inpatient, outpatient, or emergency settings.[11] In the nursing literature, the patient education process is explained as an intricate part of transmitting information based on a systematic, sequential, logical, planned course of action.[7]

## PATIENTS' RIGHTS TO OBTAIN EFFECTIVE PATIENT EDUCATION

In regard to patients' rights to obtain patient education, the consensus found in nursing (**Table 4.1**) also applies to rehabilitation care.[7] Patients must always receive education that serves their individual needs. The teaching must meet their goals and aid in their recovery. Additionally, the teaching should be organized and properly planned and be documented in the patients' records.

Patient instruction was historically considered mostly a major function of the family physician and nurses, so patient education definitions are described in the nursing literature as the process of (1) influencing patient behavior and producing changes in knowledge, attitudes, and skills necessary to maintain or improve health; (2) assisting people to learn health-related behaviors so they can incorporate those behaviors into their everyday life; and

| Table 4.1 | *Patients' Rights Regarding Patient Education[7]* |
|---|---|
| Patients have the right to patient education that provides information about their condition and interventions, procedures, possible side effects or complications of interventions, alternatives to the interventions, and prevention and health maintenance. |
| Patients should receive education based on their individual needs. |
| Patients should receive education that will help them achieve the goal to increase their health status. |
| Patients should receive education that is part of an organized and planned activity. |
| Patients should receive education that will be included in their medical records. |

(3) helping patients and clients achieve the goal of optimal health and independence in self-care.[7,11] These descriptions show that health care providers are able to apply effective patient education only through behavioral changes. It means that patients have to be motivated, feel a strong alliance with the provider through establishment of a therapeutic relationship, and be able to acquire the necessary knowledge from the provider in order to make a commitment to their behavioral modifications. The difficulty arises when the health care provider is not formally prepared to apply patient education in clinical settings.

## HEALTH CARE PROVIDERS' INSTRUCTIONAL SKILLS

Considering the professional advances of physical and occupational therapy sciences at the clinical master and doctoral levels, patient education is expected to be rendered in a proficient and experienced manner. However, although patient education is an essential aspect of care, many health care providers do not have the necessary instructional skills to provide effective patient education. For example, in physical therapy rehabilitation, therapists generally have knowledge of a specific topical area to teach procedural skills to patients, such as ambulation, therapeutic exercises, and balance. Also, they are able to provide empathy, establish a therapeutic relationship with the patients, and use proper communication abilities. Nevertheless, sometimes particular teaching and learning skills may be missing. Effective patient education requires the therapist to also be able to facilitate the learning process and the patient's attainment of knowledge. In addition to good assessment, communication, and organizational and social skills, effective patient teaching and learning also require the ability to assess the learner and his or her needs, provide an environment conducive to learning, and actively involve the learner in the education process.

In physical and occupational rehabilitation, as was discussed previously, formal patient education using teaching and learning theories is still a relatively new form of intervention. For example, physical therapy literature from the early 1990s shows that some rehabilitation providers still believed that patient education consisted only of the development of home exercise programs for their patients.[25] Some providers also assumed that the establishment of a therapeutic relationship with the patient represented a form of patient education. Although the literature found that most physical therapists teach 80% to 100% of their patients, most of the time their instruction consisted of range of motion and strengthening exercises, home programs, and treatment rationale using demonstration and verbal discussion.[25] Also, most of the therapists understood the importance of assessing the effectiveness of teaching during patient education by asking the patient to demonstrate what was taught. However, for these therapists, the teaching and learning aspects were not considered to be as important as establishment of a therapeutic relationship with the patient. Developing a trusting relationship with the patient had a relative importance of almost 100% while determining the patient's learning style had a relative importance of 79%.[25] Additionally, the most used teaching method was verbal discussion or demonstration. The effectiveness of the therapists' teaching skills was assessed having the patient demonstrate the material.[25] Approximately 76% of the time, the therapists used objective standards to assess patient improvement because of their teaching efficiency.[25]

Rehabilitation providers such as physical and occupational therapists are constantly aware that patient education is important for successful rehabilitation. Nevertheless, many therapists are not formally prepared to apply teaching and learning concepts to their clinical skills. One study found that in the early 1980s, only 65% of physical therapy education programs included some preparation for teaching activities.[26] The major skills incorporated in the physical therapy courses were writing objectives, planning experiences, lecturing, demonstrating, giving and receiving feedback, writing home programs, and assessing learning expectations. In modern health care, teaching and learning are improving considerably. Contemporary rehabilitation clinicians believe that clinical expertise involves, among other skills, being able to properly provide patient education in the clinical settings. For example, studies from 2000 and 2003 established that physical therapy clinicians who were considered experts in the profession valued the most the ability to provide successful patient education.[27,28] These rehabilitation clinicians assumed a patient-centered approach to care that improved both the effectiveness of care and patient satisfaction. They also understood the significance of teaching methods in patient education and the relationship between patient instruction and patient empowerment.[28]

##  Constructing a Definition of Patient Education

When constructing a definition of patient education, the rehabilitation literature provides a great deal of input. For example, literature from the early 1990s found that patient education consisted of five educational elements:[25]

1. Teaching and informing the patient about the illness

2. Instructing the patient to perform home exercises

3. Giving advice and information about illness-related behavior

4. Providing general health education

5. Counseling the patient about stress-related problems

These five general elements used in daily private physical therapy practices for individual patients coincide with some of the patient instruction basics suggested by the *Guide to Physical Therapist Practice*.[22] Another report from the mid-1990s described patient education as consisting of:[2]

- A description of the illness (causes, prognosis, diagnosis, and complaints)

- Instructing the patient to perform home exercises

- Advice and home information (regarding rest, correct posture, work, sports, hobbies, self-care, health services, and aids and appliances)

- Providing general health education

- Counseling the patient about stress-related problems

The most current patient-related instruction from the *Guide to Physical Therapist Practice* describes patient education as a process of informing, educating, or training patients, clients, families, significant others, and caregivers to promote and optimize physical therapy services.[22] Patient education in physical therapy must be relevant to the current patient's condition and all other patient variables such as impairments, functional limitations, disability, risk factors, wellness, and fitness (**Table 4.2**).

Patient-related instruction may include education and training of patients, clients, family and/or caregivers regarding the following:[22]

- Current conditions such as the pathology and pathophysiology of the disease (disorder or condition)

- Impairments, functional limitations, and disabilities

- Performance enhancement

- Plan of care

- Health, wellness, and fitness programs

- Risk factors for pathology and pathophysiology of the disease (disorder or condition)

- Patient's transitions to new roles

- Patient's transitions across care settings

| Table 4.2 | **Specific Requirements of Patient Education in Physical Therapy[22]** |
|---|---|
| Patient education must be related to the current conditions. |
| Patient education must be related to specific impairments and functional limitations or disabilities. |
| Patient education must be included in and correlated to the plan of care. |
| Patient education must be associated with the need to enhance the patient's performance. |
| Patient education must be related to patient's transition to a different role or setting. |
| Patient education must be related to risk factors for developing a problem or dysfunction. |
| Patient education must be able to improve the patient's health, wellness, and fitness. |

There are several specific benefits of patient teaching and learning in physical and occupational rehabilitation settings (**Table 4.3**). These benefits assist patients or clients to acquire the best possible rehabilitative health care.

Patient education must be appropriate for individuals with impaired arousal, attention, or cognition that may have an impact on learning and memory, and for those with sensory impairments (such as vision or hearing loss) that may affect learning and skill acquisition. Patients may also require instructional or educational assistive technology (such as large print cards) or environmental accommodations or modifications (such as enhanced lighting or using sign language). In occupational therapy, similar to physical therapy, patient education must be individualized and appropriate for the patient's psychological readiness and acceptance level. Also, patient instruction should be suitable to the educational and cognitive levels of the patient and family members, and be sensitive to and understanding of the patient's sociocultural issues, cultural background, and preferred methods of learning. All these elements and contemporary trends in rehabilitation helped this author

| Table 4.3 | *Specific Benefits of Patient Education in Physical Therapy* |
|---|---|
| | Patient education optimizes patient's interventions and decreases impairments, functional limitations, and/or disabilities. |
| | Patient education affects patient's personal goals for improved performance. |
| | Patient education reduces the risk factors that caused the pathology and pathophysiology of the disease (disorder or condition), and the impairments, functional limitations, and/or disabilities. |
| | Patient education identifies and addresses prior to and throughout the interventions the patient's potential learning barriers (such as beliefs, language, and cultural expectations). |
| | Patient education identifies the patient's impairments, functional limitations, and/or disabilities that need assistance (such as caregiver, family member, or equipment) in order to achieve effective learning and skill acquisition. |
| | Patient education provides instruction and education about the plan of care to the patient's support system. |
| | Patient education improves health, wellness, and fitness programs. |

create the consistent definition of patient education in physical and occupational therapy rehabilitation (**Table 4.4**).

# *Establishing a Plan of Care for Patient Teaching*

In order for teaching activities to be appropriate for each learner, the therapist needs to have an examination and evaluation tool that can be used to determine the patients' impairments and functional limitations, but also to determine the patient's teaching and learning needs. For example, in nursing care, the patient education process starts in the patient examination procedures by establishing the patient's learning needs, readiness to learn, and learning styles.[11] The same process can be applied to the initial examination and evaluation in rehabilitation. For example, in physical therapy, the determination of physical therapy diagnosis and plan of care (POC) can include the development of a *teaching POC* based on a patient/therapist-generated teaching and learning plan. The teaching POC may consist of development of teaching and learning activities mutually predetermined with the patient, or if not cognitively possible, with the patient's family, significant other(s), or caregiver(s). During the intervention process, the planned and organized teaching activities can take place using specific instructional methods and tools appropriate to the patient. The modification and redirection of interventions will also take into consideration (in addition to the patient's changes in condition/disorder) the patient's changes in regard to knowledge, skills, behaviors, and beliefs conducive to rehabilitation and general health. The modified ASSURE paradigm model used in nursing care can also be applied to the dynamic process of physical and occupational therapy examination and evaluation when designing the teaching POC for/with the learner as well as during the procedural interventions (**Table 4.5**).

Establishment of a teaching POC (designed with/for the learner) in the initial examination and evaluation can also contribute to improvement of patient education, as well

| Table 4.4 | **Definition of Patient Education in Physical and Occupational Rehabilitation** |
| --- | --- |
| | Patient education in rehabilitation consists of patient-centered, -designed, and -organized teaching and learning activities appropriate to the needs and goals of the learner and intended to facilitate the patient's voluntary adoption of skills, behaviors, or beliefs conducive to high quality rehabilitation and good health. These teaching and learning experiences are part of the rehabilitation interventions across all settings for all patients. |

| Table 4.5 | Modified ASSURE Acronym for Physical/Occupational Rehabilitation[11] |
|---|---|
| **A**nalyze the learner. | |
| **S**tate the teaching POC (designed with/for the learner). | |
| **S**elect teaching methods and educational materials for the learner. | |
| **U**se teaching methods and educational materials during interventions. | |
| **R**equire learner performance. | |
| **E**valuate and re-evaluate the teaching POC. | |

as to patient readiness to assume greater responsibility for his or her care. Patient-centered POC including the teaching POC means care and instruction that is respectful of and responsive to individual patient preferences, needs, and values, which are some of the key ingredients of health care quality. As a result, patients will increase their motivation, performance, and adherence with interventions.

# PREDICTORS OF EFFECTUAL PATIENT EDUCATION

## Objectives

After completing Chapter 5, the reader will be able to:

- Recognize the importance of adherence in the health care delivery system.
- List the major adherence variables in physical therapy research.
- Compare and contrast the three predictors of adherence in patient education (motivation, self-efficacy, and locus of control).
- Understand the complexity of patient satisfaction in patient education, especially in relation to patient participation in the goal-setting process.
- Determine a patient-centered approach to patient education that achieves patient empowerment.
- List the challenges of patient-centered education and patient empowerment.

## The Importance of Adherence in Patient Education

Patient education has been shown to improve patient adherence with interventions, outcomes, and satisfaction. When teaching and learning principles are applied correctly, patient education becomes more effective at increasing patient adherence. In addition, when other tools such as personal counseling, verbal instruction, referral to education specialists, written materials, and audio- and videotapes are applied to patient education, patient adherence also is increased. In the medical context, the term *adherence* (or *compliance*) refers to a patient both agreeing to and then undergoing some part of his or her treatment program as advised by the doctor or other health care provider. Adherence also is a means to an end, an approach to maintaining or improving health as well as managing symptoms and signs of disease/ disorder. Adherence is a complex behavioral process strongly influenced by the environments in which patients live, health care providers practice, and the health care systems that deliver the care exist.

In the medical literature, adherence or compliance most commonly applies to patients taking their medication (drug adherence); however, adherence also relates to the use of surgical appliances, chronic wound care, rehabilitative interventions such as exercises or gait training, and forms of behavioral therapy such as counseling.[29] In regard to the term *compliance*, the literature explains it as an act of submission or yielding to predetermined goals.[7] Some health care providers view noncompliance as a health care professional's term for disobedience, likening the provider-patient relationship to that of a parent and child. The provider's expectation that the patient surrenders to the medical model is still a central problem with the way some health care professionals think about adherence, especially when patients are unwilling or unable to follow the health care provider's instructions. The contemporary theories of health communication do not view the patient as a generic, rational receiver of care and information, but rather as a complex individual who constructs very personal and unique meanings about health and disease.[30] The contemporary health care trends also give patients the right to their own health care decisions and to not follow predetermined courses of action. Patients are the best source of information about attitudes, beliefs, and lifestyle issues affecting their acceptance of medical treatments. Many health care providers prefer to use the term *adherence* instead of *compliance*. Nevertheless, some health care literature suggests that *compliance* is a constructive term comparable to achievement of a goal based on a preset regimen.[7] Compliance may also convey the extent to which a patient follows recommendations given by his or her health care professional.[31] For these reasons, the terms *adherence* and *compliance* are used interchangeably in the health care literature and research. In this text, for reasons of consistency, the term adherence will be used throughout.

In health care, adherence is significant for many reasons, including in the treatment of older people or people with chronic diseases who need to manage aging changes or chronic conditions. Other reasons include using adherence when trying to prevent developing diseases or complications of diseases and when trying to reduce the risk of injuries. Because of cost containment, adherence is also important for patients who are discharged early from hospitals and need to learn how to manage their conditions and treatments at home. Patients' adherence with treatment recommendations, especially when trying to control chronic disease, has been shown to decrease morbidity and permanent disability.[7] A patient's failure to adhere to the recommended treatments can result in disease progression, development of complications requiring expensive and prolonged hospitalization, and even possibly increased morbidity and mortality.

Another consideration regarding adherence is patients' failure to keep initial appointments and the follow-up engagements. Failing to show up to a scheduled appointment can have serious consequences for the patient and the health care provider. The patient can lose the time that was put aside for tests or other diagnostic procedures and the opportunity to receive a correct diagnosis and prognosis. On the other hand, the provider will be anxious that they missed the problem-solving aspect of proper diagnostics. As a result, a patient arriving late or totally ignoring an appointment increases the risk of early stages of disease going undetected or of a simple medical problem becoming a major one for lack of early intervention. In American health care, typically patients' failure to keep follow-up appointments after discharge from inpatient facilities is the reason for more frequent readmissions and rehospitalizations than occurs with patients who visited their physicians for a regular follow-up check-up.[30] Missed specialist referral appointments cause postponement of diagnosis regarding grave diseases and illnesses that, in the long run, may increase patients' morbidity and mortality.

## CLASSIFICATION OF NONADHERENCE

There are three classifications of nonadherence or noncompliance in health care: type I, type II, and type III (**Table 5.1**). Nonadherence types I and III can originate from an essential misunderstanding between the health care professional and the patient. Type I occurs because the patient does not understand the provider's instructions or recommendations at all, whereas type III occurs because the patient does not understand the rationale behind the instructions and is also unwilling to blindly comply. Type III nonadherence takes place mostly when a patient's beliefs about interventions or medications clashes with the health care professional's recommendations. For example, the parents of children with asthma often do

| Table 5.1 | *Classifications of Nonadherence*[32] |
|---|---|
| Type I | Unwitting nonadherence when the patient does not understand the medical advice that he or she is given. |
| Type II | Erratic nonadherence when the patient understands and wants to adhere to the interventions or therapy but has difficulty doing so because of personal circumstances, a complicated regimen or program, or just forgetfulness. |
| Type III | Nonadherence as a result of health beliefs in which the patient or patient's family considers the health professional's instructions incorrect and is thus trying to alter or discontinue the interventions. |

not want to administer medication to their children to prevent asthma attacks, preferring to conserve the drug to administer it during the attack.[29] In this example, the patient viewed the physician's prescription as a guideline rather than a treatment standard. In nonadherence type II, the patient wants to comply with the health care provider's suggestion, but often the conditions or the environment surrounding the patient may be in conflict with his or her adherence.

## ADHERENCE IN HEALTH CARE

When patients do not adhere with health recommendations, both patients and the health care system suffer. The worst examples of nonadherence in health care are related to the patient not taking a prescribed medication. For example, acute conditions such as infections can often be cured with short courses of medications as a required treatment. Typically, antibiotics function to kill the bacteria causing the infection. Because the symptoms of an infection may disappear altogether even if a certain amount of bacteria remains in the system, many infected individuals discontinue the antibiotic use early in the treatment.[29] As a result, the surviving bacteria become resistant to the antibiotic, proliferating succeeding generations of bacteria that are more resistant to the already used antibiotic medication. Eventually, the bacteria will evolve into a strain completely immune to that particular antibiotic. This causes antibiotic-resistant infections that can lead to illnesses that are extremely difficult to cure.[29] Additionally, in the area of communicable diseases such as tuberculosis or human immunodeficiency virus (HIV), society as a whole is at risk when a patient fails to adhere to treatment, resulting in the development of resistant strains that may prove incurable.[29] Patients with psychiatric illnesses such as schizophrenia or bipolar disorder may feel entirely well when they are stabilized on medication but are at risk of relapse if they discontinue the medicine.[32] Patients taking antihypertensive medications may experience severe high blood pressure if they discontinue the medication abruptly.

In the United States, at least half of the patients who have been given a prescription do not receive the full benefit of the medication because they do not take the medication at all, do not take the recommended dosage, or stop the medication prematurely.[33] Poor adherence to medication is a recognized medical problem costing an estimated $100 billion per year.[34] Also, poor medication adherence causes approximately 125,000 unnecessary deaths and over 1 million hospitalizations annually.[30] Patients with chronic diseases such as arthritis, diabetes, or hypertension have the worst medication compliance. For example, drug nonadherence for arthritis is between 50% and 71%; for diabetes it is between 40% and 50%, and for hypertension it is 40%.[33] Medication or treatment nonadherence increases morbidity, exacerbates the disease, adds to the number of needed physicians' visits and hospitalizations, and raises mortality rates. As a result, nonadherence increases use of health care services, decreases productivity through lost work days, and ultimately escalates health care and insurance costs.[7] The National Pharmaceutical Council and the Institute of Medicine report that the health expenditure attributable just to patient nonadherence is between $75 billion and $100 billion annually.[33] These figures do not include the cost increases associated with bacterial resistance (because they are difficult to accurately quantify).

## ADHERENCE IN REHABILITATION

In rehabilitation, in regard to terminology, the physical therapy literature prefers to use the term *adherence* instead of *compliance*.[35,36] The terms *adherence* and *cooperation* appear in the literature as a better choice (instead of compliance) to avoid considering patients as passive recipients of rehabilitative care. Adherence is described as a complex concept affected by over two hundred factors. The major factors encountered in physical therapy may include attitudes, knowledge, beliefs, needs, rewards, and barriers to interventions, such as pain or difficulty performing the activities.[5] Rehabilitation research shows that adherence is affected by several variables such as the patient's attitude toward the illness or disability, the relationship between the therapist and the patient, the type of disease or condition, the patient's impairments and functional limitation, the complexity of the rehabilitation program, the patient's coping mechanisms, and the degree of lifestyle disruption that affects adherence.[5,35–40] In physical therapy rehabilitation, it seems that the most important adherence variables are the patient's illness, his or her beliefs and attitudes, the therapist's behavior, and various sociodemographic factors (**Table 5.2**).

When relating adherence to certain sociodemographic characteristics, the results of studies were found to be contradictory.[37,38,41] For example, the results of one study indicated that educated young women are less compliant with home exercise programs (HEPs) than less educated ones.[35] Among young men, adherence is not related to education; highly educated and less educated young men are equally adherent with interventions.[41] Other findings were that patients with trauma or postoperative conditions adhere to rehabilitation better than do patients with systemic conditions or back, neck, or shoulder pain.[38] Also, patients with a high degree of disability adhere better with HEPs than patients with less interference from the illness.[37] Most of the time, patients' beliefs and attitudes are found to be the biggest nonadherence factors.[40,41] The belief that the interventions or prevention strategies are not important cause the patient not to come back to physical therapy

| Table 5.2 | *Adherence Variables in Physical Therapy Rehabilitation* |
| --- | --- |
| | Factors related to the patient's sociodemographic characteristics. |
| | Factors related to the relationship between the patient's beliefs and attitudes and adherence. |
| | Factors related to physical therapists' behavior such as establishing a therapeutic relationship or offering positive feedback. |
| | Factors related to the patient's perceived barriers and helplessness. |

or to stop the exercises altogether. Pain or discomfort during exercises or activities also may cause nonadherence issues. Physical therapists' behaviors are significant variables in patients' adherence, especially when offering positive feedback with interventions (such as exercises and activities) and being able to establish a therapeutic relationship with the patient.[38,40]

Other major variables causing nonadherence in physical therapy are the barriers and problems that patients may perceive, lack of positive feedback, and patients' perceived helplessness.[38] The strongest of these factors are the barriers that patients may perceive. In relation to exercises, these patients' perceptions are that the exercises are time consuming, are not adjusted to their particular situations, and do not fit into their daily routines.[38,39] Some patients admit that their nonadherence to exercises is caused by forgetfulness. Tiredness at the end of the day, a busy schedule in general, and complaints of pain with exercises are other variables found in physical therapy literature in regard to nonadherence. Additionally, patients' attitude toward the illness and the type of disease can be a problematic factor of adherence, especially when patients have chronic diseases or injuries. During periods of disease remission, when the symptoms are absent, patients lack relevant cues to continue with treatment.[38,41] When patients perceive that the disease or the injury is serious, they feel vulnerable and perform the prescribed interventions more readily.

Adherence to physical therapy rehabilitation is also enhanced when patients establish a positive relationship such as a partnership with the therapist. Furthermore, an adherence variable can also be related to the extent to which patients perform the clinical and home prescribed intervention programs. In addition, patients with an external locus of control (believing that health and illness only slightly depend on their own behavior) appear to be less adherent to interventions than those with an internal locus of control.[37] (Locus of control is discussed in more detail in the following section.)

In physical therapy rehabilitation, therapists should be able to use clinical patient education and health education to restore, maintain, and promote not only each patient's optimal function, but also optimal wellness, fitness, and quality of life as they relate to movement and health. Adherence can be a major element to accomplish these goals, both during the rehabilitation process and after rehabilitation during the continuity of care phase.

Similar to health care, older adults have difficulty adhering to treatments prescribed in HEP regimens.[37] The reasons for nonadherence are explained by the patients as insufficient time, lack of social support, no place to exercise, no transportation to an exercise site, fear of falling and injury while exercising, and insufficient funds to buy exercise equipment or join an exercise facility.[37,38] However, apart from patients' individual rationalizations, the main factors for adherence in physical therapy from the patients' perspective seem to be psychological predictors such as motivation and motivating factors.[37,38]

## *Predictors of Adherence in Patient Education*

In patient education, the variables that most influence adherence are psychological factors such as motivation, self-efficacy, and locus of control.[41–43] Patients will have difficulty establishing goals without being motivated or becoming confident in their ability to learn new skills and behaviors. In patient teaching, the rehabilitation provider can use motivation to guide the patient to participate in the learning process and to sustain his or her enthusiasm for acquiring new skills. Self-efficacy allows the patient to successfully produce behaviors leading to successful outcomes. Patients with low efficacy expectations will have difficulty performing tasks and learning new information. As a result, they will try to avoid situations in which they feel unable to cope. Patients who believe in their ability to learn to perform specific skills or behaviors will be able to accomplish their actions. The term *locus of control* often is used interchangeably with *self-efficacy*; however, the terms are not equivalent. Whereas self-efficacy focuses on the perception of ability to act competently and effectively, locus of control focuses on the perception of control. A patient with an internal locus of control will believe that the rehabilitation outcomes are related to his or her behavior and active participation in the learning process. Patients with an external locus of control will consider that their abilities in physical therapy performances are controlled by outside forces such as luck or the power of prayer.

The following sections will discuss these three elements of adherence in more detail.

## ADHERENCE AND MOTIVATION

Evidence of motivation can be assessed by the patient's willingness or readiness to take the necessary action (**Table 5.3**). Motivation is also a process in which internal and external factors direct and strengthen thoughts, feelings, and actions.

Motivation is what encourages an individual to move in the direction of meeting a goal. This can derive from a combination of personal and social factors, including personal goals or incentives, expectations of personal efficacy, movement-related perceptual and affective experiences, and social and physical features of the environment.[41] Motivation is a crucial predictor of adherence in many areas of health care research including nursing,[34] cardiac rehabilitation,[41] pharmacology,[42] physical therapy,[38,43–45] ophthalmology,[46] psychiatry,[47] and psychology.[41,48] These literature search results are explained by the fact that, in general, adherence with medical recommendations is based mostly on the patient's motivation or readiness to act.

Motivation as a predictor of adherence is dependent on several types of variables, including cognitive, affective, physiological, and environmental. As examples, the cognitive variables for motivation are the patient's capacity and determination to learn including constructive attitude, desires, inquisitiveness, and willingness to acquire positive

Table 5.3

### *Definition of Motivation*[41]

Motivation is a psychological force that moves a person to take action in the direction of meeting a need or goal.

behavioral outcomes. A patient's perception of the importance of interventions is also a cognitive variable in determining whether to follow or not to follow the recommendations.

Affective elements contributing to motivation are the relationship and interaction between the patient and the health care provider. The significance here is based on the provider's empathy, partnership, and establishment of a therapeutic relationship with the patient. Patient satisfaction with the provider's explanations and treatment is also a positive feature of patient-provider interaction.

Physiological variables of motivation are related to the characteristics of the disease. Asymptomatic types of diseases and sometimes poor functional capacity of the patient in severe diseases lead to poor motivation and decreased adherence with interventions.[38] Opposite to it, the higher the patient's perception of the gravity of the disease consequence, the greater his or her motivation may be.

Environmental factors affecting motivation are sociodemographics such as age, gender, education, and household income. As an example in pharmacology, older patients showed higher motivation to adhere to medications than did younger female patients, especially those with low education status and low family income.[42] However, sociodemographic variables are contradictory in research and do not always have a strong predictive relationship to motivation.

## ADHERENCE AND SELF-EFFICACY

In addition to motivation, self-efficacy (**Table 5.4**) is another essential factor that affects a patient's adherence.[41]

According to social cognitive theory, self-efficacy is a proximal, direct predictor of a person's behavior.[41] Self-efficacy is a construct based on cognitive and behavioral concepts and also describes an individual's perception of his or her skills and abilities and whether the skills/abilities produce effective and competent actions.[41] Self-efficacy influences perceptions of actions and coping behaviors and the choice of environments and situations in which the individual will attempt to access.[41] Psychologists believe that there is a reciprocal relationship between cognitive process and behavior change in self-efficacy theory.[41]

The concept of self-efficacy encompasses two components—efficacy expectations and outcome expectations. Efficacy expectations refer to an individual's conviction that he or she can successfully produce the behaviors that will lead to a desired outcome; outcome expectations refer to an individual's belief that a particular course of action will produce a certain

| Table 5.4 | **Definition of Self-Efficacy[41]** |
| --- | --- |
| | Self-efficacy is a person's belief or confidence in his or her ability to succeed at making a change. |

outcome.[41] Efficacy expectations have an effect on one's choice of settings, behaviors, and persistence. For example, in physical therapy, a patient with diabetes and low efficacy expectations will likely avoid seeking exercises as interventions because he or she feels unable to follow them. Instead, the patient will seek out situations he or she feels able to handle, such as taking medication for the diabetes.

Persistence in producing behaviors is also affected by efficacy expectations. Individuals who have high levels of efficacy expectations will be more likely to persist with behaviors when they become difficult and will therefore be more likely to execute the behavior successfully, which in turn increases their efficacy expectations even more. On the other hand, individuals with low levels of efficacy expectations will be more likely to cease production of behaviors once the behaviors become difficult, which will in turn reinforce their already low efficacy expectations. The concept of self-efficacy is also situation-specific, meaning that an individual will have a range of both high and low self-efficacy expectations at any one time depending on the specific situation, task, or behavior.

Psychological research in cardiac rehabilitation found that patients' self-efficacy beliefs about their ability to exercise in spite of various barriers (such as bad weather or lack of time) predicted their adherence to the recommended exercises.[41] Self-efficacy is also cognitively dependent on the importance of the task. Depending on the health scenario and the importance of the action for adherence, patients may exhibit different levels of self-efficacy. For example, a patient who has diabetes and is overweight may be convinced of the importance of losing weight but has a low level of confidence based on previous failure to lose weight or keep weight off. By contrast, a patient who has hypertension may be confident that taking the antihypertensive medication will lower blood pressure, although he or she is not convinced of the importance of the action. A deficiency in the importance of the action or task can lead to a patient's unwillingness to commit to change and be motivated.

For long-term maintenance related to either exercises or keeping weight off, the literature shows that the power of self-efficacy or task importance becomes weak.[40,41] The same happens in regard to responsibilities that patients find to be very complex. As an example, maintenance of regular physical activity for 3 months in cardiac rehabilitation after a myocardial infarction was found to be a complex task when related to the exercise intensity and frequency.[41] The reason is that physical activity requires not only the patient's motivation, but also self-efficacy with respect to self-regulation of action in the face of barriers that occur when an individual has to reschedule and reorganize his or her daily life. Psychologists found that patients' strong beliefs about their ability to maintain the tasks and recover from a decline in task performance help to increase their motivation and self-efficacy with cardiac rehabilitation.[41,48]

Cognitive social theory says that two factors can modify an individual's behavior—belief in the efficacy of the proposed intervention and belief in self-efficacy for the acquisition of a given behavior.[42] The strongest factor is the intensity of belief in self-efficacy. This factor determines the initiation of behavior modification and the effort required to modify the behavior. Perceived self-efficacy derives from four sources (**Table 5.5**): personal experience, the experience of others, persuasion, and physiological and affective states.[41]

| Table 5.5 | *Sources of Self-Efficacy*[41] | |
|---|---|---|
| Personal experience | In terms of success, relates to personal accomplishment or mastery. | |
| Experience of others | Knowing another individual in the same situation who successfully mastered a difficult situation. | |
| Persuasion | Experienced through verbal persuasion by others, in which experts or others try to convince the individual that he or she can be successful. | |
| Physiological and affective states | Involve emotions, such as anxiety during a threatening situation, that make the individual incapable of mastering the situation. | |

Physical indicators of efficacy are particularly pertinent in dealing with physical challenges. Among all these sources of perceived self-efficacy, the most powerful factor described in physical therapy is the personal experience, when an individual's own actual performance history can affect the interventions.[49] To improve a patient's perceived self-efficacy, physical and occupational therapists can use therapeutic programs that build on a base of successively more difficult performance accomplishments. These intervention programs help to promote a patient's sense of personal responsibility for his or her accomplishments.

The literature reveals that perceived self-efficacy is also associated with the modification of numerous behaviors, such as perseverance in smoking cessation, weight control, and adhering to preventive behaviors.[48,50] Perceived self-efficacy has a positive impact on adjustment to illness and to the interventions. In rehabilitation, perceived self-efficacy can improve adherence to interventions in the clinic and at home.

In nursing, self-efficacy is increased through establishment of a therapeutic relationship with the patient.[34] In rehabilitation, the therapeutic relationship allows the patient and the therapist to agree from the beginning of treatment to short- and long-term goals that need to be achieved over a defined period of time, while taking into account the preferences, constraints, and skills of the patient. Moreover, patient achievement of the goals is an important source of self-efficacy. At this point of success, the patient is ready to undertake more difficult behavioral modifications that would help the interventions. Even before the patient successfully meets the goals, the fact that the goals, preferences, and capacities are taken into account when establishing a contract with the patient in the initial evaluation is a significant source of self-efficacy for the patient.

## ADHERENCE AND LOCUS OF CONTROL

Another predictor of adherence is *locus of control*, also called health locus of control (**Table 5.6**).[50] The concept of locus of control was developed in psychology and transposed to the field of health science under the name of health locus of control.[50] Locus of control can be either internal or external. Individuals with an internal locus of control believe they control their own destiny. They also believe that their experiences are controlled by their own skill or efforts. Individuals with an external locus of control believe that someone or something else more powerful controls their destiny.

In regard to health locus of control, individuals believe that their health is controlled by either internal or external factors. Patients or clients with an internal locus of control believe their health is determined by the actions they take.[50] Those with an external locus of control believe their state of health is determined by chance or by influential people, meaning health care professionals.[50] In general, the development of locus of control stems from family, culture, and past experiences leading to rewards. Most of the individuals with an internal locus of control (ILC) have been shown to come from families that focused on effort, education, and responsibility.[50] On the opposite side, most of the individuals with external locus of control seem to come from families of a low socioeconomic status where there may be a lack of life control.

Several studies found that internal locus of control is a predictor of greater adherence to medical recommendations or the adoption of preventive measures.[42,48,50–52] Patients with an ILC are more confident in the effectiveness of the proposed interventions. In occupational therapy, ILC is also a predictor of adherence in patients with diabetes, as well as for patients with upper-extremity amputations who were treated with HEPs.[53] In physical therapy, patients with an external locus of control (ELC), who believe that health and illness hardly depend on their own behaviors, are less adherent with interventions than those with an ILC.[54]

In patient education, motivation, self-efficacy, and locus of control can be facilitated through effective patient instruction. Establishing a therapeutic partnership between the health care provider and the patient is one of the most important factors in regard to patient teaching and learning. The therapist must carefully listen to patients and recognize the patients as experts in relation to their own lives. The therapist must not criticize patients' efforts or their failure to follow recommendations as anticipated. In some cases, patients

| Table 5.6 | *Definition of Locus of Control*[50] |
|---|---|
| | An individual's generalized expectations concerning control over future events. |

may have their own rationale for not following specific recommendations. Understanding patient resistance, lack of motivation, and nonadherence can help the health care provider work more effectively in helping patients achieve their goals.

## *Patient Education and Satisfaction*

The health care literature shows that patient education is strongly related to patient satisfaction.[55,56] Throughout the entire American health care delivery system, health care providers are highly accountable for patient satisfaction. Additionally, patient satisfaction is a worldwide concern in virtually every health care specialty. The concept of patient satisfaction is that it reflects the overall experience of an individual receiving an examination and treatment in a specific environment in a particular period of time. Patient satisfaction is also continuously viewed from the perspective of quality of care and customer service. For example, the research shows that people who are satisfied with health care are more likely to complete a course of treatment, improving their overall outcomes over those of people who do not return for prescribed care.[55–57] Furthermore, patient satisfaction is linked most of the time to both adherence to treatment and cost effectiveness.

Patient education methods are constantly being revised to increase patient satisfaction. In the current health care market, patients are faced with many different options when deciding on a specific health care provider. Also, for many health care organizations, quality patient service is a readily understood health care standard. A health care organization's reputation for its commitment to quality and patient-centered service represents one of the main criteria for individuals choosing a health care service provider. The measurement of patient satisfaction and creating a culture where service is deemed important are strategic goals for most American health care organizations.[58–60] As a result, health care industry leaders are focusing their attention on improving patient satisfaction through various initiatives, including patient education.

In contemporary health care, patients are no longer considered submissive, but are regarded as individuals who make the best choice regarding the services and providers that most meet their health care needs. The health care delivery system must accommodate the busy schedules of patients, providing them useful information and encouraging their involvement in the decision-making aspects of care. Appropriate patient instruction increases patient satisfaction and adherence, especially when treating chronic conditions. For example, patients with chronic pain who received patient education from their physicians had increased satisfaction while getting pain management interventions.[55] Patient perception of being educated by their physician was the strongest predictor of increased patient satisfaction. Patient satisfaction is also an important quality indicator of care in hospitals and outpatient department. In the current health care system, all health care institutions must recognize the benefits of patient education in increasing patient safety and satisfaction and assisting in meeting compliance goals. As a result, the rising costs of American health care can be tremendously reduced.

In physical therapy, as described in the *Guide to Physical Therapist Practice*, patient satisfaction is taken into consideration from the initial examination and evaluation and continues through interventions, reexaminations, discharge, and continuity of care.[22] In the initial examination and evaluation, the physical therapist must establish with the patient and his or her family short-term and long-term goals for the plan of care that take into account patient education and satisfaction.[22] These anticipated goals and expected outcomes are a high priority for the physical therapist and are crucial in setting up a patient/family education program that addresses risk reduction, prevention, impact on societal resources, and patient satisfaction.[22]

In health care, patient instruction containing adequate explanations and a sense of caring were found to cause patient satisfaction in emergency departments, plastic surgery consultations, and primary health care settings.[58] Patients who are well informed and have high satisfaction with care are adherent to treatment and take an active role in their health care. A patient's understanding of explanations by the health care provider is a major predictor of adherence to return visits. In addition, a patient who is well informed through patient education is likely to have high satisfaction with care, be adherent to treatment, and in general, take an active role in his or her health care.

In physical therapy rehabilitation, patient satisfaction in the initial examination and evaluation is highly correlated with patient participation in the goal-setting process.[57] The highest correlation of satisfaction is dependent on the therapist–patient interaction, when the physical therapist treats the patient with respect, explains the treatment, and answers patient questions.[57] The patient-therapist interaction is also characterized by seeing the same provider over a period of time and developing a relationship based upon trust. In physical therapy outpatient departments, similar to primary medical care settings, patient satisfaction is greatly associated with longitudinal continuity of care.[56] Nevertheless, in today's competitive health care environment some facilities may use a production model of health care delivery with daily exchangeable patients and therapists. Even with a production model, the therapists are still able to establish a trusting relationship with their patients, thus increasing patient satisfaction. The therapist should demonstrate empathy, warmth, and sincere concern for the patient and use effective communication techniques. In health care, it is recognized that patient satisfaction with the instructional aspect of medical interventions increases when the health care provider offers enough information to the patient, invites the patient to participate in decision-making, and has a good and trusting relationship with the patient and the patient's family.[58]

## THE THERAPEUTIC RELATIONSHIP AND PATIENT SATISFACTION

Research advises that establishing a special relationship with the patient is one of the most important variables to affect patient satisfaction and adherence.[56–59] For example, to change a patient's behavior in the context of smoking cessation or diabetes management requires the health care provider to intervene in such a way that makes it meaningful to the patient and generates a sufficient sense of urgency to compel the patient to take action.[59] Patient satisfaction increases when the health care provider initiates and maintains a partnership with the patient that is based on trust and understanding. Specific variables (**Table 5.7**) related to the establishment of a therapeutic bond between the patient and the provider can help improve their general relationship.[59] Factors such as trust, perceptive listening, careful observation, understanding the patient's goals, and determining the patient's needs can create a favorable atmosphere to affect patient education, patient satisfaction, and the patient's adherence with interventions. Perceptive listening allows the provider to understand the patient's values, goals, challenges, and interests. The provider must also determine the patient's actual needs by asking questions with a spirit of curiosity and with a goal of trying to be aware of how others perceive the world around them. This could be the most critical skill of a health care provider. Only through effective inquiry about patients' needs and goals can providers establish themselves as trusted partners of care.

Effective inquiry methods need the provider to focus his or her attention on the patient by smiling and looking at the patient. This encourages the patient to feel free to talk. Attention must also be given to the patient's nonverbal communication, such as facial expressions, gestures, tone of voice, and body posture. The provider must ask questions to clarify the meaning of the patient's words and the patient's feelings. The patient's message can be repeated in a reflective way to show correct understanding of the patient's ideas. The provider's nonverbal gestures, such as nodding the head, keeping eye contact, or keeping hands at the side, indicate direct involvement in the patient's message.

Most cases of patient dissatisfaction can be traced to an inadequate discovery of patient needs. As an imaginary example, a patient is seeing a physical therapist for the first time because she has back problems. However, during the initial examination, the patient mentions that she keeps getting these strange twinges of pain in her left shoulder and arm, especially in the afternoon. Given the hectic nature of the day, the physical therapist might be tempted to ignore the patient's remarks and complete the initial examination and evaluation of her back; however, suspecting that this would not meet the patient's needs and that it also could be significant for the patient's general health and perhaps her back pain, the physical therapist responds with interest. As the conversation unfolds, the patient proceeds to tell the therapist that she tried on her own to perform a Pilates technique for her

| Table 5.7 | **Variables Affecting Patient Satisfaction[59]** |
| --- | --- |
| Establishment of a sense of trust between the patient and the health care provider. |
| Perceptive listening and careful observation of small details that give a glimpse into the life of the patient. |
| Determining the patient's needs. |

back when she heard a click in her shoulder. She did not mention this to her physician because he was very busy. By taking the time to listen and probe deeper, the therapist can better help the patient and also create a foundation for a stronger long-term therapist-patient relationship.

It is recommended that providers have a dialogue with patients and not attempt a didactic monologue.[59] Patients dislike people who dominate the interaction, trying to give prescriptive and paternalistic advice. Instead, the provider can ask questions, explore values, and make a connection with every patient. Rather than hearing the patient's complaints and immediately responding with a solution, the provider needs to investigate deeper with probing questions. It is important to find out how the patient's problem affects their daily life, how he or she approaches the problem, and what the results are. The patient's internal knowledge must be supported, recognizing that patients often know their own bodies. Only after they finish speaking should the therapist address other options. Physical and occupational therapists should always ask the patient how the other options sound in the context of their overall goals.

Additionally, patients cannot be forced to make commitments for interventions before they are ready to do so. If the therapist is busy and in a hurry, pushing the patient to make a commitment too soon will cause mistrust and anger. For example, in physical therapy, a patient may need to start a HEP from the first visit but says he is too busy to exercise. The therapist may have to wait until the second or third visit, or may try to negotiate the HEP with the patient. When negotiating, the therapist may need to offer a simple activity that will help the patient in the same way as the HEP. Also, the patient must be able to enjoy the activity and not spend too much time performing it. If the proposal is acceptable to the patient, then a commitment can be confirmed; if not, another negotiation must be requested. Following up with the patient by checking on them by phone or email is also important. Asking patient permission to contact them at home during their treatments is essential. If the therapist has no time to call, their staff should call to ask how things are going, whether their goals are progressing, and whether they would like to make another appointment to see the rehabilitation provider. Sending birthday cards, emailing health tips, and pursuing other avenues of contact with patients is necessary. These procedures build a therapeutic relationship and demonstrate the therapist's commitment to help his or her patients.

# Patient Education and Empowerment Using a Patient-Centered Approach

Patient education and empowerment requires patients to be actively involved in the decision-making process of care from the beginning to the end of interventions and throughout the continuity of care process. Empowerment is a patient-centered, collaborative approach tailored to match the fundamental realities of patient care.[60] Patient empowerment through instruction involves helping patients discover and develop their inherent capacity to be responsible for their own life. Health care providers are experts on different areas of health care, whereas patients are experts on their own lives. A patient-centered approach recognizes that knowing about an illness is not the same as knowing about a person's life and that, by default, patients are the primary decision makers in control of the daily self-management of disease or illness.[60]

Physical and occupational therapists need to recognize and accept that patients are well-informed, active partners or collaborators in their own care. The therapists' role is to help patients make informed decisions to achieve their goals and overcome barriers through education, appropriate care recommendations, expert advice, and support. Nevertheless, many patients prefer to adopt the old passive system of care in which they accept the provider's recommendations without question. In this case, the decision-making aspect is totally in the hands of the provider. Many times, patients also do not want involvement or to accept providers' instructions because they are searching for better ways outside of the health care system to solve their medical problems. On other occasions, patients present to providers decisions that are totally unrealistic in relation to the pathology and the outcomes.

In contemporary health care, the goal of physical and occupational therapists as rehabilitation providers is to use patient education to help patients in their decision-making and to increase their awareness of rationalizations and justifications. This requires a special patient-provider relationship based on respect, honest communication, trust, empathy, and compassion. The patient-provider relationship is considered the very heart of the health care delivery system (**Table 5.8**).[60] This relationship not only gives patients access to health care, but also can promote patient empowerment and healing. The effectiveness of the patient-provider relationship is related to health outcomes. To be a successful rehabilitation provider requires a foundation of mutual responsibilities that need to be shared equally by the patient and the therapist. The therapeutic relationship between the patient and the provider often extends to the patient's family members, friends, patient advocates, and other health care providers or professionals.[59,60] In this context, patient education can influence behavior and produce changes in knowledge, attitudes, and the skills needed to maintain and improve health.

The Joint Commission and the Commission on Accreditation of Rehabilitation Facilities (CARF) require health care providers and professionals to involve patients in the decision-making aspects of care and the establishment of intervention goals.[60,61] Therefore, all health care providers' teaching objectives must include patients' participation in decision-making and helping patients develop the necessary skills to actively take part in their treatment and continuity of care (**Table 5.9**).

The Joint Commission promotes the concept of patient-centered education that involves patients as significant members of the health care team.[60–63] Collaboration by the entire health care team is vital for effective patient and family education. Patient education promoted by most health care providers requires an interdisciplinary approach that includes the patient, the family, and other disciplines as part of the health care team.[63] Patient education must be ongoing, interactive, and consistent with the patient's plan of care, educational level, and needs for continuity of care.

| Table 5.8 | **Elements of an Effective Patient-Provider Relationship[60]** |
|---|---|
| A mutual understanding of the patient's expectations of the therapist and the therapist's expectations of the patient. ||
| A strong basis for discussing options to achieve expected goals of care. ||
| A resource of learning from each other. ||

## THE SIGNIFICANCE OF PATIENT-CENTERED CARE

The health care literature indicates that patients who are actively involved in their care through the patient-centered approach become empowered to make decisions, change behaviors, and better manage their health.[60–63] The purpose of patient education within the empowerment philosophy is to help patients make decisions about their care and obtain clarity about their goals, values, and motivation. Approaches to patient education within the empowerment approach incorporate interactive teaching strategies designed to involve patients in problem solving and address their cultural and psychosocial needs.

As a result of being empowered, patients can maintain better health with fewer complications (**Table 5.10**). In addition, they require less hospitalizations, emergency department visits, and clinic and physician visits.

| Table 5.9 | **The Provider's Educational Objectives for Patient Decision-Making Skills[61]** |
|---|---|
| To promote the patient's participation in decision making and health care options. ||
| To increase the patient's potential to follow the health care plan. ||
| To help the patient develop self-care skills. ||
| To improve the patient's and family's coping skills. ||
| To increase the patient's participation in the continuing of care. ||
| To encourage the patient to adopt a healthy lifestyle. ||

| Table 5.10 | *Definition of Patient Empowerment*[61] |
|---|---|
| Patient empowerment involves educating and encouraging patients to expand their role in decision-making, health-related behaviors, and self-management of care. |

Patient-centered care is still a new concept in the American health delivery system. Even today, some health care providers are continuing to use the old, disease-centered model in which the provider makes almost all treatment decisions based largely on clinical experience and data from various medical tests. The reason for using the old model may be that the patient-centered model is still a new concept that has been gradually incorporated into medical care over the last 10 to 15 years.[63] The foundation of patient-centered came from psychotherapeutic interventional care. It involves six interactive components of care: (1) exploring the disease or disorder with the patient; (2) understanding the patient as a whole person; (3) finding with the patient a common ground regarding their management of the disease, disorder, or illness; (4) incorporating prevention and health promotion; (5) enhancing the patient-provider relationship; and (6) being realistic.[63]

The first interactive component of the patient-centered care model involves exploring the meaning of the disease or disorder with the patient. To be able to effectively perform this investigation, the health care professional can use differential diagnoses and inquiry about the dimensions of the disorder or disease from the patient's perspectives (such as the patient's ideas, feelings, expectations, and effects on function).[63] The second interactive component of patient-centered care, understanding the whole person, means to consider the patient's life history, his or her personal and developmental needs, and the context of family, physical environment, and anyone else involved in or affected by the patient's disorder or disease.[63] The health care provider who understands the whole person recognizes the impact of the family in ameliorating or aggravating the disorder. The patient's cultural beliefs and attitudes can also influence care. For health care providers, an understanding of the whole person can deepen their knowledge of the nature of the patient's suffering and the patient's response to the illness.[63]

During the third interactive component of patient-centered care, the clinician must find common ground with the patient and openly discuss problems and priorities, goals of interventions, and the role of the patient and the health care provider in the patient's health management.[63] Furthermore, developing an effective management plan requires the provider and the patient to reach an agreement in three areas: the nature of the problems and priorities, the goals of interventions, and the roles of the provider and the patient. Often, health care professionals and patients have widely conflicting views in each of these areas. The process of finding a satisfactory resolution involves moving toward a meeting of minds and discovering common ground.[63] This practice encourages the provider to incorporate patients' ideas, feelings, expectations, and function into the plan of care.

Prevention and health promotion strategies represent the fourth interactive component of care. This component of patient-centered care includes health enhancement, risk reduction, early detection of diseases or disorders, and ameliorating the effects of disease or disorder. In the fifth interactive component, enhancing the patient-provider relationship, the provider must form a therapeutic relationship with the patient using nurturing and sincere caring, share control of the management with the patient, connect with the patient in an empathetic and healing manner, and encourage self-awareness.[63] Disease prevention requires a collaborative and ongoing effort for both the patient and the provider. This process is important to enable patients to take control over and improve their health and also encourage continuity of care and screening practices for health promotion.

The realistic component of the patient-centered model is the last part, and it includes clinical considerations of team building and the needed time and resources.[63] Frequently, health care providers experience competing patients' demands for their time and energy. This approach requires them to learn to manage their time effectively for the benefit of their patients. Resource allocation and teamwork are important issues, and providers must develop skills for prioritizing and considering community resources.[63]

For modern health care in the United States, patient-centered care is a critical multi-faceted component that involves many significant variables such as respect for patients' values, preferences, and expressed needs; coordination and integration of care, information, communication, and education; emotional support and physical comfort; involvement of family and friends; and transition and continuity of care.[63] The American health care vision for the future predicts that by the year 2015, at least 50% of patients will participate in patient-centered care, including shared decision-making processes that lead to a measurable improvement in decision quality.[60]

Care that is truly patient-centered considers patients' cultural traditions, their personal preferences and values, their family situations, and their lifestyles.[30] It makes patients and their loved ones an integral part of the health care team who collaborate with health care professionals in making clinical decisions. Patient-centered care puts the responsibility for important aspects of self-care and monitoring in patients' hands, along with the tools and support needed to carry out that responsibility.[30] Patient-centered care ensures that transitions between providers, departments, and health care settings are respectful, coordinated, and efficient. When care is patient-centered, unneeded and unwanted services can be reduced. In this context, patient-centeredness includes both the patient's experience of care and the presence of an effective partnership between the clinician and patient and the patient's family, when necessary.

## PATIENT-CENTERED CARE AND PATIENT EDUCATION IN PHYSICAL AND OCCUPATIONAL REHABILITATION

The patient-centered care approach has been part of physical therapy[28,35,57,64–66] and occupational therapy[67,68] for a long time (**Table 5.11**). Patient-centered physical therapy achieves

| Table 5.11 | **Definition of Patient-Centered Care Related to Patient Education[68]** |
|---|---|
| | Patient-centered care requires educating patients as partners of care, involving them in planning their health care, and encouraging them to take responsibility for their own health. This process can increase patient empowerment, motivation, and satisfaction with interventions. |

effective patient education and increases patient adherence with interventions, as well as patient satisfaction and empowerment. Patient-centered occupational therapy can provide a more efficient framework for understanding, evaluating, and interpreting a patient's occupational performance.

From a clinical perspective, the patient-centered care model is valuable because it is explicit about the therapist's necessary behavior in relation to patient management, including patient teaching and learning aspects.

In physical rehabilitation, researchers found that patients made the greatest gains when the goals and interventions became meaningful to them and made a difference in their lives.[64–66] Patient motivation and empowerment was achieved from the beginning of physical therapy programs through establishment of a patient-centered functional goal program.[66] In a patient-centered model, patients become active participants in their own care and receive services designed to focus on their individual needs and preferences, in addition to advice and counsel from rehabilitation professionals. To achieve motivation, patients must be considered collaborators and partners for health. When patients establish their own goals in a patient-centered approach, the whole concept of adherence to interventions becomes relevant to them.[66] Also, when patients work toward their own goals, their motivation is intrinsic. Because true and lasting motivation comes from within, patients are able to make and sustain changes in their behavior.

Listening to patients' meanings and values is the starting point to gain patients' adherence. When occupational and physical therapists work with patients to reach an agreement on a plan of care (that also makes sense in the context of the patient's life), they facilitate patients' adherence to self-management and continuity of care. Patient adherence with interventions should be based on two very important medical models—patient-centered care and patient empowerment.[64–68] The rehabilitation provider remains a great source of knowledge for the patient, but his or her role is more of a teacher or mentor. The patient visits the therapist to access and receive teaching and learning regarding interventions, technical resources, rehabilitation expertise, and psychosocial support. However, the patient maintains the responsibility for managing his or her disorder or disease. In this context, adherence becomes less an issue of obedience and more an issue of setting and working toward realistic and relevant rehabilitative goals.[67]

In the patient-centered model, in order to achieve a patient's adherence and motivation in patient education, the rehabilitation provider should establish four important conditions in the teaching and learning process: patient-shared values, language, learning, and mutual respect (**Table 5.12**).[66–68]

True partnership with the patient requires the health care provider to learn to listen to the patient and family member(s) on issues that are both broad and specific. Effective listening is the primary skill when interacting with a patient. It is also a pathway to engage in a therapeutic relationship, build trust, and promote the patient's cooperation with treatment.[63,64] In addition, a physical therapy patient-centered plan of care is essential when encouraging the patient always to have the last word in the plan of care.[66] In one example found in the literature, expert physical therapy clinicians used a patient-centered approach in their clinical practices.[28] In this model, patients were viewed as active participants in therapy, and the primary goal of care was to empower patients to make decisions in their care.

The patient-centered model can have excellent results based on the therapist's appropriate clinical reasoning, values, virtues, and style of practice.[64–68] The successful rehabilitation clinician using a patient-centered approach to practice should also have a strong clinical knowledge base and skills in differential diagnosis and self-reflection.[66] Information and skills are necessary so that the therapist can empower the patient and facilitate

| Table 5.12 | *Key Variables in Patient-Centered Teaching*[66–68] |
|---|---|
| Patient-shared language and communication | Listening to the patient's feelings, language, and values; communicating in simple layman's terms; helping the patient understand; showing empathy; establishing a partnership with the patient. |
| Patient-shared values | Considering the patient's unique views on health and disease; reaching an agreement with the patient about the plan of care; setting goals with the patient. |
| Patient-shared respect | Demonstrating respect for the patient's knowledge, values, and feelings; acknowledging in a respectful way differences in values or points of view. |
| Patient-shared learning | Supporting the patient's teaching and learning; facilitating the patient's problem solving; acknowledging patient difficulties; providing different teaching styles. |

patient-therapist collaborative problem solving to enhance the patient's abilities to make autonomous decisions. The patient-centered approach increases the clinician's appreciation of and respect for patient individuality while also building the patient's motivation, satisfaction, and trust. In such a collaborative patient-therapist relationship, patient education goals can become patient-centered and increase the patient's motivation.[64–66]

Patient participation in goal setting as patient-centered care is emphasized by the APTA and is included in schools' curricula requirements. The APTA's *Guide to Physical Therapist Practice* recommends that the plan of care must be established by the physical therapist in collaboration with the patient, taking into consideration the expectations of the patient and appropriate others.[22] The essential skills that every physical therapist graduate must have at the completion of his or her professional education consist of designing a plan of care that is mutually agreed upon with the patient and identifying and considering patients' goals and expectations.

The patient-centered care model gives physical and occupational therapists the opportunity, in the initial examination and evaluation, to better understand their patients or clients in relation to their motivational characteristics and their roles and capacities to perform activities or tasks. For example, it was proposed that in their initial examination, occupational therapists use the nine dimensions of the client-centered performance context:[67]

1. Temporal dimension (client's past and present, and their possibilities and hopes for the future)

2. Environmental dimension (the client's physical space and environment to perform the task)

3. Cultural dimension (client's shared beliefs, values, customs, tools, materials, and cultural group)

4. Societal (institutional) dimension (community resources, economic factors, rules and regulations, and medical precautions)

5. Social dimension (client's relationship with others and cooperation with occupational therapist)

6. Role dimension (client's perceived role and the role behavior expected by the client and society)

7. Motivational dimension (client's values, interests, and goals that give meaning to the task and provide motivation)

8. Capacity dimension (client's broad clinical description of physical potentials for change, delimiters to progress, or precautions toward interventions)

9. Task dimension (the task to be performed and the client's perceived constraints)

To establish these interrelated dimensions and better construct an interventional plan of care for their clients, therapists can perform an informal observation of the client and also use a comprehensive interview process.[67,68] Using these dimensions in a client-centered context may allow occupational therapists to conceptualize the tasks that are most important to the client, the meaning of those tasks for the client, and the nature and time and effort required to complete these tasks from both the client's and therapist's perspective.[67,68]

In regard to patient education in physical therapy rehabilitation, patient teaching and learning in a patient-centered care model should be customized according to the patient's needs and values. Teaching and learning must include knowledge that is shared and information that flows freely. Decision-making should be evidence-based. In addition, in patient-centered care, patient safety becomes a system requirement for education and care, cooperation among clinicians is a priority, the patient's needs are continuously anticipated, and waste is constantly decreased. Using patient experiences as part of the curriculum helps to individualize educational programs and ensure that the content provided is relevant to the learner's needs. In patient-centered care within physical therapy, patients should be encouraged to participate in the goal setting of their learning process (**Table 5.13**).

Similar to the interventions, the process of goal setting may contain five steps. The first two steps need the health care provider to define the patient's needs and motivation to learn and change (including self-efficacy, locus of control, and learning styles) and ascertain the patient's beliefs, thoughts, and feelings that may support or hold back the selection of the learning goals.[66] The third step is to identify short- and long-term goals of acquiring the knowledge towards which patients will work.[66] The fourth step is for patients to choose and commit to making a behavioral change that will help them achieve their short- and long-term goals. The final step is for patients to evaluate their efforts and identify what they learned in the process.[66] This goal-setting approach eliminates the concepts of success and failure. Instead, all efforts are opportunities to learn more about the true nature of the problem, related feelings, barriers, and effective strategies. The therapist's role in the teaching and learning aspect of care is to provide information, collaborate during the goal-setting process, and offer support for each patient's effort.[66–68]

| Table 5.13 | **The Goal-Setting Process in the Patient-Centered Care Teaching Model[66]** |
| --- | --- |
| 1. | Define patient's learning goals (dependent on patient's needs, motivation, self-efficacy, and locus of control). |
| 2. | Ascertain patient's beliefs, thoughts, values, and feelings. |
| 3. | Identify patient's short- and long-term goals for teaching and learning. |
| 4. | Facilitate patient's commitment to learn and change. |
| 5. | Facilitate patient's self-evaluation of teaching and learning process. |

## STRATEGIES IN PATIENT-CENTERED TEACHING AND LEARNING

Physical and occupational therapists actively try to involve their patients and families in the goal-setting process of rehabilitation. Sometimes, because of time constraints, the patient's age, or their cognitive status, patient participation is not maximized during rehabilitation.[68] Many patients also still perceive their role as a passive recipient of care and do not want to participate in the goal-setting process. In addition, some patients may have unreasonable or unachievable desired outcomes that therapists cannot include in the plan of care as truly patient-centered goals and outcomes. Because a patient-centered approach is part of the plan of care in the 21st century, physical and occupational therapy professionals have been searching for new methods to maximize and improve the patient-centered model of care. The patient's functional goals were identified as the most meaningful and feasible patient-centered goals for the teaching and learning aspect of interventions (**Table 5.14**).[66]

A patient-centered evaluation tool was created for physical therapy to acknowledge the views, experience, and perspectives of all participants involved in rehabilitation. The Rehabilitation Problem Solving form (RPS form) used in cardiovascular, neurologic, and musculoskeletal problems in Europe was successfully applied in research to physical therapy rehabilitation in a patient-centered model of care.[64] The RPS form was shown to help therapists involve patients actively in the rehabilitation process and better communicate with patients.[64] Also, a more recent study proposing a decision-making framework using a patient-centered approach was suggested in neurologic physical therapy rehabilitation.[65] This framework adds a patient enablement perspective and hypothesis-generation methods to the previous disablement model used in the *Guide to Physical Therapist Practice*. The study also recommended using the Hypothesis-Oriented Algorithm for Clinicians (HOAC) to allow rehabilitation professionals to better explore a patient's concerns and problems that are not identified by the patient (but by the clinician and caregivers).[65] Using the new models, rehabilitation clinicians can assist neurologic patient integration in the decision-making aspect of patient-centered care.

Table 5.14

### *Methods to Identify a Patient's Functional Goals*[66]

Determine the patient's desired outcome of therapy.

Develop an understanding of the patient's self-care, work, and leisure activities, and the environments in which these activities occur.

Establish goals with the patient that relate to his or her desired outcomes.

# THE EVOLUTION AND CHALLENGES OF THE PATIENT-CENTERED APPROACH

Using a patient-centered approach within the field of patient education is still new and relatively untested method. The patient-centered model is evolving in the contemporary health care system. As mentioned earlier, the American health care system is experiencing a slow and subtle shift from a professionally driven approach to one that is patient-centered (also called consumer-centered).[60] This advancement stems from a growing recognition that incorporating an individual patient's perspectives and encouraging greater involvement in his or her care results in better health outcomes and quality of care.[60] However, populations such as low income individuals, uninsured persons, immigrants, racial and ethnic minorities, and many elderly face greater barriers to patient-centered care. Additional research is needed in every area of health care to include new methods and models of patient participation in the delivery of care, especially for these underserved populations.

Patient education and empowerment methods are also needed to educate and encourage vulnerable populations in a patient-centered approach of care for decision-making, health-related behaviors, and self-management. Physical and occupational therapists and assistants need increased teaching and learning competence in patient and health education to better understand and consider all the complexities involved in the teaching and learning aspects of care (**Table 5.15**).

| Table 5.15 | *Suggestions to Enhance Patient Education Using a Patient-Centered Approach*[65–68] |
|---|---|
| Adapt patient education by considering different teaching and learning styles and preferences. ||
| Adapt patient education by considering the patient's culture, including ethnic traditions, homelessness, and addiction. ||
| Adapt patient education by considering the patient's economic and educational status. ||
| Adapt patient education by considering the patient's health literacy level. ||
| Adapt patient education by considering the patient's family patterns and situations. ||
| Adapt patient education by considering the patient's traditions, including alternative and folk remedies. ||
| Adapt patient teaching to allow better communication with the patient (in a language and at a level that the patient understands). ||

Other challenges for patient education, especially for underserved populations, are coordination and integration of care requiring assessment for formal and informal services that will have an impact on health and interventions and advocacy for the patient and family. Patient privacy, emotional support, physical comfort, and involvement of family and friends must also be considered. In the future, the entire American health care system and public policy structures will need to reset priorities in terms of reimbursement by Medicare, Medicaid, and private insurance and place greater emphasis on wellness and prevention as well as treating of diseases (disorders). Additionally, physical and occupational therapists, assistants, and all health care providers should take a more proactive role at the federal and state levels to promote legislation, policies, and increased funding to support the patient-centered care approach.

# CONCLUSIONS

## Section I Summary

This section discusses basic concepts of patient education perceived to be critical to understanding the importance of patient education in the health care delivery system, including rehabilitation. In modern health care, patient and health education are promoted at the governmental level and are embraced by all health care providers. Patient education and teaching and learning are part of the curricula of rehabilitation professional schools. Rehabilitation research has been investigating various methods for teaching and learning, increasing patient adherence and satisfaction, and implementing patient-centered care for patient empowerment. However, formal patient education using teaching and learning theories is still a relatively new form of intervention. Also, developing a plan of care that is patient-centered is a critical and complex part of health care involving several variables.

The APTA's *Guide to Physical Therapist Practice* recommends a plan of care be established in collaboration with the patient. The literature shows the need for rehabilitation professionals to maximize the patient's (and the patient's family's) participation in the patient-centered model of care. More research is necessary to examine new approaches for better patient education and patient care.

Rehabilitation professionals' roles are growing to include complex and demanding teaching that goes beyond the disease pathology, wellness, fitness, and prevention. Concepts introduced in this section such as a patient-centered approach to care, adherence, motivation, satisfaction, and empowerment make up the core of contemporary patient teaching and learning in clinical patient education and health care education.

# Section I Case Study

## PATIENT EDUCATION FOR PATIENT-CENTERED CARE

Per the APTA's *Guide to Physical Therapist Practice*, the patient physical therapy diagnostic classification pattern is:[22]

Impaired motor function and sensory integrity associated with acute or chronic polyneuropathies

ICD-9-Cm Codes: 250.6 Diabetes with neurological manifestations

The APTA's *Guide to Physical Therapist Practice* recommendations for patient-related instruction:[22]

Instruction, education, and training of patient and caregiver regarding:

- Current condition (pathology/pathophysiology, impairments, functional limitations, or disabilities)
- Enhancement of performance
- Health, wellness, and fitness programs
- Plan of care
- Risk factors (pathology/pathophysiology, impairments, functional limitations, or disabilities)
- Transitions across settings
- Transitions to new roles

### Patient Description

Patient is a 68-year-old man with a medical diagnosis of polyneuropathy secondary to diabetes mellitus. He has a 12-year history of impaired glucose tolerance. He also has hypertension. He complains of fatigue and has slight ataxia. The patient has been retired for approximately 1 year from an office job with the government. He uses no alcohol. Ten years ago, when his diabetes was discovered, he received diabetes education and learned home glucose monitoring. Since his retirement he has been leading a sedentary life, watching television most of the time and staying home. He also stopped playing golf. He gained weight. Five months ago he noticed some burning and tingling in his feet. Walking gradually became a significant chore. For the past 3 weeks he has had burning pain in both feet and is using a walker (that belonged to his mother) to be able to go shopping. The patient did not want to see a doctor. His wife convinced him to seek medical attention.

At the doctor's office, he denied chest pain or shortness of breath. He denied any other symptoms and had no fever or chills, cough, bloody stools, or hematuria. He had gained 15 pounds. A review of his blood glucose log revealed fasting and premeal blood glucose levels generally < 150 mg/dl. Postprandial glucose levels were almost always > 186 mg/dl.

Laboratory studies revealed normal chemistries except for a fasting blood glucose of 157 mg/dl. A complete blood count, lipid panel, liver screening, and renal profile were all normal, as was a prostate-specific antigen (PSA) test. A thyroid-stimulating hormone (TSH) test was included to rule out thyroid disease, and $B_{12}$ and folate were measured to rule out pernicious anemia. The physician recommended nerve conduction studies. EMG and nerve conduction studies showed sensorimotor neuropathy.

After he received the results, the physician explained to the patient that he has diabetic neuropathy and that his treatment begins with glycemic control. In the physician's office, the patient was started on repaglinide (Prandin), 0.5 mg twice a day taken with breakfast and the evening meal to better regulate his glucose levels. Also, the doctor recommended duloxetine (Cymbalta) 60 mg once daily to decrease the pain in his feet. He continued his glucose monitoring and was asked to fax in his blood glucose levels every 2 weeks for the next 2 months. He was encouraged by his physician to restart his exercise regimen and received a referral for physical therapy.

In physical therapy, the patient presents with bilateral burning foot pain and tingling. He also has bilateral weakness of the lower extremities. He has no open lesions on either foot and has intact protective sensation for both feet. His reflexes are normal and pedal pulses are palpable. He has a slight ataxic gait.

### Guiding Ideas to Write a Patient-Centered Education Plan of Care

1. The physical therapist has to establish a partnership with the patient (and patient's family) showing support for the patient's self-management efforts in cases of chronic diseases (such as diabetes). As an example for this patient, the therapist may want to say in the beginning of the examination and evaluation:

   > I understand that living with diabetes is difficult. You have many decisions to make each day that will have an impact on your future health and well-being. We are here to help you. You know a great deal about diabetes and how to care for it. You know yourself better than anyone. You know what you want and what you are able and willing to do to care for your diabetes. Caring for your diabetes will help your weakness, pain, and tingling sensations in your feet. By combining what you know about yourself with what we know about diabetes and your physical discomfort, we can come up with a plan of care that will work for you. We are partners and we need to work together.

   Also, the therapist needs to begin each visit with an assessment of the patient's (and patient's family's) concerns, questions, and progress toward the goals. Some professionals use a form for patients to complete containing one to three open-ended questions to ascertain any problems or concerns that need to be addressed during the visit.

2. The physical therapist has to find out more about the patient and his methods of managing his diabetes. The therapist also has to listen to the patient's (and family's) fears and concerns. As an example, the patient stated that over the years, he was doing very well caring for his diabetes. He was very active, played golf regularly, and walked

one mile at least four times a week. However, after retirement he lost his social friends and became sedentary, also eating "bad stuff." In addition, he disliked visiting with health care professionals. He stated that every health care provider wanted to give him advice without listening to him. All rushed him through the visits, asking and talking only about his blood glucose level. Nobody cared how he felt psychologically or even physically. Everyone's interest was just the blood glucose level. He felt that he was viewed by every health care professional as just a "blood glucose number." For that reason, he preferred not to see a health care provider even when he had pain.

3. The physical therapist has to generate options for the patient and negotiate reasonable goals and intervention options. For example, the therapist asked questions in regard to the patient's previous management of glucose level and also about his level of function including exercises and hobbies. The patient and his wife knew how important controlling the glucose level was. The patient was proud to be able to manage his glucose in the past. He admitted that his lifestyle changed after retirement, and he was staying home most of the time. He wanted to go back to playing golf and walking with his wife. He also acknowledged that he needs to see a dietician to help him manage his food intake. His short-term goal was to stop the burning pain in his feet, especially at night, and be able to walk at least a few steps without getting so tired and using the walker.

4. The physical therapist has to decide with the patient and the patient's wife on mutually agreeable and feasible goals and interventions. As an example, the patient wanted to come to therapy 4 days per week to get stronger faster. His wife wanted him to come only 3 days per week to have 4 days to go back to playing golf. The therapist, the patient, and the patient's wife agreed to 3 days, while on the fourth day the patient had to do a few more repetitions of the HEP for strengthening.

5. The physical therapist has to take advantage of teachable moments that occur during each patient visit, assisting the patient in solving problems and overcoming barriers to self-management. The therapist needs to provide and coordinate system-specific strategies (such as referral to other providers) to promote patient self-management. The therapist may need to create a team with other health care professionals in the area (or system) who have additional training in the clinical, educational, behavioral, and psychosocial aspects of care.

The following discussion ideas can connect the patient with the therapist and the intervention goals:

- Share with me your greatest concern in regard to your health.

- Share with me your goals to progress toward your improvement. Could you be more specific?

- We can look together at the progress you achieved in the past and work in that direction.

# Section I References

1. Drench ME, Noonan AC, Sharby N, Hallenborg Ventura S. *Psychosocial Aspects of Health Care*. 2nd ed. Upper Saddle River, NJ: Pearson Education; 2007.

2. Gahimer JE, Domholdt E. Amount of patient education in physical therapy practice and perceived effects. *Phys Ther.* 1996;76(10):89–96.

3. Muma RD, Lyons BA, Newman TA, Carnes BA. *Patient Education: A Practical Approach*. Stamford, CT: McGraw-Hill/Appleton & Lange; 1996.

4. Berry L, Seiders K, Wilder SS. Innovations in access to care: a patient-centered approach. *Ann Internal Med.* 2003;139(7):568–574.

5. May BJ. Patient education: past and present. *J Phys Ther Ed.* 1999;13(2):1–7.

6. Kovner A, Jonas S. *Jonas and Kovner's Health Care Delivery in the United States*. 6th ed. New York: Springer; 1999.

7. Falvo DR. *Effective Patient Education: A Guide to Increased Compliance*. Sudbury, MA: Jones and Bartlett; 2004.

8. LaLonde M. *A New Perspective on the Health of Canadians*. Ottawa: Government of Canada; 1974.

9. U.S. Surgeon General. *Healthy People: The Surgeon General's Report on Health Promotion and Disease Prevention*. Washington, DC: Department of Health, Education, and Welfare; 1979.

10. U.S. Department of Health and Human Services, Office of Disease Prevention and Health Promotion. Healthy People 2010. Available at: http://www.healthypeople.gov. Accessed June 2007.

11. Bastable SB. *Essentials of Patient Education*. Sudbury, MA: Jones and Bartlett; 2006.

12. Hayne CR. The preventive role of physiotherapy in the national health service and industry. *Physiother.* 1988;74:2–3.

13. Sluijs EM. A checklist to assess patient education in physical therapy practice: development and reliability. *Phys Ther.* 1991;71(8):17–25.

14. Murphy W. *Healing the Generations: A History of Physical Therapy and the American Physical Therapy Association*. Alexandria, VA: American Physical Therapy Association; 1995.

15. Commission on Accreditation in Physical Therapy Education, American Physical Therapy Association. Evaluative Criteria for PT Programs: 2006. Available at: http://www.apta.org. Accessed June 2007.

16. Jensen GM. Patient education [editorial]. *J Phys Ther Ed.* 1999;13(2):1–2.

17. Vanderhoff M. Patient education and health literacy. *PT Mag Phys Ther.* 2005;13(9):42–46.

18. McEwen IR. "STEPS" in practice [editorial]. *Phys Ther.* 2004;84(7):606–607.

19. Deusinger SS. Teaching is easy? [editorial]. *J Phys Ther Ed.* 1999;13(2):1.

20. Shepard KF, Jensen GM. *Handbook of Teaching for Physical Therapists*. 2nd ed. Woburn, MA: Butterworth-Heinemann; 2002.

21. Jette DU, Bacon K, Batty C, et al. Evidence-based practice: beliefs, attitudes, knowledge, and behaviors of physical therapists. *Phys Ther.* 2003;83(9):786–802.

22. American Physical Therapy Association. *Guide to Physical Therapist Practice*. 2nd ed. Alexandria, VA: Author; 2001.

23. American Occupational Therapy Association. *Occupational Therapy Practice Framework: Domain and Process*. Bethesda, MD: American Occupational Therapy Association Press; 2002.

24. Venes D, ed. *Taber's Cyclopedic Medical Dictionary*. 20th ed. Philadelphia: F.A. Davis; 2005.

25. Chase L, Elkins JA, Readinger J, et al. Perceptions of physical therapists toward patient education. *Phys Ther.* 1993;73(11):57–66.

26. May BJ. Teaching: a skill in clinical practice. *Phys Ther.* 1983;63:1627–1633.

27. Jensen GM, Gwyer J, Shepard KF, et al. Expert practice in physical therapy. *Phys Ther.* 2000;80(1):28–43.

28. Resnik L, Jensen GM. Using clinical outcomes to explore the theory of expert practice in physical therapy. *Phys Ther.* 2003;83(12):1090–1106.

29. O'Conner P. Improving medication adherence. *Arch Intern Med.* 2006;166:1802–1804.

30. Stone MS, Bronkesh SJ, Gerbarg ZB, et al. Meshing patient and physician goals. *Strat Med.* 1998;1:1–7. Available at: http://www.hsmgroup.com. Accessed June 2007.

31. Lutfey KE, Wishnet W. Beyond compliance: is adherence improving the prospect of diabetes care? *Diabetes Care.* 1999;22:635–639.

32. Ayalon L, Areán PA, Alvidrez J. Adherence to antidepressant medications in Black and Latino elderly patients. *Am J Geriatr Psychiatry.* 2005;13:572–580.

33. Lowes R. Patient-centered care for better patient adherence. *Fam Pract Manage.* 1998;3:1–7.

34. Kyngäs H. Patient education: perspective of adolescents with a chronic disease. *J Clin Nurs.* 2003;12(5):744–751.

35. Sluijs EM, Kok GJ, van der Zee J. Correlates of exercise compliance in physical therapy. *Phys Ther.* 1993;73:771–782.

36. Guccione AA. *Geriatric Physical Therapy.* St. Louis, MO: Mosby-Year Book; 1993.

37. Henry KD, Rosemond C, Eckert LB. Effect of number of home exercises on compliance and performance in adults over 65 years of age. *Phys Ther.* 1998;79(3):270–277.

38. Bassett SF. The assessment of patient adherence to physiotherapy rehabilitation. *NZ J Physiother.* 2003;31(2):60–66.

39. Forkan R, Pumper B, Smyth N, et al. Exercise adherence following physical therapy intervention in older adults with impaired balance. *Phys Ther.* 2006;86(3):401–410.

40. Bassett SF, Prapavessis H. Home-based physical therapy intervention with adherence-enhancing strategies versus clinic-based management for patients with ankle sprains. *Phys Ther.* 2007;87(9):1–12.

41. Luszczynska A, Sutton S. Physical activity after cardiac rehabilitation: evidence that different types of self efficacy are important in maintainers and relapsers. *Rehab Psych.* 2006;51(4):314–321.

42. Poirier P, Turbide G, Bourdages J, et al. Predictors of compliance with medical recommendations regarding pharmacological and nonpharmacological approaches in patient with cardiovascular disease. *Clin Invest Med.* 2006;29(2):1–12.

43. Mayoux-Benhamou MA, Roux C, Perraud A, et al. Predictors of compliance with a home-based exercise program added to usual medical care in preventing postmenopausal osteoporosis: an 18-month prospective study. *Osteopor Int.* 2005;16(3):325–331.

44. Mori DL, Sogg S, Guarino P, et al. Predictors of exercise compliance in individuals with Gulf War veterans illnesses: Department of Veterans Affairs Cooperative Study 470. *Milit Med.* 2006;171(9):917–923.

45. Alexandre NM, Nordin M, Hiebert R, et al. Predictors of compliance with short-term treatment among patients with back pain. *Rev Panam Salud Publica.* 2002;12(2):86–94.

46. Searle A, Norman P, Harrad R, et al. Psychosocial and clinical determinants of compliance with occlusion therapy for amblyopic children. *Eye Sci J Royal Coll Ophthalmol.* 2002;16(2):150–155.

47. Donohoe G, Owens N, O'Donnell C, et al. Predictors of compliance with neuroleptic medication among inpatients with schizophrenia: a discriminant function analysis. *Eur Psychiatry.* 2001;16(5):293–308.

48. Nielsen B, Nielsen AS, Wraae O. Factors associated with compliance of alcoholics in outpatient treatment. *J Nerv Ment Dis.* 2000;188(2):101–107.

49. Lewthwaite R. Motivational considerations in physical activity involvement. *Phys Ther.* 1990;70(12):808–819.

50. Abella R, Heslin R. Health, locus of control, values, and the behavior of family and friends—an integrated approach to understanding preventive health behavior. *Basic Appl Soc Psychol.* 1984;5:283–294.

51. Kristiansen CM. A 2-value model of preventive health behavior. *Basic Appl Soc Psychol.* 1986;7:173–183.

52. Schneider A, Körner T, Mehring M, et al. Impact of age, health locus of control and psychological co-morbidity on patients' preferences for shared decision making in general practice. *Patient Ed Counseling.* 2006;61(2):292–298.

53. Chen CY, Neufeld PS, Feely CA, et al. Factors influencing compliance with home exercise programs among patients with upper-extremity impairment. *Am J Occup Ther.* 1999;53(2):171–180.

54. Sluijs EM, Kok GJ, van der Zee, J. Correlates of exercise compliance in physical therapy. *Phys Ther.* 1993;73(11):41–56.

55. Worcester S. Patient education improves satisfaction with chronic pain care: physician involvement. *OB/GYN News.* 2003;August:1–21.

56. Beattie P, Dowda M, Turner C, et al. Longitudinal continuity of care is associated with high patient satisfaction with physical therapy. *Phys Ther.* 2005;85(10):1046–1052.

57. Baker S, Marshak HH, Rice GT, et al. Patient participation in physical therapy goal setting. *Phys Ther.* 2001;81(5):118–1127.

58. Saultz JW, Albedaiwi W. Interpersonal continuity of care and patient satisfaction: a critical review. *Ann Fam Med.* 2004;2(5):1–9. Available at: http://www.annfamed.org. Accessed July 2007.

59. Pawar M. Five tips for generating patient satisfaction and compliance. *Fam Pract Manage.* 2005;12(6):44–46.

60. Agency for Healthcare Research and Quality. Expanding Patient-Centered Care to Empower Patients and Assist Providers. Available at: http://www.ahrq.gov. Accessed July 2007.

61. O'Connor AM. Patient education in the year 2000: tailored decision-support, empowerment, and mutual aid. *Qual Health Care.* 1999;8:1–5. Available at: http://www.qshc.bmj.com. Accessed July 2007.

62. Deakin T. Structured patient education: who are the x-perts? *J Diabetes Nurs.* 2006;10(10):375–379.

63. Stewart M, Weston WW, Brown JB, McWhinney IR, McWilliam CL, Freeman TR. Patient-centered Medicine: Transforming the clinical method. Thousand Oaks, CA: Sage Publications; 1995.

64. Steiner WA, Ryser L, Huber E, et al. Use of the ICF model as a clinical problem-solving tool in physical therapy and rehabilitation medicine. *Phys Ther.* 2002;82(11):1098–1108.

65. Schenkman M, Deutsch JE, Gill-Body KM. An integrated framework for decision making in neurologic physical therapist practice. *Phys Ther.* 2006;86(12):1681–1702.

66. Randall KE, McEwen IR. Writing patient-centered functional goals. *Phys Ther.* 2000;80(12): 1197–1204.
67. Fisher AG. Uniting practice and theory in an occupational framework. *Am J Occup Ther.* 1998;52:509–521.
68. Jamieson M, Krupa T, O'Riordan A, et al. Developing empathy as a foundation of client-centered practice: evaluation of a university curriculum initiative. *Can J Occup Ther.* 2006; 73(2):76–85.

# PATIENT EDUCATION VARIABLES: ADHERENCE, COMMUNICATION, AND BEHAVIORAL MODIFICATIONS

Section II of this book, "Patient Education Variables: Adherence, Communication, and Behavioral Modifications," describes adherence approaches and specific communication strategies to be used in patient teaching and learning. Appropriate communication methods for verbal, nonverbal, and written patient education materials are recommended, taking into consideration literacy, numeracy, and health literacy. Section II concludes with descriptions of behavioral modification techniques applied to physical and occupational therapy using the five stages of change model and motivational interviewing.

Section II is divided into the following three chapters:

- Chapter 6: Patient Education and Adherence Variables

- Chapter 7: Patient Education and Communication Variables

- Chapter 8: Patient Education and Behavioral Modification Variables

# PATIENT EDUCATION AND ADHERENCE VARIABLES

## Objectives

After completing Chapter 6, the reader will be able to:

- Recognize how strongly patient education can impact adherence.
- Understand the effects of adherence on interventions.
- Discuss various basic teaching and learning strategies to affect adherence.
- Describe socioeconomic barriers and their importance to adherence.
- Determine patient education approaches for patients who are homeless.
- Explain general adherence strategies for a variety of cultural beliefs.

## The Importance of Patient Education for Adherence with Interventions

Health care literature describing adherence indicates that between 10% and 90% of patients do not fully follow their health care provider's instructional recommendations related to therapeutic regimens.[1-7] Most of the literature agrees that at least half of all patients do not adhere with prescribed regimens including prescription drugs.[1,3–7] In rehabilitation, adherence to lifestyle regimens such as exercises and activities is probably far worse. In regard to pharmacotherapy, it is difficult to predict who will adhere to a given course of medication and who will not because adherence does not correlate with age, sex, race, occupation, education, income level, or socioeconomic status. Even homelessness is not an indicator of a low likelihood of adherence in all patients. Individuals who are homeless can be adherent when given appropriate access to treatment, encouragement, and rewards. The most stable indicator of future adherence seems to be the patient's behavior regarding past interventional regimens.[2]

In pharmacotherapy, adherence to prescription drug regimens can save patients' lives.[3,4,7] The five most common types of nonadherence with medications are: (1) failing to have a prescription filled, (2) taking an incomplete medication dose, (3) taking the medication at the wrong time, (4) forgetting to take one or more medications, and (5) stopping the medication.[1] Each of these behaviors requires individual consideration in order to formulate strategies to enhance patient adherence. Furthermore, failure to consult a health care provider and ask for a medication is especially problematic in patients with asymptomatic conditions, such as hypertension or latent tuberculosis.[7] In many situations, the health care provider must reinforce the importance of taking medications daily—even if the patient does not "feel sick"—in order to prevent the effects of target organ damage or developing resistant strains of an infection. Once a patient obtains a medication, the two most common nonadherence behaviors are omitting one or more doses or taking a medication at the wrong time.[7] These behaviors have been termed *partial adherence*.[7] Although partial adherence is intentional in a minority of patients, in others, such as in older individuals, it is often unintentional. Forgetting to take a medication is the most common cause of taking insufficient medication in this population, and it is attributed to a variety of factors including using more than one pharmacy, seeing different physicians, confusion regarding the regimen, inaccurately labeled containers, and the inability to open childproof containers.[1]

Health care providers have been searching for decades to learn new methods to influence patients to become or remain adherent to good behaviors and self-care. In contemporary medical care, through patient teaching and learning, health care providers play a unique and significant role in assisting patients' adherence with interventions and behavioral changes. Most health care practitioners are aware that compliance or adherence depends not only on the patient's acceptance and understanding of education but also on the provider's ability to persuade the patient that the intervention is meaningful.[1] The patient's perception of the provider's concern, interest, empathy, and credibility also affects adherence.[1,2] Nevertheless, patients and providers view adherence through very different outlooks. Whereas providers value adherence as a necessary factor in maintaining health, patients may value convenience, money, cultural beliefs, habits, and any number of other factors that may take precedence over health care goals.[1] Also, what providers call nonadherence may actually be a patient's expression of disagreement about treatment goals.[2]

# *General Patient Education Strategies to Increase Adherence*

Adherence with medical recommendations is a major concern in medical care. For the most part, when it comes to patients with long-term or chronic medical conditions, adherence is essential to maximize the benefit of the medical interventions.[2] For adherence, in general, both the health care provider and the patient need to work together to achieve the common goal of patient health. The health care provider can enhance adherence by using four simple, general approaches: (1) clarifying and tailoring the intervention regimen to the individual patient, (2) recognizing the patient's teaching and learning needs, (3) identifying behavioral problems, and (4) enlisting and encouraging family members to participate and be supportive.[1,2] However, when relating to the patient, adherence includes many complex variables. For example, for patients who need to enter and remain in care, to take medications, or to modify their lifestyle, several factors can be involved. These factors vary from patient to patient and within individual patients. Issues such as the recommended behavioral modifications, the complexity of the regimens, and the ease with which patients can incorporate those recommendations into their daily routine can significantly affect adherence. A patient's observance of medications or other therapeutic regimens also depends on the patient's ability to pay for care.

## ADHERENCE AS A MULTIFACTORIAL BEHAVIOR

Adherence to medical interventions is a multifactorial behavior and requires a multifactorial response.[1,3,4] Therefore, patient education strategies to encourage adherence must not only address intrapsychic factors such as knowledge of the regimen, belief in the benefits of treatment, subjective norms, and attitudes toward accepting intervention behavior, but also environmental and social factors such as the interpersonal relationship between the health care provider and the patient and social support from family members and friends. Educational approaches to enhance teaching effectiveness and adherence generally begin with providing the patient with a basic understanding of the importance of the medical recommendations.[2] However, verbal information delivery and task demonstration may not be sufficient to sustain or reinforce a behavior over time. Health care providers who employ a combination of verbal and written instructions and demonstrations coupled with behavioral modification resources often see enhanced levels of adherence among their patients.[1] This also can be true for disadvantaged populations and for individuals with low health literacy skills, who often benefit from tailored educational messages regarding the duration of treatment, dosage, frequency, or purpose of intervention. It also has been established that personalized teaching and learning and following up on a patient's observance of therapeutic regimens can result in increased rates of adherence.[1,3–8]

## MULTICOMPONENT ADHERENCE STRATEGIES

When trying to increase adherence, especially with medications, many successful behavioral strategies are available. Multicomponent strategies, however, are much more effective than single component approaches. Some of the most effective behavioral strategies include tailoring the medical regimen to the patient's daily routine and lifestyle, developing cues and rewards, and contingency contracting (**Table 6.1**).[6–8]

Cues, or prompts, are often one of the most effective and efficient behavioral strategies to enhance medication adherence and other types of intervention, including rehabilitation.[5] Another strategy found to be quite successful in improving and maintaining high levels of adherence to medical recommendations is social support, either from a health care professional or within the patient's personal environment. Other factors that can positively impact adherence include direct assistance from the health care provider, patient general satisfaction with the medical visit, and the support of family members in the home environment.[4,5]

Health care providers need to be able to assess patient's adherence with therapeutic regimens. However, in clinical settings, proper assessment of adherence is difficult to perform. The main reason is because of the need for valid and reliable methods to complete such assessments, especially when using direct and indirect approaches.[1,2] An example in physical therapy of direct assessment with adherence would be to have the patient wear a heart rate monitor at home to show adherence with exercises; an indirect assessment could be employed by asking the patient's spouse if the patient is doing the exercise daily. Additionally, when assessing adherence, health care providers must be able to distinguish between patients not using a recommended treatment and those not responding to a given treatment. The basic methods of adherence assessment in health care involve interviews, appointment reviews, prescription refill examinations, analyses of health services utilization, and demonstration of a procedure (**Table 6.2**).[1–8]

The most common forms of adherence assessment in health care, including in physical and occupational rehabilitation, are the interviews of the patient and the patient's family/friends. The clinical interview can be adjusted to the patient's education needs, establishing a patient-centered relationship with the patient (and patient's family/friends) and

| Table 6.1 | Adherence Behavioral Strategies[6–8] |
|---|---|
| | Adjusting interventions to a patient's routines/lifestyles. |
| | Using reminders or cues for interventions (such as emails, phone calls, or postcards). |
| | Using verbal contracts. |

Table
6.2

## *Basic Adherence Methods in Health Care[1–8]*

Interviewing patients and patients' family/friends.

Assuring appointments are made and kept.

Assuring prescriptions are filled and refilled.

Counting pills.

Assessing utilization of health care.

Assessing patient's home-performance of exercises/activities using heart-rate monitor.

asking open-ended questions. The interview can also use the recall interview method. The literature indicates increased adherence to diabetic and pediatric antiretroviral regimens when the provider uses the 24-hour recall interview.[3,4]

Health care providers, especially in pharmacotherapy, are responsive to the fact that detection of nonadherence is a necessary prerequisite for adequate treatment and patient safety. As mentioned before, the two general patient assessment methods for adherence are the indirect and direct approaches.[3,4,7] The *indirect* approaches are most utilized not only in pharmacotherapy, but also in other health care therapeutic regimens. Indirect approaches include the patient self-report, the interview, and the therapeutic outcome. In pharmacotherapy, the computerized medication adherence monitors are the most recent and reliable of the indirect detection methods.[3] The *direct* methods are often used for tracking adherence with prescription drug regimens and include biologic markers, tracer compounds, and biologic assay of body fluids. The direct methods of detection have a higher sensitivity and specificity than the indirect methods. Yet, the direct approaches are more difficult to use in rehabilitation because of the cost of the equipment (such as a heart-rate monitor) and patient's problematic use of such equipment.

Also in pharmacotherapy, use of adherence aids such as medication calendars; special containers, caps, and dispensing systems; and/or adherence packaging are also indicated. In addition, there is an "intelligent" tablet bottle that, unknown to the patient, electronically records the times of opening to assess the adherence of patients with prescribed oral medication.[3] Although the "intelligent" tablet bottle is an expensive method of assessment, in situations such as when providing chemotherapy orally, it could be a life-saving adherence approach. Additional strategies for improving adherence with health care interventions include: (1) identification of risk factors for nonadherence; (2) development, with the patient's participation, of an individualized treatment plan that simplifies the regimen as much as possible; (3) education of the patient, including information about his or her illness; (4) detailed instructions on how to accomplish the therapeutic regimen; and (5) an explanation of the benefits and possible adverse effects of the therapy.[2–4,7,8]

Some of the listed adherence strategies have been used for decades in rehabilitation. For example, physical and occupational therapists always interview patients about their exercise programs, educate them about their illness or disorders, and explain to them the benefits, the adverse effects, and the alternatives to interventions (**Table 6.3**).[5]

In the area of adherence and patient education, rehabilitation providers are aware that determining which factors impede adherence is essential when searching for strategies to improve it. These strategies are dependent on the patient's goals regarding health outcomes. Almost all research on adherence focuses on a health outcome and presumes that adherence to selected recommendations facilitates achievement of the desired outcome.[1,3–9] Therefore, patient education and establishment of therapeutic goals with the patient are extremely important. For example, adult patients with diabetes who have knowledge of therapeutic goals are typically adherent with cholesterol-lowering medications.[10]

Many other variables and predictors can be involved with adherence. In regard to predictors, patient adherence during the first month of treatment is a predictor of long-term continuity of the therapeutic regimen.[1,4] Nevertheless, the literature shows that adherence routinely decreases over time.[4–7] The behavior of the health care providers and the method of delivery of medical care are two important contributors to a patient's adherence. When the rehabilitation provider sincerely believes in a specific method of intervention, the patient's adherence increases.[4] Also, the quality of the patient-provider relationship can

| Table 6.3 | ***General Adherence Strategies Within Physical and Occupational Rehabilitation***[1,5,6] |
|---|---|
| Considering the patient's desired health outcome. |
| Prioritizing the patient's needs. |
| Using specific intervention(s) proven to help the patient. |
| Establishing a therapeutic relationship with the patient. |
| Assessing and positively responding to additional adherence variables of the patient, such as physical, cognitive, social, economic, and cultural. |
| Cooperating with the health care team (and organization) to increase patient satisfaction. |
| Conducting an efficient patient interview. |
| Using effective teaching and learning techniques. |

determine the patient's adherence to interventions. A satisfactory therapeutic relationship and partnership among the patient, the therapist, and the health care organization (including the health care team) are significant factors in health care adherence. As examples, patients who have diabetes and are satisfied with their relationship with their health care providers show better adherence to diabetes regimens.[4] Patients with chronic diseases who have a negative view of others and do not trust others rate their adherence as poor because they do not have confidence in their health care provider or health care organization.[6] These patients also have low adherence to medication use.

Being able to properly distinguish between behavioral and nonbehavioral causes of nonadherence also represents a strategy for adherence improvement.[2] This process of differentiation may include examining whether the patient's behavior contributes directly to the nonadherence or whether there are other factors beyond the patient's control such as physical or cognitive impairments or even social and cultural issues. Social factors can impact a patient's ability or readiness to follow recommendations. A patient's social support system, such as family or friends, can encourage or discourage adherence. Ethnic or religious influences also can significantly affect adherence, as can adequate or inadequate housing, transportation, or resources.

Health care providers must be able to understand each specific patient's requirements from the initial examination and the beginning of interventions so they can help them adhere to therapeutic regimens. For example, in cases of diabetes, the health care provider who initially diagnosed the patient should evaluate whether the patient has financial resources to modify his or her dietary needs or to buy all the necessary antidiabetic medications and testing supplies.[4] A patient's specific performance and needs must be ranked in their order of importance. Although the majority of patients with diabetes may be able to receive help with drug prescriptions, the patient's priority will always be the ability to buy the antidiabetic medications and testing supplies before modifying his or her dietary needs. In addition, each patient's behavior must be rated according to changeability. Theoretically, in rehabilitation, the patient with diabetes may be more likely to adhere to the daily dietary instructions than follow the physical therapist's recommendations with home exercises. Ultimately, the therapist should prioritize the patient's adherence behaviors, considering their importance and changeability. Then, the patient's education goals and strategies should target those selected adherence behaviors that will help the patient succeed. Collecting this data about the patient requires that the therapist use sensitivity and skill and, most importantly, teaching and learning techniques.

## Specific Patient Education Strategies to Increase Adherence

Identifying adherence factors can help the health care provider to assess a patient's needs in regard to knowledge, skills, or attitudes, which will maximize the potential for positive interventional outcomes. Because patient education includes a relationship between the provider and the patient, specific patient needs should be considered prior to starting the patient education process.[2] Patient education is not a method of only giving information to the patient, but also involves receiving information from the patient. During patient teaching and learning, there should be a continuous search on the part of the health care provider to identify and correct probable causes that may impede the educational process and adherence. Some of these causes can be categorized as socioeconomic and cultural, specific physical impairments (such as an older adult's problems with vision, hearing, or cognition), and behavioral factors.[2,9]

## STRATEGIES RELATED TO SOCIAL SUPPORT VARIABLES

A patient's socioeconomic barriers to adherence may include his or her family relationship and social support, practical and logistical issues such as lack of transportation and health insurance, the inability to take time off from work to keep medical appointments, and a lack of medical continuity (not always seeing the same health care provider).[11] The patient's family and friends are social groups that can influence, both negatively and positively, the patient's ability to follow therapeutic regimens. For example, in situations where the patient may be willing to adhere to specific interventions, the family could have a negative impact on the patient's adherence if they do not understand the importance of the interventional regimen.[11,12] In contrast, research indicates that spouse and family member support increases intervention adherence.[4–7,11,12] Patients who receive social support from the community, family, spouse, friends, companions, or caregivers have better adherence with health care and medication regimens.[11,12]

In regard to exercise, the support of the spouse is a significant predictor of adherence, especially for male patients.[12] Social support is also a strong predictor of exercise tolerance in cardiac rehabilitation.[11] Patients and their spouses need collective teaching and learning to assume responsibility for and adopt exercise programs or activities. Patients or clients who have low levels of family conflict and high levels of cohesion, organization, and good communication patterns within the family are associated with better adherence.[11] Consequently, the role of the health care provider in patient education is to be able to understand the individual patient and that patient's relationship to the social group represented by family and/or friends, and their influence on the patient. Teaching and learning should be adapted not only to the patient, but also to the patient's social group.[12]

One example of a patient adherence strategy, the 90 Second Intervention (90 SI), can be employed as a way to increase a patient's social support from family or friends.[8] The 90 SI uses the therapeutic relationship between the health care provider and patient and enlists family and friends to maintain the patient's adherence with the therapeutic regimen.[8] It is based on the premise that social support plays a key role in promoting health, decreasing susceptibility to disease, and facilitating recovery from illness. The method is simple: the health care provider asks the patient to identify who in their life loves or cares for them and would help them adhere to the intervention regimen. To implement the 90 SI, the health care provider instructs the patient to telephone, in his or her presence, the identified helper(s) who then agree to support the patients' therapeutic interventional regimen.[8] Health care providers have used the 90 SI to help patients improve and control their hypertension.[8]

In physical and occupational therapy, the 90 SI can be used to support patients in a home exercise program (HEP). The helper would need to come to therapy with the patient and receive the necessary patient instruction, including diagrams, pictures, and directions regarding the HEP. The physical or occupational therapist would need to call the helper daily and check on the patient's progress with the HEP. When necessary, the therapist may need to offer more information or clarification to the helper to improve patient success with the HEP regimen. The idea of the 90 SI also was applied in a nursing research study that evaluated assisted walking and walking combined with conversation as compared to a conversation-only intervention in nursing home residents with Alzheimer's disease.[9] The conversation component of the combined walking and conversation treatment can improve patient adherence with the intervention and the outcome.[9] This result shows that having another individual, such as a member of the family or a friend, helping the patient with physical or occupational therapy interventions can increase patient adherence.

## STRATEGIES RELATED TO HOMELESSNESS

Patient education and adherence in the homeless population is a major challenge for health care providers. People who are homeless have the same health problems as people with homes, but at rates three to six times greater than housed people.[13] Without a home, there is no place to recuperate from an illness or to treat an injury, and health problems tend to get far worse before they get better.

Homelessness is a social problem of epidemic proportions worldwide. In the United States, estimates of the homeless population range between 3 and 13.5 million, and as much as 7.4% of the general population will experience homelessness in their lifetime.[14] Homelessness affects a diverse population of all ethnic groups and includes urban and rural families, the elderly, children, veterans, migrant farm workers, persons with mental illness, and individuals with substance use disorders.[14] Minority groups are overrepresented in this population, most likely due to disparities in economic opportunities. Causes of homelessness are related to divorce or separation, domestic violence, pregnancy, adolescent runaways, substance use, eviction, acute or chronic unemployment, and the deinstitutionalization of persons with mental illness. A disparity between the need for low-income housing and its availability has also contributed to the epidemic of homelessness. A large segment of the population who is homeless consists of families with children. Each year, more than 1.35 million children and youth experience life without a home, living in shelters, vehicles, and parks.[15] One out of seven of those treated by homeless health care projects is a child under age 15.[15] Forty percent of men who are homeless are veterans, although veterans comprise only 34% of the adult male population.[16]

People who are homeless suffer from a variety of medical problems such as hypertension, diabetes, seizures, arthritis, pulmonary diseases, and musculoskeletal disorders.[17] The severity of the disease or disorder for individuals who are homeless is very high. The majority of homeless individuals may not seek medical care. The reasons can be addiction disorders, mental illness, or the inability and unwillingness to visit a health care provider and adhere to treatments.[17] As a result, it is not unusual to see younger individuals developing the health impairments and disabilities common in older people.[17] Conditions such as hypertension, diabetes, and anemia are often inadequately controlled and may go undetected for long periods of time.[17] Other common health problems in homeless individuals are pulmonary disorders, venous stasis, and skin infections. Additionally, because of inadequate footwear, prolonged exposure to moisture, and long periods of walking and standing, homeless people may have various foot disorders (such as tinea pedis, onychomycosis, and corns and calluses).[17] Proper foot care requires early detection of problems, education regarding foot hygiene, and the provision of adequate shoes and socks.[17]

People who are homeless are at increased risk of contracting tuberculosis (TB).[17] The transmission of TB, especially among high-risk groups also who may be infected with HIV, may go undetected and untreated for years.[18] Consequently, TB should be tested for in any person who is homeless, especially those who have a fever and a persistent cough.[17] The majority of TB cases among the homeless are diagnosed as primary tuberculosis. Treatment of active TB can be complicated because of nonadherence to medication therapy and the development of drug resistance.[17] Many individuals who are homeless, especially younger people, are also infected with HIV.[17] Common risk factors for HIV infection in young individuals may include prostitution, multiple sexual partners, inconsistent use of condoms, and injection drug use.[16] Similar to nonadherence with TB treatment, the homeless population infected with HIV is at high risk for poor adherence to highly active antiretroviral therapy (HAART).[19] A study found that one-third of the homeless and marginally housed persons receiving HAART discontinued therapy during the follow-up period.[19] This, in the homeless population, can cause a development of drug-resistant strains of HIV.[19]

Typically, individuals who are homeless do not have health insurance. The federal Medicaid plan, together with individual state programs, has been providing coverage for many women and children who are homeless as well as for some disabled men. Similar to other health care providers, physical and occupational therapists must include the following considerations when examining and evaluating patients who are homeless: information regarding the place where the patient lives, eating habits, access to food and water, sexual history, medications, use of illicit drugs or tobacco and alcohol, literacy level, friends and extended family, and walking activity as well as the condition of their footwear (**Table 6.4**).[20]

At each visit the health care provider should:[20]

1. Reassess the patient's current living situation including where they live, how long they have lived there, who lives with them, and their relationship to that person.

2. Reassess the psychological, sociological, and economic factors that may affect the plan of care.

3. Refer the patient to community resources, as needed (such as the Department of Social Services).

4. Reassess food sources.

5. Obtain an emergency contact with a phone number.

6. Obtain a phone number for the patient if possible. Some patients have cell phones, voice mail numbers, or can receive messages at shelters or programs.

| Table 6.4 | *Patient Education Considerations for Homeless Patients*[20] |
|---|---|

Assess where the patient is living (such as in a shelter or on the street).

Inquire as to when the patient last had a permanent or regular place to live, and if they have ever had their own apartment or home.

Inquire about the patient's eating habits and patterns including nutrition status, weight history, and food sources (such as soup kitchens). Many food sources supply only one meal a day, so the homeless person must visit multiple places for food.

Inquire as to whether the patient has access to food and water when they want or need it.

Assess and reassess how much walking the patient is doing as well as the condition and fit of footwear.

Inquire as to whether the patient has ever had foot sores, ulcers, or any other problems with their feet.

Obtain a sexual history including contraception and reproductive history.

Ascertain the patient's current medications and how they are obtained.

Explore the use of tobacco, alcohol, and illicit drugs, and the frequency and route of use. Assess the patient's readiness to change this behavior.

Assess the patient's literacy level.

Be aware of the term *doubled up*, referring to a situation where individuals are unable to maintain their housing situation and are forced to stay with a series of friends and/or extended family members.

In regard to patient education, many patients who are homeless are dependent on tobacco, alcohol, or illicit drugs, and may not be ready or able to abstain from these substances. Helping the patient move in that direction may be the final goal. Many therapeutic interventions can help to decrease the person's health risks until the individual is ready to change their behavior. Motivational interviewing is a successful technique to reduce risk of complications. Self-management goal setting also can be a useful method to involve patients in their health care.[21] Allowing the patient to decide what is important in the contribution to his or her health is considered another adherence strategy, even if the goal is not directly related to a diagnosis of their disease or disorder. This first step for the health care provider's patient education is to give the patient the confidence to make further changes as necessary. Providing culturally suitable patient education that involves the patient in the learning process is also critical.[21,22] Successful approaches to teaching people who are homeless may include peer interaction and support groups. Unfortunately, regarding physical and occupational therapy, unstable living conditions or homelessness can have a large negative impact on therapeutic interventions and adherence (**Table 6.5**).

In physical therapy, an important aspect when treating homeless patients is an assessment of the patients' feet. Foot problems in homeless patients often result from prolonged standing and walking. When combined with diabetes, the patient is at high risk for foot ulcers. The same as when treating diabetic patients, physical therapists should apply the following patient instructions:

1. Keep feet dry and take shoes and socks off at night.

2. Wash socks every night, if possible, and dry thoroughly.

| Table 6.5 | *Teaching and Learning Strategies for Those Who Are Homeless or in Unstable Living Conditions*[13] |
|---|---|
| The health care provider should involve family members in the intervention or refer the patient to a support group. | |
| The health care provider should help the patient meet the fundamental needs for housing and food. | |
| The health care provider should help the patient address comorbid conditions such as psychiatric illnesses and substance abuse. | |
| The health care provider should offer incentives for adherence and encourage routine participation in health care visits. | |
| The health care provider should provide information about interventions. In cases of medication adherence, the health care provider should directly observe medication administration and provide information about medications and side effects. | |
| Patient education ensures continuity of care and reduces the complications related to illness and incidence of disorder/disease. | |
| Patient education maximizes the individual's independence with home exercise programs and activities that promote independence in activities of daily living as well as continuity of care. | |

3. Examine feet; if they cannot see the bottom of their feet, teach patients how to use a mirror.

4. Visit the clinic immediately if the patients have open foot sores or areas of redness.

5. Elevate legs to a level at or above their heart whenever possible to prevent/alleviate fluid stasis in lower extremities; this is especially important for patients who are sleeping in chairs.

Additionally, physical therapists must identify community resources to acquire free shoes and socks and also refer patients, as needed, to medical intervention. For example, a patient with diabetes and foot problems should be referred to a podiatrist for relief of diabetic foot conditions.

## STRATEGIES RELATED TO CULTURAL VARIABLES

Demographic factors such as being an ethnic minority, having a low socioeconomic status, and having a low level of education have been associated with low regimen adherence, especially in chronic diseases such as diabetes.[4] Health, morbidity, and mortality are also related to income and education factors.[21] For example, life expectancy, deaths from cancer and heart disease, incidences of diabetes and hypertension, and use of health services have been correlated to family income.[21] In regard to ethnicity, many African American patients view receiving health care as a degrading or humiliating experience.[21] Some patients fear or resent health clinics because of the long waiting times, feelings of racism or segregation, use of medical terminology by the health care providers, loss of identity, and feelings of powerlessness and alienation in the system. Also, among Native Americans, mistrust of mainstream institutions such as hospitals or health care establishments is common.[21]

For physical and occupational therapists working as rehabilitation providers, building trust with the patient and his or her family is an important step in patient adherence and education. The therapist's cultural competence plays a very significant role in adherence. Cultural beliefs can dictate how medical information is disseminated and received. For example, in some Arab cultures, it is preferable for a family or community member to act as an intermediary communicating directly with the health care provider and then discussing the findings with the patient.[21,22] When considering cultural communities, the lesbian, gay, bisexual, and transgender (LGBT) community should also be included. Trust in the rehabilitation provider can encourage LGBT older adults to act on health messages and promote compliant behavior.[21] Welcoming language and respect for privacy and confidentiality can generate trust and reliability. Using terms such as *partner* instead of *family* and avoiding heterosexual relationship terms can increase a patient's feelings of trust and adherence.[22]

Cultural competence takes time to acquire as physical and occupational therapists and assistants learn new skills, change attitudes, and grasp new knowledge. Examining personal biases and stereotypes as an initial step is extremely important to enhance quality cross-cultural care.[23] Increasing the therapist's ability to recognize different cultural values, beliefs, and practices and to address these factors in interventions can lead to successful outcomes.[23] Rehabilitation providers should always consider that culture impacts how patients comprehend and apply health information. Patients apply their individual experiences and customs to each health situation. For example, many patients from parts of the world where health resources are inadequate may not understand or comply with preventive measures such as blood pressure checks or mammogram and Pap smear screenings.[23] Cultural differences are also apparent when working with patients from different regions of the United States; for example, individuals living in the south of the country may have different health concepts and intervention preferences as compared to those living in the north.

Because it is almost impossible to meet all of a patient's cultural needs, all health care providers including physical and occupational therapists and assistants have to continuously learn to become culturally competent and help their patients to the best of their abilities. The development of cultural competence depends more on attitude than on specific knowledge of the culture. Appropriate patient interaction and education can only be applied using respect of and sensitivity for each patient's cultural background. In general, cultural competence can be addressed through awareness, acknowledgment, acceptance, and respect of a patient's racial characteristics, national origin, religious affiliations, physical size, spoken language, sexual orientation, physical and mental disability, age, gender, socioeconomic status, political orientation, geographic location, and occupational status.[23] Therapists should continuously try to achieve the ability and availability to effectively work within the cultural context of a patient including the patient's family and the community. Using a cultural desire concept of wanting to become culturally knowledgeable (see Chapter 16), therapists should be open and flexible with patients, accept patients' cultural and social differences, learn from their patients, and show genuine commitment to care and help all their patients. Through patient education, physical and occupational therapists and assistants should be able to create a better fit between the needs of their patients and specific adherence methods to meet those needs (**Table 6.6** and **Table 6.7**).

Creating a welcoming atmosphere is important for patient education and adherence to show patients that they are appreciated and respected. Despite cultural and linguistic differences, rehabilitation providers should use communication methods that their patients can understand. For example, they can use translated signs or display multicultural artifacts in their offices. Also, greeting patients in their native language and trying to pronounce their names correctly conveys the willingness to communicate with patients despite linguistic differences.[22] Using trained interpreters is also important for patient education, not only from the aspect of communicating properly, but also from the ethical, confidential, and cultural beliefs aspects.[22] The interpreter can act as a cultural broker when presenting information by maintaining the patient's own cultural beliefs and practices.[21]

In rehabilitation, as in other areas of health care, physical or occupational therapists and assistants benefit from understanding and preserving a patient's cultural beliefs during the rehabilitation process. Applying interventions while accepting and complying with a patient's cultural norms is a gradual and slow learning process for therapists. Rehabilitation providers continuously need to learn from their patients, trying to understand their culture and apply interventions that take into consideration their traditions, customs, and norms. As an example in physical therapy, a physical therapist was treating a patient after a

| Table 6.6 | **Basic Patient Education Adherence Strategies for Cultural Belief Barriers[23]** |
|---|---|

Establish a relationship with the patient characterized by trust and support.

Determine the patient's preferences regarding teaching and learning.

Seek an understanding of the causes of illness from the patient's cultural point of view.

Elicit and understand (in a nonjudgmental way) information about the patient's use of nontraditional interventions.

When providing patient education, consider whether the primary importance is placed on the patient or on the community; the roles that are generally accepted in regard to women, men, and children; whether the preferred family structure is nuclear or extended, and one generation or multigenerational; and who receives the information.

Acquire the skills and competencies necessary for quality cross-cultural care.

| Table 6.7 | **Basic Patient Education Adherence Strategies for Patients with Limited English Language Proficiency[22]** |
|---|---|

The therapist should use a translator. The therapist should try not to use a family member or a companion to translate to the patient or for the patient.

The therapist should always provide direct communication to the patient and not the family member or companion.

The therapist should not talk loudly or exaggerate his or her speech.

The therapist should use nonverbal cues and body language.

The therapist should use diagrams, pictures, or pictograms to help communicate information.

The therapist should reinforce the information with a family member or a companion, if available and appropriate.

The therapist should verify patient understanding by having the patient "teach back" the instructions he or she received.

cerebral vascular accident (CVA) who had come to the United States from India.[23] Although the therapist applied the best methods of intervention, the patient cancelled the therapy sessions and ended the program. The reason for termination was that the patient became offended by having his feet touched during therapy. The therapist approached the patient from the perspective of the culture of rehabilitation, assuming that the manner of intervention is secondary when reaching the patient's goals and outcomes.[23] In this example, the therapist had to stabilize the patient's feet in order to increase his balance and coordination in standing. In the patient's culture, the feet are considered dirty and touching them meant a significant invasion of his sense of body space.[23] If the therapist had a prior understanding of the patient's cultural taboos there would have been a better outcome, preserving the patient's adherence and motivation.

Additionally, the written materials for patient education should be culturally appropriate, including graphics and examples that the patient can relate to and accept. The therapist and the translator must work together to develop written rehabilitative information that is accurate and adapted to patients' linguistic and cultural differences. Many translated documents can lose their meaning when important accent marks are omitted. For text translations, the provider can translate the materials from English to the new language, translate back the information from the new language to English (for accuracy), design and lay out materials to enhance understanding, test the material with the patient, and make any necessary revisions.[22] When two languages need to be used on the same document (such as English and Spanish), the therapist may consider the fact that one sentence in English can be three to four sentences in Spanish. In that case, the material should be written using a small number of words and more illustrations to avoid having the page look crammed full of text. Consideration should be given to a patient's culture, age, and interests. For example, in rehabilitation, a home exercise program should include pictures of activities that a patient may be more familiar with rather than complicated exercises.

Verbal communication with patients who speak limited English should focus on the most essential skills and behaviors. Physical and occupational therapists and assistants should ensure understanding of the patient's goals, taking into consideration the patient's age, degree of anxiety, and level of understanding; the presence of a language barrier; and specific cultural customs.[22] Speaking clearly and concisely in a normal tone of voice is very important. Communication should be at a slower pace, pausing for 2 to 3 seconds after asking questions or providing new information.[22] Therapists should not use a loud voice in their communication because it may be interpreted as anger. The tone and volume of voice are qualities that all health care providers, including those involved in rehabilitation, must be constantly aware of during verbal communication and patient teaching and learning. They also should remember that a patient's limited English proficiency is not a reflection of the patient's level of intellectual functioning or the patient's ability to communicate in his or her native language.[22] In general, technical jargon or technical terms should never be used in communication with patients.

# 7 PATIENT EDUCATION AND COMMUNICATION VARIABLES

## Objectives

After completing Chapter 7, the reader will be able to:

- Discuss the general importance of communication skills in patient teaching and learning.
- Identify the importance of verbal and nonverbal communication in patient education.
- Identify health communication issues and strategies.
- Recognize the significance of literacy, health literacy, and numeracy in the process of communicating between the health care provider and the patient or client.
- Define literacy, illiteracy, numeracy, and health literacy.
- Describe low literacy barriers and strategies to improve patients' teaching and learning.
- Recognize the importance of proper communication in the instruction of patients with low health literacy.
- Assess the role of the Internet as a communication tool to provide health information.
- Evaluate the importance of written communication in patient education.
- List methods for evaluating the readability level of written patient education material.

- Compare and contrast three readability methods: the Flesch Reading Ease test, the Gunning Fog formula, and the Flesch-Kincaid test.

- Apply the SMOG formula of readability to written patient education material.

- List general guidelines for written patient teaching and learning information.

- Describe the most important readability design strategies.

- Compare and contrast *concept words* with *category words* and *value judgment words*.

- Identify basic communication strategies regarding teaching and learning for patients with visual, cognitive, and hearing impairments.

- List patient education strategies that can be applied with patients who have limited English language proficiency.

# *General Communication Skills/Strategies Used in Patient Education*

In health care, one of the key features of patient education and adherence with interventions is the health care provider's ability to effectively communicate with the patient or client (and family). Good communication enhances the relationship between the provider and the patient. The tasks of effective communication include giving and receiving appropriate information.

## EXPRESSIVE AND EMOTIONAL SKILLS

Two communication skills required to convey information are expressive and emotional skills. Expressive skills are an individual's ability to give information verbally to others regarding their behaviors and also to articulate his or her beliefs and feelings.[24,25] Emotional skills are an individual's ability to take responsibility and make difficult decisions when transmitting a message to another person.[24] Skills involving emotions also can be considered interpersonal skills. Emotional skills can be used to speak about information that is difficult to express but needs to be said. Another communication skill is the ability to listen and obtain information from others.[24] When receiving information, the listener's emotional skills allow him or her to expressively understand the other person's concerns and feelings and agree (or disagree) with the social interaction rules. These rules are ways people behave as they interact with each other.[25] Expressive verbal skills are considered the simplest forms of communication to interact with people. Expressive verbal skills are typically performed in three stages: (1) getting the other person's attention, (2) conveying the information, and (3) checking the other person understanding.[25] Listening skills are a mirror image of the verbal expressive skills. They are more difficult than expressive skills, however, because they depend on a foundation of emotional skills.

## ACTIVE LISTENING SKILLS

A health care professional with good listening capabilities in patient education can place him- or herself 100% at the speaker's disposal.[26] Only through active listening can physical and occupational therapists and assistants offer effective patient teaching and learning. Active listening encourages the establishment of a therapeutic relationship with the patient, and is a skill the therapist can learn and practice.[26] It requires effort, honesty, commitment, and sometimes changing the therapist's personality to learn compassion and empathy (**Table 7.1**).[26]

Active listening in physical and occupational rehabilitation practice includes the following actions:[26]

1. The therapist focusing their attention on the patient.

2. The therapist helping the patient feel free to talk and express opinions (by smiling and looking at the patient).

3. The therapist being attentive to the patient's nonverbal communication, such as gestures, facial expressions, tone of voice, and body postures.

4. The therapist asking the patient to clarify the meanings or feelings involved in the message or to expand on the statement.

5. The therapist repeating the patient's message to verify the meaning and the content.

6. The therapist taking notes to help remember and document the patient's information.

7. The therapist using nonverbal communication (such as facial expressions, tone of voice, and body language) as necessary to show involvement in the patient's message.

| Table 7.1 |
| --- |
| **Effective Listening Skills[26]** |
| Listening to the other person with undivided attention. |
| Using verbal and nonverbal expressions when listening. |
| Acknowledging the other person's whole message. |
| Checking with the other person to verify correct understanding of the meaning of the message. |
| Asking the other person questions to clarify the meaning. |

8. The therapist giving the patient adequate time to present the full message.

9. The therapist genuinely empathizing with the patient.

Acknowledgement is one of the most important aspects of good listening skills. The therapist's ability to recognize and acknowledge the significance of the patient's message can increase or decrease the effectiveness of the communication process.[26]

Additionally, in rehabilitation, proficient listening skills are critical elements of the initial examination and evaluation. The therapist's listening skills could create—from the beginning of rehabilitation—a good interpersonal relationship with the patient. This relationship is characterized by the therapist showing empathy, courtesy, friendliness, reassurance, support, and encouragement as well as offering explanations and positive reinforcement.[27] In the primary care practice, the establishment of an interpersonal relationship with the patient has been linked with increased patient adherence with interventions and patient satisfaction.[27]

## NONVERBAL COMMUNICATION SKILLS

The communication process includes nonverbal expressions, such as a person's facial expression, direction of gaze, posture, gestures, and proximity between speaker and listener.[26] It also involves elements of verbal communication such as the characteristics of a person's speech, tone of voice, pace, pause, inflection, volume, and timbre. Nonverbal communication allows someone to make a general judgment about how genuine the other person is based on the amount of agreement between what a person's words state and what his or her body language shows.[26]

There are three basic body language patterns (**Table 7.2**). The *aggressive pattern* is characterized by a large silhouette posture, forward movement gestures, a demanding tone of

| Table 7.2 | *Body Language Patterns*[27,28] | |
|---|---|
| Appeasing pattern | Negative pattern expressing shy and nervous behavior; part of an individual's self-defense mechanism. |
| Aggressive pattern | Negative pattern expressing hostile and antagonistic behavior; also part of an individual's self-defense mechanism. |
| Non-defensive pattern | Positive pattern expressing trust and control. |

voice, an angry expression, and sustained eye contact.[28] The *appeasing pattern* is character-ized by a small silhouette posture, shy gestures, a soft or tremulous tone of voice, an appre-hensive expression, and minimal eye contact.[27] The *nondefensive pattern* is characterized by normal posture and gestures, usual expression, and frequent eye contact.[27] The nondefen-sive pattern typically is an intermediate between the appeasing and aggressive patterns.[27] Aggressiveness and appeasement are both self-defense mechanisms that show defensive-ness in the other person.

It is difficult for someone to change their nonverbal behavior because it requires con-scious control. As a result, physical and occupational therapists and assistants have to be aware of their own body language patterns and also recognize and empathize with their patients' nonverbal communication. For example, in health care, aggressive behaviors may be caused by lack of training in leadership roles, ambiguous roles and responsibilities, and standard operating procedures.[28] For therapists, the best communication pattern is non-defensive behavior characterized by openness, sincerity, responsiveness, understanding, and exploration of other points of view.[26] Listening and summarizing the patient's position as well as being open-minded, flexible, and appreciative of people's opinions could help to achieve goals and outcomes and also demonstrate concern and responsiveness to the patients or clients.[26]

## COMMUNICATION PRIORITIES IN PATIENT-CENTERED CARE

The entire communication process needs to be prioritized by health care providers. Typi-cally, a rehabilitation provider should first address the patient's highest priority issue; then, the provider's main concern or questions can be expressed and resolved. During the com-munication process, effective decisions should be made by the therapist and the patient if the appropriate information was given and received. For the therapist to make effective decisions that are patient-centered, the following patient priorities should be understood: feelings, information, decisions, and outcomes (FIDO; see **Table 7.3**).[2,5]

| Table 7.3 | *Patient's Priorities for Care Using Modified FIDO[2,5]* |
|---|---|
| **Feelings** of the patient towards outcomes. |
| **Information** given by the patient that is specific, accurate, and relevant to the outcomes. |
| **Decisions** expressed by the patient. |
| **Outcomes** expressed by the patient that are to be accomplished. |

## COMMUNICATION BARRIERS AND STRATEGIES

Patients, the same as health care providers, need to learn communication methods to be able to interact with providers. Unfortunately, many patients still exhibit the passive approach to health that existed in the United States before the 1960s. For centuries, the prevailing view was that normally competent adults become vulnerable and childlike when afflicted with an illness. Wrongly, it was believed that illness changes people into individuals who are unable to understand anything about their medical condition or what to do about it. In that very old approach, the health care provider–patient relationship mirrored the parent-child relationship. In addition, because in the past the majority of providers were men (physicians), the relationship was called paternalistic. In the late 1960s and early 1970s, this view began to change due to advances in science and medical technology. Patients and their advocates understood that illness does not automatically render them incompetent to make decisions, and they should have the opportunity to give their informed consent to interventions.[29] As a result, for more than 30 years, health care providers have been experiencing patients changing from submissive to assertive. Nevertheless, sometimes patients may confuse assertiveness with aggressiveness. They feel they need to challenge health care providers and not actively participate in their care. These patients or clients need education to understand that they are partners in their health care, exploring outcomes and making informed decisions regarding their goals. At the same time, some health care providers, especially those whose education was rendered either years ago or in other countries, need to change their attitudes, biases, and past practices. They should maintain objectivity and deliver health care in a friendly and respectful climate.

The business model of care also can cause problems regarding the patient-provider relationship and also the patient teaching and learning aspect of modern health care. In this model, patients are considered to be consumers of care and not participants in care. The business model of health care is wrongly marked in American culture by a "buyer beware" warning that encourages distrust of the health care provider and creates a very unfriendly climate. In this environment, patients' opinions or requests are misinterpreted and challenged and health care providers are perceived as angry and confused. For patients who are involved in this type of situation, it is best to look for another provider who will better understand them and offer what they want. Patients should present themselves and be recognized as equals and experts in their own right.[26] They need to learn from the beginning of their visit with the health care provider that they are considered partners whose views and questions deserve consideration and not automatic dismissal.[26] Patients also need to learn that they can be active, assertive partners, exploring the best outcomes with their health care providers, and not necessarily telling them what to do.[26] Patients must determine that their interest is in understanding and not in challenging the provider. Additionally, the role of the patient is to explain and not to apologize. By becoming partners with their health care providers, patients are able to transition from a paternalistic relationship to a collaborative one.

Modern health care relies more and more on objective, evidence-based knowledge. Many health care providers and professionals from various health care disciplines prefer to treat patients using objective knowledge, dismissing as unproven a patient's subjective information. This is a 21st-century phenomenon in which providers use medical technology for diagnostic purposes, ignoring the subjective patient interviews. Many health care professionals prefer to use just the "science of medicine," instead of the "art of medicine." The science of medicine represents a systematic and objective basis for understanding the human body and its afflictions whereas the art of medicine is composed mostly of subjective patient data.[29] Following the scientific trend, some health care providers ignore the art of medicine to obtain patient symptom information. Some patients are happy with these new methods of diagnosing and providing interventions; however, most patients prefer health care professionals and providers who combine the science with the art of medicine. Physical and occupational rehabilitation providers are able to harmoniously unite the evidence-based science with the art of medicine. The patient's subjective communication is added to the objectivity of tests and measures, combining to create a patient-centered plan of care for optimal patient rehabilitation outcomes.

Another barrier in patient communication that may affect many areas of health care delivery is the time issue. Insurance reimbursement systems, where insurance companies negotiate fees for various health care services, have affected several areas of the health care industry. Primary care as a point of consultation and evaluation is one of these areas because insurers do not pay providers for listening to patients. As a consequence, some primary health care providers must see more patients, spend less time with them, and neglect the importance of the listening aspects of the examination.[29] Unfortunately, these providers are not aware that inviting patients to speak, listening to them, and acknowledging their concerns have been shown to minimally increase time spent. Nevertheless, the majority of health care providers and professionals are responsive to patient information, understanding its value in successful interventions.[29] Listening skills associated with the art of medicine are extremely important for the patient-provider relationship and outcomes.

Physical and occupational therapists should establish a therapeutic relationship with the patient by asking nonjudgmental questions, listening to the patient and family, and encouraging the patient in problem solving and decision making (**Table 7.4**).[26]

When asking nonjudgmental questions, the therapist should encourage the patient to be honest and open about their beliefs and concerns. Many cultures place a different value on time than the Western health care provider. Acting in a hurried or impatient manner may seem like a sign of disrespect. The therapist needs to take time to ask questions and listen to the patient to learn more about their disease or disorder. A patient who feels respected will be more likely to respond honestly and completely. Listening attentively to the patient without interrupting shows genuine interest in the patient's replies.[26] Rephrasing the patient's comments demonstrates that the therapist is listening and gives the patient an opportunity to understand that the provider heard them correctly or to explain again if necessary.[26] Many misunderstandings are common even when the patient and the provider come from the same culture. When a patient and a provider come from different cultures, the likelihood of miscommunication is greatly increased.[23]

Changing patient behavior is challenging for everyone. Patient education can be improved when the therapist considers the social and family contexts of the patient and

| Table 7.4 | *Communication Skills that Promote Therapeutic Relationships*[26] |
|---|---|
| | Asking the patient nonjudgmental questions that help the provider understand the patient's perspective on the disease (disorder), its causes, and its possible interventions. |
| | Carefully listening to the patient's replies, trying to pick up clues to the patient's understanding as well as his or her ability to adhere to a recommended intervention. |
| | Working with the patient and family members (as appropriate) to set realistic goals for behavior change, if needed. |
| | Involving the patient in active problem solving. |

adjusts the recommendation for interventions accordingly. In addition, for many patients, a "lecture" from the health care provider (or a family member) is not the most effective method for receiving or acting on a health message and adhering with interventions. Most patients would be more attentive and remember instructions much better if they were actively involved in identifying their problems and seeking practical solutions with the provider.

# Patient Education and Health Communication Factors and Strategies

In contemporary health care, patients are expected to be active and assertive partners in health.[26] Health care providers need to explore facts with their patients, but not tell the patients what to do. The health care providers' role is to understand the patients, not to challenge them. In this collaborative model of care, the health care providers apply evidence-based interventions to their patients. Inviting patients to speak, listening to them, and acknowledging their concerns increases the success of interventions.[26] Communication, and specifically health communication, is an intricate part of patient education and encompasses the study and use of communication strategies to inform and influence the individual and his or her decisions that enhance health.[30]

## THE IMPORTANCE OF HEALTH COMMUNICATION FOR PATIENT TEACHING AND LEARNING

Health communication is increasingly recognized as a necessary element of efforts to improve personal and public health.[30] It can contribute to all aspects of disease prevention and health promotion and is relevant in a number of contexts, including:[30,31]

- Health care provider–patient relationships

- Individuals' exposure to, search for, and use of health information

- Individuals' adherence to clinical interventions and regimens

- The construction of public health messages and campaigns

- The dissemination of individual and population health risk information, that is, risk communication

- Images of health in the mass media and the culture at large

- The education of consumers about how to gain access to the public health and health care systems

Additionally, health communication is used regularly in clinical patient education and in the area of health education for prevention and health promotion.

For patients or clients, effective health communication can: (1) help raise awareness of health risks and solutions, (2) provide the motivation and skills needed to reduce these risks, (3) help them find support from other people in similar situations, and (4) affect or reinforce their attitudes.[30,31] Health communication also can increase demand for appropriate health services and decrease demand for inappropriate ones. It can make available information to assist the patient in complex choices, such as selecting health care plans, health care providers, and interventions. For the community, health communication can be used to influence the public agenda, advocate for policies and programs, promote positive changes in the socioeconomic and physical environments,[30] improve the delivery of public health and health care services, and encourage social norms that benefit health and quality of life. Other benefits of health communication are described in **Table 7.5**.

The practice of health communication has contributed to health education through health promotion and disease prevention in several areas. One of these areas is the improvement of interpersonal and group interactions in clinical situations such as between the provider and patient, between two or more providers, and among members of a health care team through the training of health care professionals and patients in effective

Table 7.5

### *Benefits of Health Communication for Patients*[30,31]

| |
|---|
| Enhances the relationship between patient and health care provider. |
| Adds to the patient's knowledge about health issues. |
| Decreases the patient's health risks. |
| Increases the patient's adherence to health education. |

communication skills. Collaborative relationships are enhanced when all parties are capable of good communication. Another area is the dissemination of health messages through public education campaigns that seek to change the social climate to encourage healthy behaviors, create awareness, change attitudes, and motivate individuals to adopt recommended behavior. Public education campaigns traditionally have relied on mass communication such as public service announcements on billboards, radio, and television, and educational messages in printed materials (pamphlets) to deliver health messages.[31] Other campaigns have integrated mass media with community-based programs. Many campaigns have used social marketing techniques. Contemporary health improvement activities are using digital technologies, such as CD-ROMs and the World Wide Web, which can target audiences, tailor messages, and engage people in interactive, ongoing exchanges about health.[31]

An emerging area where physical and occupational rehabilitation professionals are being encouraged to be more involved is using health communication in communities.[30] In addition to traditional practice areas, specialized physical and occupational therapists of the 21st century will increase their focus on the health effects of rising obesity and diabetes rates as well as health care disparities affecting interventions and services. They will also help individuals redesign their lifestyles, modify homes and businesses to enhance wellness and health promotion, and use teaching and learning opportunities for job and life modifications. Injury prevention programs in the workplace, functional capacity evaluations, work site analyses, and management of workplace injuries are areas of occupational health physical therapy that are expanding rapidly. As a key societal need, disease prevention will require physical and occupational rehabilitation providers to better attend to the education needs of their patients and clients to be sure they adequately understand the information to promote self-reliance and maintenance of a healthy status over an extended lifespan. All the new opportunities in wellness, health promotion, and disease prevention can support and enhance communities' health. This trend can emphasize the empowerment of individuals and communities to effect change on multiple levels.

## BASIC STRATEGIES TO IMPROVE HEALTH COMMUNICATION

Generally, there are at least eight basic strategies to improve health communication with patients and enhance teaching and learning aspects of physical and occupational rehabilitation (**Table 7.6**). The first strategy requires the therapist to know and be familiar with his or her audience. This includes learning about the patient's literacy level, language, culture, and age.[30,31] The therapist should also be sensitive to the patient's disability and emotions.[26]

The second strategy requires the provider to tailor his or her communication to meet the needs of each patient. For example, the physical therapist may need to draw pictographs for a patient who speaks limited English or teach just one concept at a time to a patient who has trouble concentrating. Additional learning resources can be offered to patients who want to learn more.

The third strategy involves creating a welcoming and supportive environment.[30,31] Whether the environment is in a physical or occupational therapy office or in cyberspace, the therapist must ensure that it is safe, feels private, and encourages thought and reasoned action. Furthermore, the environment can set a tone for patients to feel comfortable to ask questions, disagree, and inform the therapist when they do not understand the information.

The fourth strategy relates to communicating with patients in whatever ways work best for them.[30,31] For example, outside of just talking or using written materials, the therapist may consider options such as metaphors, objects, models, videos, and computer technology. Nevertheless, plain language should be applied to all forms of health communication. This includes using words that patients already know, teaching terms they need to learn, and presenting information from the patient's perspective.

The fifth strategy of health communication is to confirm the patient's understanding.[30,31] Communication is effective only when the other person understands. When there are gaps, the information must be rephrased and not just repeated. The sixth strategy requires the therapist to communicate to the patient information he or she needs to know at the time.[30,31] For later or more advanced learning, evidence-based resources can be provided. Providing a large amount of information at once can lead to confusion.

The seventh strategy is for the therapist to consider the ethics of simplicity by conveying the necessary information to the patient in clear and simple terms.[26,30] The role of the health communicator is to interpret complex scientific and medical information into words and concepts that patients and families can understand. This is difficult to do, especially

| Table 7.6 | **Summary of Basic Strategies of Health Communication**[30,31] |
|---|---|
| | Knowing the audience. |
| | Tailoring the communication to the patient's needs. |
| | Creating a welcoming and supportive environment. |
| | Using plain language and presenting information from the patient's perspective. |
| | Confirming the patient's understanding. |
| | Offering basic needed information required for that session. |
| | Keeping the information simple. |
| | Collaborating with patients, families, other providers, and the community. |

when information is ambiguous or conflicting. When deciding which information to offer or to omit, the implications of these choices for the patient should be considered. The eighth and final health communication strategy is to collaborate with patients and their families, colleagues, and the community to improve health understanding.[26,30]

Another important strategy in health communication requires the health care provider to ensure that patients receive accurate health information (**Table 7.7**).[26,31] The educational material must be easy to access and understandable, and the data should be consistent over time and evidence-based. Furthermore, the health care provider must consider the cultural competence of the material and the readability requirements of his or her patient population.

Physical and occupational therapists and assistants also need to consider that often people with the greatest health burdens have the least access to information, communication technologies, health care, and supporting social services. Even the most carefully designed health communication programs will have limited impact if underserved communities lack access to crucial health professionals, services, and communication channels that are part of a health improvement project. Typically, low-education and low-income groups remain less knowledgeable and less likely to change behavior than higher education and income groups.[31] This creates a knowledge gap and leaves some people chronically uninformed. For these reasons, health literacy is increasingly vital to help people navigate a complex health system and better manage their own health. Differences in the ability to read and understand materials related to personal health as well as to navigate the health care system appear to contribute to health disparities.[31] People with low health literacy are more likely to report poor health, have an incomplete understanding of their health problems and treatment, and be at greater risk of hospitalization.

# *Patient Education Related to Literacy, Health Literacy, and Numeracy*

Literacy is a social determinant of health when a mismatch exists between an individual's literacy skills and the literacy demands of the health context.[31] Poor communication based on faulty assumptions, incomplete disclosure, inappropriate language, or hidden confusion causes problems for patients, clients, and health care providers and professionals. In addition, limited health literacy can be difficult to detect if the individual patient does not want to acknowledge reading or vocabulary limitations. Many people feel shame or mask these difficulties to maintain their dignity and pride.[32] Also, many people feel that their health literacy skills are adequate when they are not.

## THE IMPORTANCE OF LITERACY AND HEALTH LITERACY IN PATIENT TEACHING AND LEARNING

The *Healthy People 2010* report identifies health literacy as an important component of health communication, medical product safety, and oral health.[31] Health literacy is a patient's ability to read, understand, and take action in regard to health information to make

| Table 7.7 | *Characteristics of Teaching and Learning Effective Health Information*[26,31] |
|---|---|
| Accuracy | Characterized by valid health information, without errors of fact, interpretation, or judgment. |
| Availability | Characterized by health information that is delivered or placed where the audience can access it. The placement of information varies according to the audience. |
| Balance | Characterized by having health information that presents the benefits and risks of potential actions or recognizes different and valid perspectives on the issue. |
| Consistency | Characterized by providing health information that remains internally consistent over time or consistent with information from other sources. |
| Cultural competence | Characterized by health information that is designed, implemented, and evaluated for special issues for selected population groups, educational levels, and disabilities. |
| Evidence-based | Characterized by health information based on relevant scientific evidence and a rigorous and comprehensive review to formulate practice guidelines. |
| Reliability | Characterized by the information coming from a credible source and containing updated content. |
| Repetition | Allows the health information to impact given audiences over time. |
| Target | Characterized by reaching the largest possible number of people in the target population. |
| Timeliness | Characterized by health information being applied when the audience is the most receptive or in need of specific data. |
| Understandability | Characterized by the health information being provided using a language level and format appropriate for the specific audiences. |

appropriate health care decisions.[33] Health literacy is linked to many issues of critical importance to national health policies.[32] The public health mandate of protecting the health of the nation relies on communication strategies for a variety of issues ranging from bioterrorism to obesity. Health literacy is so complex that many people with strong literacy skills may have difficulty obtaining, understanding, and using health information.[33] For example, an accountant may not know when to get a mammogram, a science teacher may not understand information sent by a doctor about a brain function test, or a surgeon may have trouble helping a family member with Medicare forms. Health literacy is very complex because it can require a combination of education, health services, and social and cultural factors.[33] Increasing knowledge, awareness, and responsiveness to health literacy among health care providers as well as the community could reduce problems and help to promote a health-literate society.[34] Globally, health literacy is a key factor in health promotion and disease prevention. All health care providers need to work hard toward health education and health communication to promote health literacy.

Socioeconomic factors such as low literacy, lack of health insurance coverage, poor social support, family instability, and homelessness are the most consistently reported factors that impact adherence to therapeutic regimens and preventative health care.[31,33] Low health literacy and limited English language proficiency are considered important patient education and adherence barriers.

Literacy includes three basic skills (**Table 7.8**): (1) document literacy, which is required for applications, forms, graphs, and schedules; (2) prose literacy, which is required to understand and use text found in newspapers, magazines, and books; and (3) quantitative literacy, which is necessary for arithmetic operations (such as in banks or when making purchase orders).[22] Literacy also involves the ability to read and comprehend material including numbers, as well as to interpret the numbers.[22] When determining a person's literacy levels, reading, readability, and comprehension must be taken into account. Reading is the process of transforming letters into words and pronouncing them correctly. Readability is defined as

| Table 7.8 | *Fundamental Literacy Skills*[22] | |
|---|---|
| Document literacy | Being able to complete and understand the meaning of information found in applications, forms, graphs, or schedules. |
| Prose literacy | Understanding the meaning of information found in newspapers, books, magazines, and online. |
| Quantitative literacy | Understanding the meaning and being able to use basic and advanced mathematical operations. |

how easy or how difficult printed or written materials can be read based on different variables.[22] Variables affecting readability are based on the written material, such as the writing style, and also on the reader's skills, interest, or prior knowledge. Comprehension is the degree to which a person grasps the words' meaning and understands what they have read.[22] Readability and comprehension also depend on many variables related to the presented material and the reader's capabilities such as the material's significance, its legibility (such as the size or the format of the print), the length and organization of the material, the structure of sentences, and the terminology used.[22] Variables related to the reader's capability may include the reader's physical well-being, his or her educational and cultural background, ability to interpret the written message, assimilation and correlation of information, and visual acuity.

In regard to patients' reading abilities, poor health can cause stress and anxiety that may interfere with a reader's ability to fully understand the material presented to them.[22] As an example, in physical and occupational therapy a patient's readability and comprehension could be assessed by having the patient read his or her home exercise program directions. In many situations, however, the patient's ability to read the information does not necessarily guarantee comprehension.[33] Illness or other disruptive life situations could interfere with understanding and remembering what was read. A patient's reading ability and comprehension is affected by many variables not necessarily related to literacy, such as health status, effect of illness, amount of stress, physical and mental energy, behavioral conduct, and motivation (**Table 7.9**).[22,35] Additionally, a recent research study found that social behavior and literacy are also strongly connected.[36] For example, in elementary school education, students' poorer literacy achievement is associated with aggressive behavior.[36] This means that an individual's social and academic development are closely related to each other.[36]

Literacy also is related to patient education that is presented orally and to computer readability and comprehension. In health care, a patient's inability to understand the meaning of the health care provider's spoken words is extremely important for patient education and adherence. In regard to methods for teaching and learning, education transmitted only

| Table 7.9 | ***Examples of Nonliteracy-Based Variables Affecting Patient Teaching and Learning***[22,35] |
|---|---|
| Physical variables such as health, general well-being, and environmental factors. |
| Psychological variables such as stress, anxiety, and psychological stages of adjustment (denial, anger, bargaining, depression, and acceptance). |
| Behavioral variables such as motivation, aggressiveness, gentleness, offensiveness, courtesy, tardiness, and punctuality. |

in oral form is not successful because it cannot be easily remembered.[34] Written patient education is remembered better and accounts for increased patient motivation with interventions and better adherence.[34] The best results are obtained when oral instruction is combined with written instruction.[34] Additionally, computer literacy is becoming increasingly significant in health literacy and patient education and adherence.[35]

## THE IMPORTANCE OF NUMERACY IN PATIENT TEACHING AND LEARNING

In addition to reading and comprehension, numeracy is part of quantitative literacy. *Numeracy* means to be able to read and interpret numbers.[22] Persons having limited literacy skills also often have limited numeracy abilities. Basic numeracy is the ability to identify numbers and to make sense of quantitative data requiring no manipulation of numbers.[22] A simple example in rehabilitation would be identifying the time of appointments. Other numeracy abilities may include using the telephone book or correctly listing the number of pills taken daily.

Computational numeracy involves the ability to count, quantify, compute, and use simple manipulation of numbers, items, quantities, or visual elements.[22] An example in rehabilitation would be using the number of repetitions or sets correctly in an exercise program. Analytical numeracy is more complicated and includes the ability to understand higher functions such as inference, estimation, proportions, percentages, frequencies, and equivalent situations.[22] Information can be from multiple sources. An example in health care would be the ability to understand whether cholesterol level was within the normal range by evaluating a graphic representation of cholesterol levels. Statistical numeracy is a much higher proficiency that includes clear comprehension of basic biostatistics and probability statements, skills to compare different scales (such as probability, proportion, and percent), or critically analyzing quantitative information such as life expectancy or risks.[22] It also consists of concepts such as blinding and randomization. An example in health care would be making choices among interventions based on standard outcomes of relative or absolute risk.

Health numeracy is important because it allows an individual to access, process, interpret, communicate, and act on the numerical, quantitative, biostatistical, graphical, and probabilistic health information necessary for making decisions in regard to his or her health.

## BASIC TEACHING AND LEARNING STRATEGIES FOR LOW LITERACY/ LOW HEALTH LITERACY

American society demands high literacy including high health literacy. Every day, millions of adults must make decisions and take actions on issues that protect not only their own well-being, but also their family members and communities. These decisions have to be made in health care settings, as well as at homes, work, and in schools as part of the daily life of adults. For example, at home, parents should be able to calculate a child's weight and age to determine the correct dosage of over-the-counter medicine. At work, employees need to determine correct workstation placement or safe use of toxic chemicals. Safety warnings are placed in the community and at work. They are also discussed in newspapers and on television. Consumers are expected to understand the calculations of calories and sugar content of the nutritional information posted on food labels. In pharmacotherapy, clients should be able to differentiate between a cough syrup that is a suppressor and one that is an expectorant. In health care settings, health care providers expect patients to provide accurate health histories, the correct account of how an injury occurred, and precise descriptions of their symptoms. To access health programs and services, adults need to meet the demands of completing insurance forms, providing informed consent, and understanding their rights and responsibilities as related to medical procedures. The information contained in these forms and documents uses legal and scientific terms that are unfamiliar to many individuals. Inability to speak English or speaking with only limited proficiency present additional obstacles to understanding health information and accessing health care. Demands on an individual's literacy skills can create barriers to the use and understanding of health tools and information.

Low literacy refers to a person being marginally literate or marginally illiterate.[22] It means that the person can read, write, and comprehend information between the fifth- and eighth-grade levels of difficulty. Individuals with low literacy may have difficulty reading and writing common information to meet their daily needs (such as reading a television schedule). A person who is functionally illiterate has reading, writing, and comprehension skills below the fifth-grade level.[37] Individuals with functional illiteracy may have a very limited ability to communicate in writing and sometimes speaking. They do not understand basic printed instructions or audiovisual aids and are unable to read well enough to understand and interpret the information.[37] For example, a person with functional illiteracy can read the label on a soup can that directs him or her to pour the soup into the pan and heat it until hot; however, he or she is unable to comprehend the meaning and the sequence and follow through with the directions. Low literacy or illiteracy does not necessarily imply a lack of intelligence, nor does it mean a person has a low Intelligence Quotient (IQ). A person can be illiterate or have low literacy but maintain a normal IQ range.

A low level of literacy has implications for an individual's social, economic, and health status. A low literacy level typically is associated with minimum earnings, health problems, and a high rate of unemployment. Illiteracy can contribute to homelessness, unemployment, drug abuse, teen pregnancy, and even crime. The impact of illiteracy on a person's health and health care is immense.[37] A patient's ability to read and understand health information is an important part of that patient's education and his or her ability to adhere to interventions.[37] In the United States, populations identified as having poor reading and comprehension skills may include older adults, economically disadvantaged individuals, immigrants (especially illegal immigrants), racial minorities, unemployed persons, high school dropouts, prisoners, many rural residents, and people with poor health status due to chronic mental and physical problems.

Illiteracy or low literacy is a large contributor to decreased health literacy. Health literacy is the degree to which individuals have the capacity to obtain, process, and understand basic health information and services necessary to make appropriate health decisions.[22] Low health literacy is prevalent among many individuals including the elderly, individuals who have lower educational levels, those who are poor, minority populations, and groups with limited English proficiency.[33] A large number of elderly patients have low health literacy, and as a result show poor adherence, mostly in relation to prescription instructions and use of preventive medical services. This causes increased hospitalizations and visits to the emergency room, and poor management of chronic diseases.[37]

Poor health literacy also can result in impaired ability to remember and follow interventions. In regard to medication use, low health literacy and limited proficiency in English can cause serious health risks. It is estimated that more than 45% of the adult population in the United States has literacy skills at or below the eighth-grade reading level.[33] Also, inadequate health literacy increases steadily with age and is especially prevalent in patients 65 to 69 years or older.[33] Minority populations, people with limited English proficiency, and individuals with lower economic status also may lack high enough health literacy levels to be able to read health information materials, understand basic medical instructions, and adhere to medication regimens (**Table 7.10**).[37]

Health literacy in the United States is remarkably low regardless of education, race, or income.[37] More than 90 million Americans are unable to adequately understand basic health information.[34] The National Assessment of Adult Literacy (NAAL) reports that the majority of adults (53%) had Intermediate health literacy.[38] Intermediate literacy indicates skills necessary to perform moderately challenging literacy activities such as assessing reference materials to determine which foods contain a particular vitamin or identifying a specific location on a map.[38] However, 22% of adults have Basic and 14% have Below Basic health literacy.[38] Basic indicates skills necessary to perform simple literacy activities such as using a television guide to find out what programs are on at a specific time.[38] Below Basic indicates the most simple literacy skills such as signing a form or adding the amounts on a bank deposit slip.[38] Another example of Below Basic health literacy is described as not being able to locate easily identifiable simple information such as "what a patient is allowed to drink before a medical test."[37(p.340)] The majority of patients who have a Below Basic health literacy are native-born English speakers.[37] Low health literacy affects people of all ages, races, incomes, and education levels. This means that, during patient instruction, all these individuals do not receive adequate verbal communication from their health care providers. As a result, many of them are not able to adhere to interventions. Patients with low health literacy are unaware

| Table 7.10 | *Basic Patient Education Objectives That Consider Health Literacy*[22,37] |
|---|---|
| Informing the patient about his or her condition and methods of intervention. | |
| Educating the patient by using proper teaching and learning techniques. | |
| Addressing patient understanding. | |
| Ensuring that the patient has future access to the information. | |

of the health risks associated with nonadherence and often are ashamed or embarrassed to seek help (**Table 7.11**).

Despite major reports on the need to improve health literacy, little improvement has been noted in the amount of information patients understand and remember in their encounters with health care practitioners. The tools for repairing these problems are within the realms of medical patient education and clinical practices. Consequently, physical and occupational therapists and assistants should use multiple methods of transmitting information during patient teaching and learning.

The U.S. Department of Health and Human Services and other organizations such as the Partnership for Clear Health Communications and the U.S. Pharmacopeia have been working together to promote awareness of and solutions for low health literacy, especially when related to medication instructions, precautions, and/or warnings.[32] Reducing medication errors among patients with low health literacy requires a rigorous review of medication regimens, use of visual aids, and specific communication methods.[32] In addition,

Table 7.11

### *Communication Strategies for Low Health Literacy*[26,37]

| |
|---|
| Create a "shame free" safe environment that allows the patient to feel comfortable and openly discuss any issue. |
| Do not mention anything about believing that there is a reading problem. This allows the patient to express his or her own concern. |
| Never use technical terms, but only layman's terminology. |
| Provide clear and understandable verbal instructions to the patient. |
| Use diagrams, pictures, video instruction, and/or pictograms. |
| Provide written information at a fifth-grade level or lower. |
| Use large font sizes and never use italics. |
| Verify understanding by having the patient "teach back" the instructions he or she received. |
| Include a family member or friend in the educational session. |
| Call the patient to follow up on the instructions. |
| Determine the patient's condition or situation, and follow up with the intervention(s) while in his or her environment. |

rehabilitation providers should be aware that patients with low literacy levels are reluctant to ask questions for fear of appearing ignorant or lacking intelligence. If past communication experiences with other health care providers were negative, patients often will avoid getting answers to their questions and withdraw totally to prevent humiliation.

Physical and occupational therapists and assistants should be responsive to the fact that demands on a patient's literacy skills can create a barrier to the use and understanding of health tools and information. In many ways, literacy serves as a social determinant of health when a mismatch exists between the skills of the individual and the demands of the health context.[38] Poor communication, whether based on faulty assumptions, inappropriate language, incomplete disclosures, or hidden confusion, does a disservice to patients as well as to health care providers.[38] When words get in the way, the communication process fails, leading to confusion, loss of dignity, and unhealthful outcomes. The ability of patients and consumers to manage their own health and medical care can be improved through better provider-patient communication and greater inclusion of the patient in treatment decisions, such as in the patient-centered care approach.

## Patient Education and the Internet

Computer literacy is dependent on a patient's socioeconomic status, the availability of computer technology resources, and the accuracy of health information available on the Internet. As a tool for patient education, the Internet enables patients to become active participants in their care by having access to material (they want to search) 24 hours a day, 7 days a week.[39] The Internet also can provide patients with access to information that can be used to influence how decisions are made regarding their health care. For example, patients can access general medical references; recommendations for care using evidence-based medicine; or report cards on hospitals, physicians, and health plans.[39] The Internet can promote and help patient safety by allowing the patient to investigate health care providers, health plans, and hospitals in detail. For example, prior to being admitted into a hospital, a patient can visit the Joint Commission Web site, which provides guidelines for evaluating a hospital. By searching health-related Web sites, including those containing results of research studies or ongoing clinical trials, the patient has several options to help evaluate the decisions made by his or her health care professionals and providers and the recommended interventions.[39] Several Web sites supply access to updated summaries and journal articles of the best available evidence on how well a specific intervention works. This information can help patients take a more active role in the management of their health care by collaborating with their health care providers, instead of passively following their instructions. As patients become more informed, taking a more active role in their health care, medical care in the United States is moving toward a more patient-centered approach.[40]

The Internet has been changing the practice of health care from an industrial model to an information age model.[39] Patients, as health consumers, have been developing a level of expertise regarding their medical problems by using search engines and illness-specific

Web sites to locate information on their illness, identify various interventions, review their effectiveness, and participate in clinical trials.[39] Patients experience measurably better health outcomes than passive health consumers when they take initiative, ask questions, discuss and investigate options for interventions, express their opinions and concerns, and state their preferences.[39] Additionally, the Internet can be a tool to help patients find information to maintain a healthy lifestyle. Using the Web, patients can learn how to avoid the risk of disease or injury, how to detect a problem before it becomes more difficult to treat, and how they can get their health back when they are sick or injured.

Using the Internet for education allows patients to take a more proactive stance toward their health. However, learning to use the Internet to help manage health is difficult and requires specific education. Patients need detailed instructions from their health care providers on how the Internet works, how to use search engine technology, and especially how to locate accurate health-related information. In addition, techniques to evaluate information found on a Web site and guidance in finding information on the quality of hospitals, health plans, and interventions may also need to be taught. Sometimes, health care providers may be confronted by patients about specific information found on the Internet that is not necessarily true. Stories abound of health care professionals wrongly being challenged by patients asking, "Why didn't you tell me about this?" As more and more patients use the Internet to gather health-related information, health care professionals need to take a more practical role in helping patients use the Web to find the correct medical information.

In current health care, most health-related Web sites are created for patient education; very few include behavioral and cognitive treatments. These latter types of sites are customized by health care providers to provide patients with follow-up and feedback. The Internet sites containing interventions have been operationalized and specially transformed to be delivered via the Web.[39] The treatments are highly structured and can be guided totally by the patient or semi-guided by the patient and the health care provider.[39] These customized Web sites are interactive, containing graphics, animations, audio, and video. Internet sites on patient and health education are also very helpful for health promotion and follow-up with interventions. For example, in regard to following up with treatments, a continuous Internet-based education program experimentally provided patient education for children and adolescents with asthma.[41] The Internet site supplied specific self-management instructions for 6 months to 438 patients diagnosed and previously clinically treated for asthma.[41] The Internet-based education program improved patients' health outcomes by decreasing the burden of the disease, considerably reducing patients' visits to clinics, and also diminishing children's and adolescents' missed school days.[41] Consequently, the fact that the Internet educational program helped patients experience fewer asthmatic attacks reduced the costs of health services.

Health care providers have a long journey in their mission to expand the use of computer technology in patient education. It is projected that in the future, health care professionals will be building their own Web sites that contain links to recommended Web sites. On these sites, providers can build their own digital libraries that can contain links to more detailed sites and even links to articles the provider has read and believes will be beneficial to the patient's understanding of their medical problems and interventions. This method of patient education will help health care providers to better educate their patients using a medium that gives patients accurate information to make correct decisions regarding their health. In this way, the health care environment will become safer, more effective, patient-centered, timely, and equitable. Ultimately, the dynamic between the patient and the Internet can greatly impact the quality of care received, the relationship between the health care provider and patient, and patient compliance.

# Written Communication Strategies to Improve Patient Teaching and Learning

Readability is a quality and style of writing that allows something to be easily comprehended and understood. Poor reading skills may affect a person's understanding, interpretation, and vocabulary. Misinterpretation may lead to a misunderstanding of instructions. Patients who have poor reading skills may hesitate to ask questions, preferring to remain silent and not know the answer rather than expose themselves to humiliation. Also, patients who have low literacy skills tend to think in concrete, specific ways, and when presented with multiple, confusing instructions may become totally puzzled by the course of therapy or interventions and ignore the information. Comprehension tests of patients show that about 50% have serious difficulty with, or cannot read, instructional materials at the fifth-grade level.[34] Flesch (who created the readability formula) determined that the standard reading level can be at the eighth-grade to ninth-grade level.[34] However, Flesch admitted that a large amount of the population is able to read only at a fifth-grade level.[34]

## METHODS FOR IMPROVING READABILITY IN WRITTEN PATIENT EDUCATION MATERIALS

Creating readable patient education materials is an important step in improving health literacy. Readability should not be confused with comprehension or understanding. Comprehension implies that the reader has internalized the material and is measured by testing or application exercises. Readability can be determined by a number of different formulas, most of which use sentence length and word length as primary factors.

More than 40 different formulas can be used to determine readability. Individuals assessing the usefulness of health care literature have frequently chosen a particular readability formula for three reasons: longstanding use in school settings, reputation for methodical accuracy for sorting reading materials into appropriate grade-level slots, and consistency within and between various formulas when determining reading levels. The most common readability formulas used both in education and by health care providers are the Flesch Reading Ease test, the Gunning Fog index, and the Flesch-Kincaid formula. When health-based material was analyzed using these three tests, strong positive correlations of 0.93 to 0.99 were found among these three formulas.[42]

The readability tests are designed to indicate how difficult a reading passage is to understand. For example, the *Flesch Reading Ease method* determines the readability level of materials between fifth grade and college graduate.[2] Reading ease refers to the reader's ability to decode text.[2] Word length and polysyllabic words are common variables used in estimating reading level and are major contributors to increased reading difficulty.[2] The formula is based on the average sentence length (in words) of selected samples and on the average word length measured as syllables per 100 words of sample. These two factors are combined to yield a reading ease score represented by a number between 0 and 100. **Table 7.12** provides information for interpreting the score.

The *Gunning Fog formula* determines the readability level of materials between fourth grade and college.[42] This formula, considered one of the easier methods for calculating readability, is based on a short sample of 100 words and does not require counting all syllables or applying many rules.

The *Flesch-Kincaid formula* yields an index with a range from 1.0 (first-grade level) to 50 (totally unreadable).[42,43] A high readability index (over 12th grade) does not mean the writing is appropriate for college-educated readers, but rather that it is complex and difficult to read.[43]

Another common and very easy-to-use formula is the Simple Measure of Gobbledygook (SMOG) formula (**Table 7.13**).[44] This formula was developed by McLaughlin in 1969 and has been used for more than 30 years.[44] The SMOG formula can also be used by comparing

Table 7.12

### *Scores for the Flesch Reading Ease Formula[2]*

| Score | Reading Difficulty | Approximate Grade Level |
|---|---|---|
| 91–100 | Very easy | Fourth grade |
| 81–90 | Easy | Fifth grade |
| 71–80 | Fairly easy | Sixth grade |
| 61–70 | Standard | Between seventh and eighth grades |
| 51–60 | Fairly difficult | High school |
| 31–50 | Difficult | Between high school and college |
| 0–30 | Very difficult | College and higher |

| Table 7.13 |
|---|

### *Determining Readability Using the SMOG Formula*[44]

1. Choose 10 sentences in a row from the beginning, middle, and end of the document for a total of 30 sentences.

2. Every word in the chosen sentences that has three or more syllables must be counted. Read the words out loud to determine the number of syllables. Words that are repeated must be counted every time they appear in the sentence. Hyphenated words and proper nouns (that are more than three syllables) must also be counted. Additionally, abbreviations are counted as the whole word that they correspond to.

3. Calculate the square root of the total number of words with three or more syllables.

4. Add 3 to the square root. The total final number (after adding 3) represents the grade level of the document. For example, let's say 22 sentences have 48 words with three or more syllables. The square root of 48 is 6.9. Adding 3 to 6.9 is 9.9. The grade level of the document is 9.9.

the total number of words containing three or more syllables with the SMOG conversion table (**Table 7.14**).[2]

Many computer software programs also measure readability. The most simple is Microsoft Word. If the written information is in Microsoft Word (version 2003), the health care provider can do the following:

1. Click on Tools | Options | Spelling and Grammar.

2. Select the Show Readability Statistics box.

3. Click OK.

4. Select Spelling and Grammar (under Tools). Word will complete its spelling and grammar checks and then present the readability statistics for your document.

Nearly all word-processing programs will produce readability statistics. If another word-processing program is used, instructions can usually be found by searching for "readability" in the Help menu.

## WRITTEN COMMUNICATION BETWEEN PATIENTS AND PROVIDERS

Much of the communication between rehabilitation patients and their health care providers occurs verbally but often relies on written materials to augment or reinforce

Table 7.14

## SMOG Conversion Table[2]

| Word Count | Grade Level |
|:----------:|:-----------:|
| 0–2 | 4 |
| 3–6 | 5 |
| 7–12 | 6 |
| 13–20 | 7 |
| 21–30 | 8 |
| 31–42 | 9 |
| 43–56 | 10 |
| 57–72 | 11 |
| 73–90 | 12 |
| 91–110 | 13 |
| 111–132 | 14 |
| 133–156 | 15 |
| 157–182 | 16 |
| 183–210 | 17 |
| 211–240 | 18 |

verbal instructions. Patients may refer to written materials that provide instructions about treatment schedules, home exercise programs, precautions after surgeries, or preventive health care (such as for obesity, diabetes, smoking, or exercise). Patients must be able to both read and understand these written materials if there is any hope of them adhering to interventions or prevention. Because of shame and embarrassment, patients rarely admit they are functionally illiterate. They make attempts to hide their reading problems. They might have a friend or family member read documents for them, state that they forgot their glasses, or tell the provider they will read the document when they get home. However, these cues are often missed by health care providers, and these patients are usually skillful at hiding their deficiencies. To acknowledge this nationwide problem of functional illiteracy, it is recommended that patient education materials be written on a fifth- to sixth-grade reading level. However, the majority of patient education materials are written on high school or college reading levels.

Understanding the instructions that come with over-the-counter medications requires a tenth-grade reading level.[43] Reading the instructions on a frozen TV dinner requires an eighth-grade reading level.[43] An analysis of 31 Health Insurance Portability and Accountability Act (HIPAA) privacy notices found that they were written on a second- or third-year college reading level.[43] There is clearly a gap between the average person's reading ability and the reading level of many instructions and documents in society. In 2004 the Institute of Medicine (IOM) released a report about health literacy.[45] The report states that 90 million Americans have difficulty understanding and acting upon health information, and it includes specific recommendations that health care systems and providers can take to promote a health-literate society.[45]

## GUIDELINES FOR DESIGNING WRITTEN PATIENT EDUCATION MATERIALS

There are many guidelines for designing highly readable written patient education. Some are simpler than others. **Table 7.15** presents a modified list of guidelines for simpler patient education.

One important aspect of patient education, especially in written education, is interaction. Very few patient education materials include interaction. One method of including interaction when writing patient materials involves writing a short question and asking the patient to write the answer. Another method can ask the patient a few questions or pose a problem and request the patient to answer how to solve it. **Table 7.16** provides some ways to include interactivity in a written document.

When writing patient education materials, complex words should be simplified to improve readability. **Table 7.17** presents examples of difficult words and some replacements used in rehabilitation.

Some general guidelines for written patient education information are:[26]

- Write the way you talk; use active voice.
- Use common words and short sentences.
- Give examples to explain hard words.
- Include interaction and reviews.

When writing the way people talk, the material becomes easier to read, is more interesting to read, and is easier to understand.

*Concept words* should not be used in patient education because they describe a general idea or an abstract framework and are often misunderstood.[22] For example, patients with diabetes are instructed to "keep the glucose level within a normal range." A patient with low literacy skills may not know what normal is and may think that she has a "range" in her kitchen. To make sure such a concept is understood by the patient, the health care provider

| Table 7.15 | **Simple Design Guidelines for Written Patient Education**[46,47] |
|---|---|

1. The font size must be 12 point or higher. An example can be a
   **14 point Arial** type.

2. The same type of font must be used throughout the entire material. Different fonts can divert the reader from the content.

3. To achieve clarity, it is recommended to use black letters on a white background.

4. Major points can be emphasized using bold.

5. Using bullets also can help the reader follow the information.

6. The text can be divided using headings and subheadings.

7. Pictures or drawings can illustrate procedures such as exercises or activities. The pictures and drawings must be simple. A picture or drawing that shows a wrong exercise (activity) should not be used.

8. Caps must not be used. IT CAN BE VERY DIFFICULT FOR READERS AT ALL SKILL LEVELS TO READ ALL CAPS. The words become rectangular and the reading cues (supplied by the shapes of the words) are lost.

9. The page must contain a few sentences with plenty of white space (after the sentence). This allows the patient to easily follow the information. Also, the handout looks uncluttered.

10. The alignment of the text is important. The text must be written on the left side of the page (instead of the center or the right side). This allows the patient to easily follow the information.

11. Interactive elements can be used to involve the patient with the material. An example can be asking the patient to circle two exercises that he/she would prefer to perform daily at home from a group of five.

should immediately include an example such as: "This means to keep your blood sugar somewhere between 70 and 120; this is the range of sugar numbers that means your blood sugar is normal—that it's okay."

*Category words* also are difficult to understand. For example, in the *Yellow Pages*, if a person wants to rent a house, he or she won't find a category for "house" but must look under "real-estate-residential-rental." These unexplained category words can be difficult for patients

| Table 7.16 | *Examples of Interaction Methods for Written Patient Education Material[48]* |
|---|---|

Write a short question and leave a blank line for the patient to write in the answer.

Pose a problem, and ask the patient to write (or say out loud) how it can be resolved.

Ask the patient to circle one or two among four exercise pictures for the best choice.

Ask a few questions verbally after the patient has read how to lift a weight properly.

Ask a group of patients a question in writing and let them discuss their answers.

| Table 7.17 | *Examples of Difficult Words and Suggested Simpler Replacements Used in Rehabilitation* |
|---|---|

| Difficult | Simpler |
|---|---|
| Ambulate | Walk |
| Atrophy | Weakness |
| Avoid | Stay away |
| Biological | Natural |
| Bradycardia | Slow heart beat |
| Caregiver | Person who gives care (support) |
| Cessation | Stop (end) |
| Diabetes | High blood sugar |
| Disease | Illness |

*(continues)*

| Table 7.17 | **Examples of Difficult Words and Suggested Simpler Replacements Used in Rehabilitation (continued)** |
|---|---|
| **Difficult** | **Simpler** |
| Document | Paper (write down) |
| Edema | Swelling |
| Essential | Necessary |
| Etiology | Cause of illness |
| Fatigue | Tired |
| Flexion | Bending a body part |
| Fracture | Broken bone |
| Genetic | Has to do with birth of origin |
| Gerontology | Has to do with problems of growing old |
| Hazard | Danger/risk |
| Hydrotherapy | Treatment using water |
| Hypertension | High blood pressure |
| Ipsilateral | On the same side (of the body) |
| Myalgia | Pain in a muscle |
| Outcome | Result |
| Prone | Lying with face down |
| Resistance | Amount of weight to be moved |
| Supine | Lying on the spine with the face up |
| Tremor | Shaking (trembling) |
| Ventilation | Circulation of air (to bring oxygen to the blood) |

to comprehend. For example, a patient on kidney dialysis who should avoid eating poultry may not know that food such as chicken belongs to a category of food called "poultry."[22]

*Value judgment words* also are hard to comprehend because they provide vague descriptions of the amount of or thresholds for action.[22] An example in rehabilitation would be asking a patient to exercise "regularly" or not to lift anything "heavy" without explaining the meaning of these two value judgment words.

Written patient education material can be easy to read if the most important information is placed first, in the most powerful position. When writing a sentence or paragraph, the context should come first, before presenting new information.[46] In this way, the health care provider places a framework for new information to fit before it arrives. When the context is given last, the patient must carry all the information along in his or her short-term memory.[46] He or she must try to remember it all until the end of the sentence, paragraph, or list. Placing context first makes the material easier to grasp, whereas placing context last makes it more difficult (**Table 7.18**).

| Table 7.18 | **Examples of "Context First" and "Context Last" in Physical Therapy** | |
|---|---|---|
| **For a patient who has had a total hip replacement:** | | |
| Context first sentence | ***You should not cross your legs*** because your hip could dislocate and you will need another surgery. | |
| Context last sentence | In order not to dislocate your hip and need another surgery, ***you should not cross your legs***. | |
| **For a patient who needs to lower his or her cholesterol:[47]** | | |
| Context first sentence | ***You can lower the amount of cholesterol in your body*** by reducing animal food products, increasing dietary fiber in your diet, and substituting low-fat or nonfat for whole dairy products. | |
| Context last sentence | Reducing animal food products, increasing dietary fiber, and substituting low-fat or nonfat for whole dairy products ***can lower the amount of cholesterol in your body***. | |

The material should be written clearly. Physical and occupational therapists and assistants should be consistent with their words. They should not refer to "medicines," and then "medications," and then "pills;" instead, they should use the same word throughout the material. Also, the passive voice should be turned into the active voice; for example:

*Passive voice:* Your exercises should be done every morning.

*Active voice:* Do your exercises every morning.

Words that patients may not understand must be defined. Including a glossary at the end of the document may be helpful. Serif fonts (such as Times New Roman and Helvetica) are easy to read, and should be 12-point or 14-point type. The most difficult to read text styles are ALL CAPITALS, *italics*, and 10-point type. For other suggestions on creating clearly written materials, see **Table 7.19**.

Another layout feature to increase patients' perception of the importance of information is to include the patient's name at the top of the patient education material. This demonstrates that the information is valuable because it is individualized for that patient.

Patient education materials must be simple and straightforward. **Table 7.20**, **Table 7.21**, and **Table 7.22** are examples of patient education materials for total hip replacement, and they range from very difficult (college level and up) to difficult (high school and

| Table 7.19 | *Instructions for Written Material*[26] |
|---|---|
| | Write clearly and use words consistently. |
| | Use shorter words. |
| | Sentences should be 10–15 words long. |
| | Divide long sentences with commas and semicolons. |
| | Use active voice. |
| | Define words that the patient may not understand, and use a glossary if necessary. |
| | Use second person ("You") instead of first or third person. |
| | Include numerals (1, 2, 3). |
| | Use a serif font and 12- to 14-point type. |
| | Individualize patient education material by including the patient's name at the top of the material. |

| Table 7.20 | ***Very Difficult (College Level and Up) Patient Education Material*** |
|---|---|
| | A main goal in a total hip replacement is to restore maximum range of motion while also reducing the risk of dislocation. The surgeon will examine the hip during surgery to ensure this. However, the hip is at a higher risk of dislocation during recovery. Patient should avoid hip flexion and adduction. Also, patient should avoid performing hip internal rotation with a posterolateral or lateral surgical approach and hip extension and external rotation with an anterior approach. |

college level) to very easy (fourth-grade level). These three examples were evaluated using the Flesch Reading Ease formula.

However, the example of very easy patient education material (Table 7.22) can still present a problem for patients with low literacy levels. Consequently, the best patient education material for patients with literacy problems will include pictures to illustrate the movements. A picture is more important for patients than anything else. Graphic representations of a patient's positions after total hip replacement can also enhance the patient's ability to learn and avoid being uncomfortable and humiliated.

| Table 7.21 | ***Difficult (High School to College Level) Patient Education Material*** |
|---|---|
| | The main goal in a total hip replacement (as you had) is to restore maximum flexibility while also reducing the risk of hip dislocation. Your surgeon already ensured this process. However, your left hip is at a higher risk of dislocation during your recovery period. You should avoid two important leg movements called hip flexion and adduction. This means that you cannot move your affected left leg toward your body and especially toward your unaffected right leg. You need to keep your affected left leg away from the middle of your body. Furthermore, because the surgeon used a posterior and lateral surgical approach, you should avoid performing hip internal rotation. This means that you cannot move the toes of your left foot inward. When walking you must keep your left leg away from your body with the toes of your foot facing outward. |

| Table 7.22 | *Very Easy (Fourth-Grade Level) Patient Education Material* |
|---|---|
| Don't cross your legs. |
| Don't bring your knee higher than your hip. |
| Don't lean forward while sitting or as you sit down. |
| Don't try to pick up something on the floor while you are sitting. |
| Don't turn your feet inside or outside. Keep your feet straight. |
| Don't bend at the waist. |
| Don't stand pigeon-toed. |

# The Importance of Audiovisual Materials in Patient Education

In addition to verbal and written communication, physical and occupational therapists and assistants use a large amount of demonstrations in patient teaching and learning. Showing patients what to do and guiding them through the process of learning by providing practice and feedback represent important steps in understanding and ensuring correct performances of skills or tasks (see Section V). Supporting teaching and learning with demonstrations can help the learner with guidance, feedback, and practice. When returning to physical and occupational therapy, the patients display their skills or tasks, showing improvement or an increased need for practice. Audiovisual aids such as videotapes, audiotapes, and compact discs (CDs) can be loaned to patients for home use to complement clinical patient education information. The audiovisuals encourage patients to review materials at home and as often as they like. Similar to the written information, the effectiveness of audiovisuals depends on the accuracy of their content and the communication modes used for data transmission. Physical and occupational therapists should consider that commercially produced audiovisuals can easily become outdated, especially when related to evidence-based interventions. As a result, many clinical facilities in physical and occupational rehabilitation prefer to videotape an actual demonstration of a patient's performance in the clinic, offering feedback as necessary.

Audiovisuals are important tools in patient teaching and learning. They can improve learning by stimulating critical thinking and helping the development of a cognitive framework of the material. Pictorial examples and symbolic representations of concepts clarify the information and provide additional memory cues. Consequently, learners understand and remember the information better and also tend to learn the material faster. As with any teaching and learning material, audiovisuals must be related to the learning objectives. Audiovisuals also have the ability to support the main points of a presentation.

Along with being used in physical therapy educational programs, audiovisuals can also be used in clinical interventions. As an example in physical therapy research, live and videotaped demonstrations have been found to be more effective in exercise programs than written handouts alone.[49] Patients can learn better from a therapist showing the exercise as well as by watching the videotape of exercise performance. In both instances of patient education, the learners are able to model and also remember the behavior more accurately than when learning from written data alone.[49]

In physical and occupational therapy, audiovisuals should not be used without demonstrations and/or written material. Audiovisuals should always complement the therapist's clinical demonstrations, presentations, and written data. Particularly for patients with low literacy skills, the information received in the clinical settings is essential. Additionally, encouraging patients to repeat the material in their own words and perform the task or skill represent true understanding of facts. The patient's response gives the therapist the opportunity to identify any misunderstandings and offer rectifications.

## Communication with Patients Who Have Limited English Proficiency

Health care professionals and providers often encounter difficulties and inadequate funding of language services when working with patients with limited English proficiency (LEP). The increasing diversity of the United States only amplifies the challenge for health care providers. Similar to health care in general, physical and occupational therapists as rehabilitation providers must be able to determine which language services are most appropriate based on their setting, type, and size; the frequency of contact with patients with LEP; and the variety of languages encountered. Therapists should be able to deliver patient teaching and learning using culturally and linguistically appropriate methods and services. These can facilitate patients' access to care and improve delivery of interventions for patients with LEP. Effective communication with patients with LEP is essential (**Table 7.23**).

## Basic Communication Strategies in Patient Education for Older Adults

For older individuals, physical and cognitive impairments and functional limitations can increase the risk of nonadherence. For example, visual, hearing, or cognitive impairments can affect an older patient's adherence with health care interventions. The American Foundation for the Blind estimates that in the United States today there are approximately 5.5 million persons age 65 or older who are blind or visually impaired (**Table 7.24**).[50] This means that many older patients have decreased ability to perform activities of daily living as well as home exercise programs, taking medications, and following up on specific compliance safety factors.

| Table 7.23 | ***The Importance of Effective Communication for LEP*** [22,26,31] |
|---|---|

Effective communication between health care providers and patients is essential to facilitate access to care, reduce health disparities and medical errors, and assure a patient's ability to adhere to interventions.

Competent health care language services are essential elements for an effective health care delivery system in a pluralistic society.

Health care providers should advocate to the federal, state, and local governments and health care insurers for the establishment of and funding mechanisms for appropriate language services. Funding language services for patients with LEP is a societal responsibility.

All members of the health care community should continue to educate their staff and constituents about LEP issues and help them identify resources to improve access to quality care for patients with LEP. Linguistic diversity in the health care workforce should be encouraged.

Quality and risk management processes should assess the adequacy of language services provided to patients with LEP, especially in regard to outcome disparities and medical errors.

Health care providers should develop mechanisms to establish the competency of individuals providing language services for patients with LEP, including interpreters, translators, and bilingual staff and clinicians.

In the United States, the number of people with hearing loss increases with age. Hearing loss is one of the most common conditions affecting older adults. One in three people older than 60, and half of those older than 85, have hearing loss.[51] The natural aging process affects the ability to detect sounds at soft levels and also to understand speech at the usual conversational volume. This is a progressive condition that gets worse with aging. Many individuals who suffer from age-related hearing impairments report that they hear speech but have difficulty understanding, especially in the presence of background noise.[51] For example, in environments with lots of noise or echo, older individuals were found to identify fewer words correctly than younger individuals with equivalent hearing (**Table 7.25**).[51]

Impaired cognition is another barrier in patient education. Impaired cognition is strongly associated with poor adherence with interventional regimens including pharmacotherapy (**Table 7.26**).[52] Older adults with cognitive decline or memory problems may have difficulty understanding how to take their medications, may forget to take a dose, or may take too many doses.[52] This can happen with interventions such as home exercise programs or education about activities of daily living.

| Table 7.24 | **Basic Education Strategies for Patients with Visual Impairments**[26] |
|---|---|
| Give clear verbal instructions directly to the patient and not the companion. |
| Use instructions in Braille if the patient reads Braille. |
| Tape the instructions. Use audible reminders or alarm systems. |
| Use large-print written materials (with a minimum size-16 font). Use black ink on light background for high contrast. Avoid writing materials that reflect light or cause glare. |
| Encourage the patient to use bright lighting when reading and to use a magnifying device. |

| Table 7.25 | **Basic Education Strategies for Patients with Hearing Impairments**[26,51] |
|---|---|
| Do not shout or exaggerate speech, distort wording, or obscure your mouth. Use a lower voice pitch and simple language. |
| Always include the patient in the conversation, talk to the patient, and do not talk about the patient or talk to others at the same time. |
| Face the patient, use gestures, give useful clues, confirm understanding of the information, add written materials to the verbal information, and use pictures and diagrams when possible. |
| Use a quiet area for patient education. |
| Have an assistive listening device available to be used as necessary. The therapist may need to speak to the patient's better ear or ask the patient to turn up their hearing aid. |
| Repeat the information as necessary, use different words, and always confirm understanding. |

*(continues)*

| Table 7.25 | **Basic Education Strategies for Patients with Hearing Impairments[26,51] (continued)** |
|---|---|

Stand in good lighting and reduce background noises.

Do not talk down to or patronize the patient. Have patience when communicating with the patient.

If the patient prefers American Sign Language, use an interpreter, use pantomime and facial expressions, or become familiar with the manual sign language alphabet (especially when the interpreter is not available).

If the patient prefers lip reading as a method of communication, use your regular voice volume and lip movement, maintain eye contact when speaking, do not obscure the view of your face when speaking, and avoid standing in front of a light or a window (because overhead lighting can limit shadows).

If the patient prefers to communicate through writing, use short, precise phrases, pictures, and diagrams, and provide writing tools to the patient.

| Table 7.26 | **Basic Education Strategies for Patients with Impaired Cognition[26,52]** |
|---|---|

Speak slowly and clearly and use simple language.

Repeat and rephrase the information as necessary.

Confirm understanding by having the patient repeat the information.

Provide written information using simple language in order to support verbal instruction.

Establish reminder strategies tailored for the patient. These may include organizers; calendars; phone reminders; or, for medications, electronic medication dispensing devices.

Involve the caregiver in patient education.

# PATIENT EDUCATION AND BEHAVIORAL MODIFICATION VARIABLES

## Objectives

After completing Chapter 8, the reader will be able to:

- List patients' common behavioral modification variables contributing to teaching and learning.

- Determine the necessary communication behavioral strategies for patient education.

- Explain strategies for behavioral modification training necessary in health care organizations.

- Name the most common barriers for patients' change.

- Describe the Stages of Change Model (SCM) and how to use the five stages in patient teaching and learning.

- Identify the importance of the SMART goals in patient education for behavioral modifications.

- Discuss the importance of motivational interviewing during patient education for increased patient adherence in rehabilitation.

# Behavioral Modification Factors in Patient Education

The health care literature indicates that from the patient's perspective, the main factors that influence behavioral modifications, including teaching and learning, are related to the individual's emotions and acquired or learned behaviors.[1–4,6,7,32] These behavioral aspects of patient education, from the patient's point of view, can be classified as:[1,2]

1. Patient's knowledge and health beliefs (such as the seriousness of the disease/illness, vulnerability to complications, and efficacy of interventions)

2. Patient's previous levels of compliance

3. Patient's confidence in ability to follow recommended behaviors

4. Patient's perception of health and the benefits of interventions or behavioral changes

5. Availability of social support

6. Complexity of the regimen

7. Patient's relationship and communication with the provider

8. Patient's motivation and skills to undertake a recommended behavior or treatment

Increasing a patient's ability to change his or her behavior involves careful assessment of the patient's readiness to make and maintain behavioral changes. Also, building the patient's skills requires the patient to learn new strategies to help him or her adopt and maintain a newly acquired behavior, especially in situations in which daily routines are interrupted. When learning new strategies for behavioral changes (whether smoking cessation, dietary modifications, or adherence with exercises), patients need to gain knowledge of specific abilities and skills.[1]

After making the decision to make a change, to be successful, patients may need to understand the rationale and importance of the commitment, negotiate goals with the health care provider, develop skills for adopting and maintaining the recommended behaviors, use reminder systems and self-monitoring to progress toward goals, develop problem-solving skills and use social support, and steadily resolve problems that block achievement of goals (**Table 8.1**).[1,5]

Prevention is an important aspect of clinical interventions. Health care providers, including physical and occupational therapists, need to help patients integrate prevention strategies into their regular course of intervention. Behavioral modifications play an important role in prevention as well as in adherence. However, multiple skills are often necessary for patients to comply with new behaviors and maintain them over time or to give up established unhealthy behaviors.[1] In general, health care providers have difficulty trying to change a patient's way of life. Additionally, asking a patient to modify several lifestyle behaviors, especially for asymptomatic conditions such as hypertension or hypercholesterolemia,

| Table 8.1 | |
|---|---|

## *Abilities and Skills for Behavioral Modifications*[1,5]

Problem solving.

Self-monitoring.

Developing prompts and reminder systems.

Identifying a potential relapse into an old behavior.

Enlisting social support.

Setting appropriate and realistic goals.

Rewarding achievement of new behaviors.

complicates the challenge and underscores the need for long-term motivation and multiple skills. Furthermore, even patients who have motivation and skills have difficulty with adherence. The reason can be that patients make errors of omission by delaying and neglecting treatments. This is especially true and risky with pharmacotherapy.[3,7,8,52]

In physical and occupational therapy, maintaining patient adherence and including prevention in interventions face the same problems as in pharmacotherapy.[53–57] In regard to adherence with therapeutic regimens, patients had the same difficulty following them as patients who needed to take their medication consistently. As examples, in the late 1990s, reports of adherence rates for supervised exercise-based interventions associated with cardiac rehabilitation programs or other hospital- or clinic-based programs ranged from 70% to 94%.[53] Older adults had even more difficulty adhering to home exercise programs (HEPs) and lifestyle modifications for prevention.[54–56] As a result, behavioral modification methods were needed when working with patients to prevent poor patient outcomes and longer intervention periods. However, in the late 1990s, patient education and health promotion using planned learning experiences were still in the process of being developed and expanded. At that time, many therapists assumed that patients were not adherent because they did not have enough information about the disorder and intervention.[53,54] Also, physical therapists believed that patient and health education would not be beneficial, especially when related to a patient's attitudes about illness or disability or a patient's expectations toward physical therapy outcomes.[53] There were also other obstacles to patient teaching and learning, including the therapist's decreased knowledge of teaching and learning theories, not enough training in patient and health education, lack of time, and the patient's disinterest in regard to adherence and health promotion activities.[53,54]

Contemporary health care has changed for the positive since then and has become much more advanced. Increased emphasis is placed on adherence, health promotion, and disease prevention today, so therapists are better equipped to understand the behavioral factors associated with patients' willingness and ability to follow therapeutic regimens, modify lifestyles, and maintain health.[55–57] For example, in regard to health care delivery, the patient-centered care model emphasizes, in addition to patient empowerment, a collaborative model of care for behavioral changes.[58] The patient-centered care model has been very well articulated in a variety of articles regarding patients having control over their health care decisions.[59–62] This control is very important across health care, especially when dealing with chronic disorders. The patient-centered care approach involves patients in the goal-setting process, providing ongoing support for optimal patient self-management behaviors over time. Cooperation and respect are necessary in this approach, as is recognizing the patient and his or her family as the primary decision makers. The health care providers' role is to establish a therapeutic relationship with the patient; communicate clearly, conveying genuine interest in the patient; and also provide advice when the patient is ready to hear and learn more about the new recommendations.[61] Exchanging information with the patient and providing the rationale for interventions are significant for building the patient's knowledge and confidence and effecting a behavioral change.[57–61] Furthermore, emphasizing the patient's personal choices and control, reassessing his or her readiness and beliefs about the importance of behavioral change, increasing confidence, and joining the patient in his or her decision are effective ways to reduce a patient's resistance to behavioral modifications.[57,58]

Health care providers and professionals can increase patients' behavioral adherence with interventions and a prevention approach by engaging patients in their own health care decisions and plan of care with interventions. These require the provider to be trained to provide valuable patient teaching and learning using effective behavioral strategies (**Table 8.2**). For example, for patients with hypertension, morbidity and mortality were found to decrease when health care providers receive tutorials in communication and behavioral counseling, and patients are given home visits and group classes.[58]

For many health care professionals, the barriers to promoting and increasing a patient's health behaviors may be related to lack of financial reimbursement and time to incorporate the necessary strategies.[6,53–62] Effective communication between the professional and the patient depends in part on the health care professional's confidence in his or her ability to teach and enhance patient skills as well as the amount of time available to provide effective instruction. Typically, many health care professionals respond only if the patient has a complaint or question.[58] Unless the patient asks the professional about a change in lifestyle behaviors or problems with carrying out recommendations, patient education to increase adherence is not always addressed in health care practices.[58] Also, if preventive or health care education services are not an explicit concern for a clinical practice, it is unlikely that these services will be delivered.

Enhancing patient adherence with interventions is necessary for all health care organizations. Nevertheless, many clinical settings and health care providers encounter major barriers to addressing and improving patients' adherence,[1,63–69] often because the organization or provider failed to provide effective patient and health education regarding adherence

| Table 8.2 | ***Communication and Behavioral Strategies for Patient Education[58]*** |
|---|---|
| | Interpreting the patient's recommendations. |
| | Educating and motivating the patient. |
| | Monitoring responses to recommended behaviors. |
| | Providing frequent feedback. |

with interventions as well as prevention and health promotion. As an example, many emergency room departments used for primary care have decreased patient adherence because of the time barriers to integrating prevention into their treatments.[58] By contrast, health organizations and providers that regularly deliver patient and health education for disease prevention have higher proportions of patients adhering to treatments and achieving the goals set for them.[1,6,32] As another example, multiple independent physician clinics that organized a smoking cessation intervention program using education and motivational techniques increased the proportion of patients who were identified as smokers and needed support to quit.[32] The clinics successfully used behavioral modification regimens to advise patients about smoking cessation and also offered help and positive reinforcement for their attempts.[32]

Despite the desire to improve care, health care organizations often lack knowledge about how to help patients change in response to the documented need for patient education and adherence. To advance the system, health care providers need to be trained in quality improvement in order to implement effective changes in their practices for patient behavioral modifications.[1] These changes can enhance patients' adherence and health outcomes. Health care organizations such as hospitals, health maintenance organizations (HMOs), and physicians/professionals' offices influence the extent to which patient and health care education services are provided. Many times, patients who do not have health insurance must rely on primary care settings such as emergency room departments for these educational services. Health care organizations should develop environments that support prevention and interventions using increased clinical patient education and health education.

Furthermore, health care organizations must adopt systems to rapidly and efficiently incorporate innovations into their medical practices. These innovative systems to increase patients' behavioral adherence and promote prevention may include: (1) incorporation of nursing case management into their regular practices; (2) implementation of a pharmacy patient profile; (3) use of electronic transmission storage of patients' self-monitored data; (4) obtaining patient data on lifestyle behaviors before visits; and (5) providing continuous quality improvement training of professionals, providers, and staff (**Table 8.3**).[70,71]

In regard to behavioral modifications applied by health care providers such as physical and occupational therapists, these rehabilitation professionals need to use evidence-based

| Table 8.3 | Recommendations for Health Care Organizations for Behavioral Modification Training[70,71] |
|---|---|
| Develop training in behavioral science for all personnel. | |
| Use patients' pre-appointment reminders and telephone follow-up. | |
| Schedule evening and weekend office hours. | |
| Provide group and individual counseling for patients and patients' families. | |
| Develop a computer-based system containing electronic medical records. | |
| Require continuing education courses in communication and behavioral modification counseling. | |
| Develop incentives tied to desired patient and provider outcomes. | |
| Incorporate nursing case management. | |
| Implement pharmacy patient profile and recall review systems. | |
| Obtain patient data on lifestyle behavior before patients' visits. | |
| Use electronic transmission storage of patients' self-monitored data. | |
| Provide continuous quality improvement training. | |

practice and determine best methods to evaluate patients' adherence and behavioral outcomes at each visit. The therapists can also use different strategies for behavioral changes and adherence. For example, for adherence, a patient's self-report with interventions, reminder systems, and telephone follow-up may be necessary. In addition, helping patients in their commitment to behavioral modifications requires that therapists apply specific patient education behavioral strategies (**Table 8.4**). One of the most important of these strategies is to be able to incorporate behavioral modification approaches in the patient's teaching and learning plan of care.

# The Importance of Motivation in Patient Education for Behavioral Modification

The research literature overwhelmingly shows that the most important predictors of adherence in patient education are motivation, self-efficacy, and locus of control.[1,59,67,68,72] Motivation is identified as one of the most important predictors of a patient's compliance or

| Table 8.4 | **Patient Education Behavioral Modification Strategies**[1,6,7,67–69,71,72] |
|---|---|
| Foster effective communication with patients. |
| Provide clear, direct messages about the importance of a behavior change or adherence with an intervention. |
| Provide verbal and written patient instruction, including the rationale for interventions. |
| Develop skills in specific behavioral modification and counseling. |
| Include patients in decision making about prevention and treatment goals and related strategies. |
| Use tailoring and contracting strategies. |
| Negotiate goals and a plan of action. |
| Anticipate barriers to adherence and discuss solutions with the patients. |
| Incorporate behavioral modification strategies into the patient teaching and learning plan. |
| Use active listening. |
| Develop multicomponent strategies such as cognitive and behavioral strategies. |

adherence. Motivation is a critical force that can engage the patient in the task, especially when promoting adherence to chronic therapies.[1,73,74] A patient's motivation to adhere to a prescribed intervention is influenced by: (1) the patient's beliefs regarding his or her medical condition; (2) the value the patient places on interventions; and (3) the patient's degree of confidence in being able to follow the interventions (**Table 8.5**). As an example, a patient who believes that his or her condition is serious, that there could be grave consequences if the condition is left untreated, and that the intervention will be effective (treating the condition and preventing complications) may be more likely to adhere to the intervention regimen.

Motivation and readiness to change are fundamental to a patient's long-term behavioral modifications. The most common barrier to change is a lack of confidence because of past failure or critiques from family, friends, or health care providers.[1] Other barriers include ambivalence in regard to the patient's ability to choose between present comfort and long-term health, and the patient's feeling unprepared to change.[1] The unpreparedness is related to having no plan for change, lack of social or family support, and no access to adequate

| Table 8.5 | **Common Barriers to Patients' Change¹** |
| --- | --- |
| Lack of confidence. |
| Ambivalence related to the importance of the change. |
| Feeling of being unprepared to change. |

resources. Patients need to be convinced by their own personal reasons to change and not by the health care providers' (or family's) explanations. Changes in patient behavior typically occur based on the patient's own evaluation of the positive and negative aspects of change.[1] When the patient sees the positive aspects of making the change with few or no barriers, the change will take place; however, if the real or perceived negative aspects of change outweigh the positives, the change is unlikely to occur.

Because change requires action of some type, patients who seek rehabilitation (physical or occupational therapy) must be motivated to comply with interventions. As an example, in neurological rehabilitation, adherence with interventions is not sufficient for a patient if he or she does not have the necessary motivation.[74] Patients can be doing things just to please the therapist without having intrinsic motivation.[74] However, having intrinsic motivation augments patients' adherence with a desire to recover for themselves and not for the therapist. In rehabilitation, similar to health care in general, motivation is influenced by several factors such as the patient's personality, family, type(s) of illness, culture, rehabilitation providers (environment), rehabilitation goals, and forms of patient education.[74,76–78] While interviewing patients, rehabilitation providers have found that motivation is determined partly by the individual patient's personality.[74] Some patients who are described as optimists have high motivation whereas pessimists are unmotivated.[74] The patient's family also can influence motivation in a positive or negative way. For example, patients with strokes who were not required or encouraged by their family to make gains actually had reduced motivation.[74] The type of illness (such as a neurological disorder) may influence the patient's cognition and also cause depression, particularly with older individuals.

Patients' cultural norms, such as fatalistic religious beliefs, can legitimize their dependency during periods of disability. This may be extremely difficult to overcome. Additionally, some therapeutic materials oriented toward patients from Western cultures may not be appropriate for people from other ethnic backgrounds. Furthermore, rehabilitation providers' conduct in regard to labeling patients as successful or unsuccessful also can diminish patients' motivation. Studies have found that whatever sort of labels a provider wants to attach to people can become a self-fulfilling prophecy.[74–76] Also, having low expectations of how patients will perform in rehabilitation has a negative effect on motivation.

Giving patients mixed messages about their role in rehabilitation can affect motivation in a harmful way, especially if one provider encourages independence and another provider encourages dependency by doing too many things for the patient. The rehabilitation environment, such as providing a stimulating area, a well-maintained treatment room, and group treatment sessions in which patients can share beliefs about rehabilitation and observe each other's progress are suggested as positive determinants of motivation.[74]

Setting relevant rehabilitation goals and encouraging patients' involvement in these goals increase motivation. For some patients, the goals have to be small, achievable, and meaningful to demonstrate to patients that they are actually making progress. Forms of patient teaching and learning can be positive strategies for motivation if they are complete and include information about the nature of recovery (reassuring patients that they are recovering and advising against unfavorable comparison with other patients); home rehabilitation and programs, especially if no rehab gains were made; and the reasons for certain exercises and specific ways of performing them. In addition, delivering patient instruction increases motivation if there is a rapport between the patient and the rehabilitation provider and if the provider uses specific forms of instruction to culturally facilitate the patient's motivation. For example, in a stroke rehabilitation study, a rehab provider used a patient's religious beliefs to educate a patient who was unmotivated to walk because it was only the will of God that he survived.[74] The provider told him that it was also the will of God that he was in the rehabilitation unit, so he should take advantage of the opportunity that was provided for him and that it was all right to do that.[74]

The literature also indicates that motivation to change requires both the patient's conviction and confidence.[73,75,76] *Conviction* is a belief that a new behavior is important and worth the effort to achieve it.[75] *Confidence* is a belief that a person has the ability to adopt a new behavior.[75] Without these two core beliefs, patients are not motivated to take action and make changes, and are more apt to become discouraged, fall back into old behaviors, and give up.

A patient's conviction and confidence can be influenced by three factors: the health care provider, the environment, and the patient him- or herself.[75] The interpersonal skills of the health care provider significantly influence patients to change. Rehabilitation providers who express empathy and establish a supportive, knowledgeable relationship with patients are far more successful in helping people change than those who are aloof, dogmatic, and impersonal. Health care providers can offer to patients the educational and community resources available in their environment. These resources can be community and specific means offered by the health care organization. For example, in rehabilitation, the therapist can enlist community resources to offer education and any necessary supplies, organize health care organization support groups to connect patients with similar disorders (conditions), and provide crisis intervention for emergency situations through social workers and psychologists. When patients come to health care providers, they may not understand their need to change but know something is wrong and need help. They may have little conviction that a change is necessary and even less confidence that they can change. Nonetheless, the fact that patients recognize the need for change indicates that they are in the first stage of the process of change.[75]

# The Significance of Behavioral Modification Theories in Patient Education

In physical and occupational rehabilitation, the stages of behavioral change as well as the phases of psychosocial adaptation occur as a continuum. In the behavioral stages of change, the patient strives to change their behavior; in the phases of psychosocial adaptation, they try to attain an optimal state of functioning within their environment.[75,77] Patient education for behavioral change can enhance patients' motivation and adherence to rehabilitative interventions and disease prevention strategies. Patient education for psychosocial phases of adaptation to disability and chronic illness can also help a patient's coping mechanism for dealing with internal and external challenges, thus improving adherence to interventions. During both, the patient must be able to take charge of the situation and actively participate in the required changes to achieve the best rehabilitation outcomes. Patient education during behavioral stages and psychosocial adaptation phases is important to help patients meet their goals, feel confident, and have positive self-esteem. In physical and occupational rehabilitation, therapists can provide effective intervention and prevention counseling by guiding and influencing patients' behavioral choices. Understanding people's cognitive behavior and being able to apply efficient teaching, learning, and patient feedback characterize the most significant part of contemporary physical and occupational therapy practice.

Three theories of cognitive behavior can influence a patient's adherence with interventions, exercise behavior, and disease prevention and health promotion. These behavioral theories are the Health Belief Model,[78] the Social Learning Theory (SLT),[79] and the Transtheoretical Model of Change (TTM).[80] The Health Belief Model affirms that in order to make a behavioral change, an individual must believe the following:[78]

- That they are susceptible to a disease or disorder

- That the disease or disorder has serious consequences

- That making a change can reduce the threat

- That the costs of or barriers to making the change are less than the benefits

- That he or she is able to make the necessary change successfully

When applying the Health Belief Model, which can be used mostly in preventive education, the therapist should emphasize to the patient the consequences of poor adherence and the barriers and benefits of the suggested intervention. If the patient does not believe that the intervention is likely to help or believes that there are too many barriers to implement, the therapist must attempt to modify the patient's beliefs.

The SLT states that behavior is the product of a continuous reciprocal interaction between social and physical environments and psychological factors such as emotions, self-appraisals, and self-efficacy.[79] SLT can be used in rehabilitation to increase a patient's confidence to perform the interventions and to implement self-monitoring strategies for adherence. The third theory, the Transtheoretical Model of Change, will be discussed in the next section.

# Patient Education Using the Transtheorethical Model of Change

The Transtheoretical Model of Change (TTM) has been identified by psychologists as one of the most effective theories for creating an "intentional" behavioral change in an individual.[1,75–77] The TTM includes key constructs from other behavioral theories and has been evaluated in multiple clinical trials. The model has been used successfully for smoking cessation, alcohol abuse, weight control, HIV protection, organizational change, medical care adherence including pharmacotherapy, stress management, and adherence with exercises.[1,75,76,80–84] The TTM has been described as an integrative and comprehensive model of behavior change that has drawn from all major theories of psychotherapy.[1,75]

The main hypothesis of the TTM is that a person's behavioral change occurs in a series of stages or steps.[1,75] These stages are especially noticeable if the change represents a significant alteration in lifestyle. The TTM includes five sequential stages of change from old behaviors to new ones. The Stages of Change Model (SCM) is a TTM construct that represents the temporal dimensions of TTM.[1,75] SCM signifies "when" the change will take place.[1,75] The processes of change constructs of the TTM involve understanding "how" individuals change their behavior. These approaches to change include cognitive, affective, evaluative, and behavioral strategies that an individual may use to modify the problem behavior.[1,75] The major constructs of the TTM consist of: (1) stages of change (the temporal dimension of change); (2) the process of change (cognitive and behavioral mechanism to modify problem behaviors and adopt new positive behaviors); (3) decisional balance (pros and cons of a particular behavior); (4) temptation (the level or urge to engage in a negative behavior or to not engage in a positive behavior); and (5) confidence (the patient's belief in his or her ability to refrain from a negative behavior and engage in a positive behavior).[1,75,76]

## THE STAGES OF CHANGE MODEL IN PATIENT TEACHING AND LEARNING

As mentioned earlier, the TTM construes change as a process involving progress through a series of five SCM stages (**Table 8.6**).[75] These stages can be used to identify appropriate patient education interventions and foster positive behavioral change.

The SCM model has been advocated in patient education by nurses to help patients make informed decisions and keep them motivated and adherent to treatment.[2] The SCM can help the health care provider get insight into the patient's behavioral conduct when trying to acquire needed changes. The SCM proposes that there are predictable physical and psychological stages of change.[2] Additionally, the idea behind the SCM is that the behavior change of an individual does not happen in one step but by progressing through

| Table 8.6 | The Stages of Change Model (SCM)[75] |
|---|---|
| Precontemplation. | |
| Contemplation. | |
| Preparation. | |
| Action. | |
| Maintenance. | |

phases over time. Understanding the SCM phases allows health care providers to apply appropriate interventions and motivate the patient to change.[2]

In physical and occupational therapy, the use of the SCM to develop effective interventions in the exercise domain has been reported extensively.[80–86] To develop successful interventions, the therapist needs to assess the reason the patient's past interventions have failed. In the SCM, the patient's motivation is the key factor to consider, especially when past interventions may have been mismatched to the patient's actual readiness level.

The concepts of the SCM have been designed to avoid mismatching the patient and the intervention. As a result, when therapists are assessing a patient's SCM phase of change, it is imperative they recognize that all individuals differ in their level of motivational readiness to change a behavior. The therapist also should understand that strategies for promoting behavioral change vary according to the SCM stage the patient is in. Consequently, there is a need to create a "stage-matched" design and tailor each patient's interventions to the specific needs of that patient.[83] For example, exercise programs in physical and occupational therapy are action oriented, which means they should be applied when patients are in the SCM action stage of change. Attempting to begin an exercise program in an earlier stage may lead to patient nonadherence. Other patients may need to use moderate activity interventions in their initial plan of care.

Patients will be more likely to adhere to a program that has smaller, more attainable goals. For example, a cardiopulmonary physical therapy research study stated that physical therapists should educate patients on the benefits of short bouts of activity throughout the day and discourage the "all-or-nothing belief that 30 minutes"[83(p.68)] of continuous and vigorous exercise is mandatory 3 days a week to achieve physical gain.

Ultimately, the SCM phases can help therapists reduce patients' motivational barriers and improve their adherence to exercises. For example, more current research indicates the effectiveness of patient education in an interventional program for osteoporosis.[80] Similar to other studies,[80–86] the success of the educational program and the patient's motivation with interventions was based on an SCM stage-specific plan of care.

## PATIENT EDUCATION GOALS USING THE STAGES OF CHANGE MODEL

The first motivational stage of change in the SCM is called precontemplation. In this phase, the individual is unhappy with his or her current state and realizes that there may be a need to change. People may be in this stage because they are uninformed or underinformed about the consequences of their behavior. Also, they may have tried to change a number of times and become discouraged about their ability to change. Typically, they tend to avoid reading, talking, or thinking about their high risk behaviors. For example, Mrs. KS had smoked cigarettes for more than 25 years. Recently she had a heart attack and was told that she needed to stop smoking. Prior to her heart attack, she had tried to stop smoking many times but had never succeeded. In the precontemplation stage, she was not happy being a smoker, wanted to change, but viewed the task as too difficult, beyond her grasp, and not worth the effort. Typically, in the precontemplation stage, the patient does not know the specific problem behavior that needs to be changed or, as in this example, views the task as too difficult, beyond his or her grasp, and not worth the effort.[73,76]

Patients in the precontemplation stage are not ready for change and become resistant and defensive to the possibility of change. Patient education at this stage requires the provider to explain to the patient the reasons behind the needed changes. These reasons can increase the patient's perception of the risks and problems with their current behavior. Patient teaching is directed toward getting the patient to start thinking about whether the change is necessary. Patient education can increase personal awareness about the need for change, decreasing defensiveness, and rationalization of negative behavior (**Table 8.7**).[76]

In rehabilitation, the precontemplation stage may coincide with the psychosocial adaptation phase of denial that is used as a defense mechanism to alleviate anxiety and pain associated with disability and illness. Denial protects the patient from having to confront all at once the overwhelming implications of illness and injury. Denial also helps the patient to gradually understand the facts and reality of illness and injury. The rehabilitation provider should be aware that at this precontemplation or denial stage patients may be unrealistic

| Table 8.7 | **Patient Education Goals for the Precontemplation Stage**[76] |
|---|---|
| | Raise the patient's distrust in regard to their current (harmful) behavior. |
| | Decrease the patient's defensiveness and erroneous rationalization. |
| | Increase the patient's perception of risks and problems with the current behavior. |
| | Increase the patient's personal consciousness. |

about recovery goals and need time and accurate information to understand the rehabilitation facts and challenges. Therapists need to be supportive of patients and not make unrealistic predictions of goals and recovery. For example, the rehabilitation research indicates that athletes experience emotional disturbances after injuries.[81] After the initial shock, many athletes go through a denial stage, playing down the significance of the injury.[81] Physical therapists can recognize the emotion and educate the patient about the injury and the certainty of achieving their goals.

The second SCM stage is called the contemplation phase, in which the individual is more aware that changes are necessary but tends to be ambivalent about making a commitment to change (**Table 8.8**).[76]

The contemplation phase is characterized by the individual's intrinsic debate about the pros and cons of the change.[76] The person contemplates a change but at the same time may want to delay it. Patient education must concentrate on helping the patient find reasons for change as well as understand the risks for remaining in the current behavioral mode. The patient needs assistance to make a commitment to change and resolve his or her ambivalence toward the change.[76] Some people can be stuck in this stage for long periods of time. The health care provider can encourage the patient's commitment to attempt a change. For example, prior to her heart attack, Mrs. KS understood the benefits of change (to stop smoking) but was ambivalent because of her fear of failure. She was stuck in procrastination and not ready to change. In addition, many patients at this stage are open to receiving information about the necessary changes and may use instruction to reflect on their own feelings and possibility of a change. During this phase, the health care provider should avoid forcing patients into change but should support them in asking questions or expressing concerns related to the contemplated change.

The contemplation stage may coincide with anger or hostility as a response to loss and disability. The rehabilitation provider should understand the patient's anger as a normal emotion under the circumstances of disease and disability. When the anger is expressed

| Table 8.8 | **Patient Education Goals for the Contemplation Stage[76]** |
|---|---|
| | Elicit reasons for the patient to change. |
| | Explain the patient's risks for not changing. |
| | Increase the patient's confidence in his or her ability to change the current behavior. |
| | Encourage the patient to make a commitment to try to change. |
| | Help the patient resolve ambivalence. |

aggressively through physical or verbal abuse, therapists need to have the entire rehabilitation team redirect the patient's anger into productive therapeutic activities. As in the first stage, therapists need to remain supportive of patients and offer empathetic and realistic intervention goals. For example, in athletes, as the injury becomes more apparent, denial is replaced by anger directed internally toward themselves or externally towards other people.[81] Physical therapists must be aware that anger responses can vary in intensity depending on situational and personal factors. The anger reactions can be especially strong in athletes whose self-concept and personal identity are based on being "an athlete."[81] A patient with a sports injury can experience extreme grief and suffering due to loss of identity and inability to perform.[85] In this stage, physical therapists should offer realistic intermediate rehabilitation goals such as regaining full range of motion at the joint or walking without a leg brace.

The third SCM stage is called the preparation or determination stage (**Table 8.9**), when the individual already has made a commitment to change and to take action in the immediate future (perhaps next month).

Often something happens to motivate the patient to take action, such as an emotion-laden crisis, a recent illness, or a plea from an important individual in the patient's life. In Mrs. KS's case, her heart attack made her realize the importance of stopping smoking. Her confidence in her ability to do it is yet to be proved, but she is ready to take action. At this stage of preparation, patient education is the most helpful because the health care provider can help the patient outline the intervention strategies and goals that need to be accomplished. The provider should help the patient determine the best course of action for change as well as find concrete effective strategies that are acceptable to the patient. Facilitating the patient's ability to move toward the goal of making change enhances the effectiveness of patient instruction and strengthens the patient's commitment. At this stage in physical and occupational therapy, the patients should be recruited to start an exercise program or, as in the example case, referred to counseling, if necessary.

The third SCM stage may coincide with the patient's acknowledgment of the permanency of the disease or disability.[76] The patient recognizes and accepts the condition and develops new self-concepts and values while searching for new goals and meaning. Patient

| Table 8.9 | *Patient Education Goals for the Preparation Stage*[76] |
|---|---|
| | Help the patient determine the best course of action for change. |
| | Develop a plan for change with the patient. |
| | Find concrete strategies with the patient to effect the change. |
| | Reinforce the patient's commitment. |

education could help the patient find new objectives that are meaningful and long lasting. For example, following anger, the injured athlete might try to bargain or rationalize to avoid the reality of the situation. A runner may promise him- or herself to train extra hard or to be especially pleasant so he or she can recover quickly.[85] In the adaptation stage, the athlete's motivation with physical therapy rehabilitation may be reduced because of fear of re-injury.[85] Physical therapists can use verbal encouragement and reframe negative statements made by the athlete into optimistic positive ones. Realistic goal setting can also positively affect the athlete in the recovery process.

The action stage is the fourth SCM stage, when the individual is actively involved in the action of change using a variety of techniques or interventions (**Table 8.10**).[76] In nursing, patient education goals use the acronym SMART to help patients develop and work toward new positive behaviors.[2] The patient's goals in the plan of care should be specific, **m**easurable, **a**ttainable, **r**ealistic, and **t**angible (SMART).[2]

Using the acronym SMART, the therapist can establish the patient's goals regarding physical or occupational therapy. The patient's goals need to be appropriate for each patient and his or her situation, including readiness, environment, resources, conviction, and confidence. Physical and occupational therapists should be action-oriented, ready to identify specific measurable objectives for change that will help the patient reorder his or her life. A patient's high level of conviction shows that the outcome is important. A patient with a high confidence level shows that the outcome can be achieved. A patient having conviction and confidence demonstrates motivation to act and change. Methods to increase patient conviction and confidence are described in **Table 8.11**.[75]

The action stage is critical because patients are most likely to relapse into old behaviors. Patient education must help patients remain confident and convinced they really can and will be able to change their current behavior. Patient instruction is directed at helping them establish SMART goals. In this stage, patients need help to become committed to accomplish the short-term goals that would sustain their motivation and adherence throughout the change. The action stage is also the stage where vigilance against relapse is critical. The action stage is very important in physical and occupational therapy as a time to introduce exercise and activity programs that patients will be adherent to for

Table 8.10

**Patient Education Goals for the Action Stage[76]**

Help the patient identify the necessary steps to implement the plan for change.

Support the patient's confidence in making the change.

Assist the patient in developing his or her problem-solving skills.

| Table 8.11 | *Methods to Increase a Patient's Conviction and Confidence*[75] |
|---|---|
| | Create appropriate measurable objectives. |
| | Agree on objectives with the patient. |
| | Agree on assistance needed with the patient. |
| | Explore the patient's ambivalence. |

life. Additionally, teaching and learning can support patients' motivation to remain adherent with interventions not only in the clinical settings, but also at home. In the case of Mrs. KS, her goal in the action stage is to start smoking cessation counseling next week.

In the psychosocial adaptation phases, the action stage may coincide with the patient's final adjustment phase of the adaptation. This adjustment phase is characterized by the patient's new ways of interacting successfully with others and the environment. In this stage, the patient regains self-worth, understands his or her new potentials, and pursues social and vocational goals, overcoming obstacles that may arise in the attainment of these goals. In this stage, patient education is very important. Patients continuously seek support from others and are open to help. For example, in this phase, the athlete transitions from an emotional step to a problem-coping point to focus on his or her needs for help with the recovery. Physical therapists can help establish self-tasks for the athlete and encourage them to focus on intermediate goals that represent stepping stones to achieve the recovery goal. Intermediate goals usually provide direction for the day-to-day efforts of the injured athlete. These can be daily exercises that he or she should perform. The achievement of intermediate goals is also important for increasing the athlete's self-confidence. In addition, monitoring and evaluating the patient's goals are essential as is resetting goals, especially if these are too easy or too difficult to achieve in a given time frame. The importance of the psychological appraisals that athletes undertake regarding progress should not be underestimated. The therapist's support and the correct progression of exercises are identified in the literature as important determinants of attendance and adherence to physical therapy rehabilitation sessions.[84,85]

The fifth stage of the SCM is called the maintenance stage.[76] In this stage, patients work to prevent relapse (**Table 8.12**).[76] Patients are tempted to go back to their old behaviors and need ongoing support to keep them from falling back into a familiar pattern of living. The support must be enhanced by encouragement from health care providers, family, friends, colleagues, and members of support groups. In the above example, Mrs. KS joined a support group and found significant assistance in the suggestions and help of the members as she persisted in maintaining her new behavior as a nonsmoker. Patient instruction remains significant for patients who need reinforcement and a permanent commitment for sustaining

| Table 8.12 | | |
|---|---|---|
| **Patient Education Goals for the Maintenance Stage**[76] | | |
| Help the patient identify potentially tempting situations and find strategies for success. | | |
| Confirm the patient's commitment and efforts to change. | | |
| Discuss with the patient the benefits of changed behavior. | | |
| Identify and help the patient in regard to any negative consequence that resulted from the positive change. | | |

the new status quo. The health care provider should offer support, encouragement, and reinforcement to maintain the changes the patients made.

# Other Variables in Teaching and Learning Behavioral Modification

As stated previously, to facilitate behavioral change, physical and occupational therapists should establish a supportive therapeutic relationship with each patient. The general strategies to enhance patient motivation for change are the following:[76]

- Expressing empathy
- Avoiding arguments
- Developing discrepancy by pointing out to the patient the difference between the patient's behavior and his/her important personal goals
- Involving family members
- Referring the patient to a support group
- Using motivational interviewing (to increase self-efficacy and confidence)
- Recognizing small positive steps the patient is taking
- Using supportive statements
- Helping the patient set reasonable and reachable goals
- Expressing the belief that the patient can achieve the goals

Other important techniques that facilitate behavioral changes are showing nonjudgmental empathy, listening attentively and reflectively, and using proper verbal and nonverbal messages. Nonjudgmental empathy is related to the therapist establishing a therapeutic relationship with the patient based on trust, genuine interest, and consideration of the patient's feelings, ideas, desires, and actions.[26] Empathy also involves the therapist's ability to use reflective listening methods, including listening attentively to the patient and seeking to recognize not only the facts of the case, but also the overall meaning of the problem to the patient.[76] In this way, the patient feels understood and truly heard. Reflective listening also is important for the therapist to be able to express interest and be aware of what the patient is saying. The patient's tone of voice, a reply that is tentative, or certain voice inflections could demonstrate an individual's real feelings and emotions. Reflective listening demonstrates genuine concern for the patient's welfare and encourages the patient to express real feelings to the provider.[76]

## EXPLORATION OF A PATIENT'S AMBIVALENCE

In general, individuals have some degree of motivation to achieve the objective(s) related to their interventions.[76] Still, the primary reason patients are not motivated to engage in a behavior modification is ambivalence. When ambivalent, patients generally do nothing.[76] Some patients want to achieve a new behavior but realize that the process requires energy and effort that they do not have. In addition, the old behavior is familiar and comfortable. As a result, the conviction and confidence weaken. A patient's ambivalence can be overcome through reflective listening, summarizing, and acknowledging progress and responding to the positive changes. Physical and occupational therapists can reflect back the patient's words and show sincere empathy by admitting that change is difficult and takes courage (**Table 8.13**).[76,87] Summarizing the patient's accomplishments also defeats ambivalence.

If the therapist is not aware of a patient's motivational objectives, he or she will not be able to recognize motivation in that individual patient's actions. When patients visit health

| Table 8.13 | *Questions to Explore a Patient's Ambivalence*[87] |
|---|---|
| What is the down side of taking action? |
| What would you have to give up to make your goal a priority? |
| What are the good things about staying the same? |
| What are the good things about changing? |

care providers, motivation needs to be assessed from the beginning and used as a base for interventions. Motivation is a key factor in successful behavior change to promote adherence, so the SCM can be used in health care and physical and occupational therapy. Anything that moves an individual toward making a positive change should be viewed as a success. Patient education interventions that are not staged to the readiness of the individual will be less likely to succeed. Also, interventions that try to move a person too quickly through the stages of change are more likely to create resistance that will impede behavior change. For example, when trying to get a patient with hypertension to quit smoking, it is essential to know where the person is in his or her readiness to stop. A person who is not even thinking about quitting smoking (in the precontemplation phase) is generally not ready to receive information about specific smoking cessation aids. In this case, focusing the intervention on smoking cessation aids sends the message that the health care provider is not really listening. This may not only damage the rapport between the health care provider and the patient, but it also may make the patient even more resistant to quitting smoking. A more stage-specific intervention with this patient would be to try to get the patient to think about quitting (contemplation). Once the patient reaches the contemplation stage, additional strategies can be employed to continue to move the patient through the stages of behavioral change. Applying stage-specific interventions will decrease the health care provider's frustration by lessening the unrealistic expectation that change will occur with a single intervention.

## *Motivational Interviewing in Patient Teaching and Learning*

The concept of motivational interviewing evolved from experience in the treatment of problem drinkers and was first described by Miller in 1983.[1,75] The definition of motivational interviewing is a directive, patient-centered analysis style for eliciting behavior change by helping clients to explore and resolve ambivalence.[75] The central purpose of motivational interviewing is examination and resolution of a patient's ambivalence. Motivational interviewing can be used in physical and occupational therapy as an assessment and intervention strategy in order to enhance a patient's behavior and improve adherence with clinical interventions and disease prevention. Motivational interviewing determines a patient's readiness to engage in a target behavior and the choice of specific skills and strategies to apply based on the patient's readiness to create a favorable climate for change. It is also a patient-centered, directive method of communicating with the goal of enhancing a patient's intrinsic motivation to change by exploring and resolving ambivalence and resistance. Motivational interviewing can help patients identify and change behaviors that can place them at risk for developing health problems.[86,88] It can also assist patients to prevent or optimally manage chronic conditions.

## CHARACTERISTICS AND COMPONENTS OF MOTIVATIONAL INTERVIEWING

Motivational interviewing includes eight approaches that are designed to increase the level of motivation the patient has towards changing a specific behavior:[1,75]

1. Giving advice about a specific behavior that needs to be changed

2. Removing barriers (sometimes in regard to access to particular types of help)

3. Providing choice (by helping patients understand their choices to change or not to change the behavior and that the health care provider is there to encourage the change but not to insist on change)

4. Decreasing desirability (of the ambivalence towards change or the status quo)

5. Practicing empathy

6. Providing feedback (from the perspectives of family, friends, and other health care providers and giving the patient a full and accurate picture of their current situation)

7. Clarifying goals (by describing the ideal situation and providing the pathway to the patient's goal)

8. Actively helping (by expressing real interest and genuine caring and facilitating a referral, if necessary)

The goal of motivational interviewing is to identify what maintains behaviors, including the ambivalence about change, and to encourage and support patients in adopting new behaviors. Physical and occupational therapists should follow the five basic steps to help patient's change: (1) express empathy, (2) avoid argumentation, (3) support self-efficacy, (4) roll with resistance, and (5) develop discrepancy.[75]

Motivational interviewing techniques avoid telling a patient what he or she needs to do. The essence of motivational interviewing is its collaborative approach, communicating in a partnership with the patient and creating a positive interpersonal atmosphere.[75] The responsibility of change is left to the patient, and the overall goal of the therapist is to increase the patient's motivation for the behavioral change to arise from within rather than being imposed. The change must be negotiated with the patient and not dictated to the patient. Consistent with the collaborative model of change, the therapist functions not to motivate the patient but to draw out intrinsic motivation based on the patient's own personal goals and values. During motivational interviewing, the therapist should avoid argumentative persuasion but instead use the patient's subjective experiences and perspectives. This involves listening to, acknowledging, and practicing acceptance (not submission) of a broad range of patient concerns, opinions, preferences, beliefs, emotions, styles, and motivations.

The motivational interviewing approach is particularly helpful for patients who are reluctant to change and ambivalent about changing.[75] It is intended to help resolve ambivalence and get the patient moving along the path to change. For some patients this is all they really need. Once they are unstuck, they have the skills and resources they need to make a lasting change. For other patients, motivational interviewing is just a prelude to starting behavioral modification to adhere with interventions. It creates an openness to change that paves the way for more advanced lifestyle modifications. Motivational interviewing systematically directs the patient toward motivation for change, as well as creates and amplifies the patient's consciousness of discrepancy in order to enhance motivation for change (**Table 8.14**).

During motivational interviewing, the rehabilitation provider should consider that the opening of the interview, the provider's tone of voice and demeanor, and the physical circumstances significantly impact behavioral outcomes. The provider's questioning style can use: (1) open questions, (2) direct questions, (3) closed questions, and (4) leading questions.[75,89] The manner in which the information is obtained from the patient by the therapist can influence the quality of information acquired. Using the appropriate types of questions ensures that accurate information is obtained. It is known that active listening techniques often lead to unexpected and important information.[75] Summarizing and clarifying statements show the patient that the therapist is listening and is interested in understanding the patient's concerns. Also, summarizing and clarifying statements ensure that accurate information is being collected. The provider's empathetic response to the

| Table 8.14 | *Characteristics of Motivational Interviewing*[75] |
|---|---|
| Motivational interviewing relies upon identifying and mobilizing the patient's intrinsic values and goals to stimulate behavior change. |
| Motivation to change is elicited from the patient and not imposed from without. |
| Motivational interviewing is designed to elicit, clarify, and resolve ambivalence and to perceive benefits and costs associated with it. |
| Readiness to change is a patient trait but a fluctuating product of interpersonal interaction. |
| Resistance and denial are often signals to modify motivational strategies. |
| Eliciting and reinforcing the patient's belief in his or her ability to carry out and succeed in achieving a specific goal is essential. |
| The therapeutic relationship is a partnership that respects patient autonomy. |
| Motivational interviewing is directive and patient-centered analysis for better understanding and eliciting behavior change. |

patient's emotions promotes thoughtful consideration of the patient's difficulties. The therapist's attention to the patient's nonverbal cues and signs can also provide valuable information during the motivational interview. At the end of the interview, the therapist should be able to demonstrate that he or she understood the problems and has the desire and enthusiasm to help the patient in the stages of change. Ultimately, the motivational interviewing helps to explore the patient's ambivalence associated with behavior and encourage the patient to express their reasons for concerns or arguments against change.[75] As a form of assessment, motivational interviewing can also be a fast process through the use of the *READS* principles (**Table 8.15**).[75]

For the "roll with resistance" step, the resistance can take several forms, such as negating, blaming, excusing, minimizing, arguing, challenging, interrupting, and ignoring. The patient's resistance results from the interpersonal interaction between the therapist and the patient. It is not a personality flaw of the patient. Consequently, during motivational interviewing, the therapist does not directly oppose the patient's resistance but rather rolls or flows with it (**Table 8.16**).[75] Physical and occupational therapists should avoid eliciting or strengthening resistance, because the more a patient resists, the less likely any change will occur. The therapist giving up the ability to change the behavior is common where there is patient resistance.[89] By changing the style of intervention, the therapist can decrease patient resistance. Direct confrontation can create additional barriers that will make change even more difficult. A patient's resistance during motivational interviewing is expected and should not be viewed as a negative outcome. In reality, a patient who resists is providing information about factors that foster or reduce motivation to adhere to a behavioral change.

Rolling with resistance includes actively involving the patient in the process of problem solving.[75] Resistant behavior may be a signal that the patient does not believe or accept information that has been presented. The therapist should give the patient information and alternatives, and explore possible solutions. Exploring the reasons behind the resistant behavior can lead the patient to seriously consider possibilities for change.

| Table 8.15 | |
|---|---|
| **The READS Acronym**[75] | |
| 1. **R**oll with resistance. | |
| 2. **E**xpress empathy. | |
| 3. **A**void arguing. | |
| 4. **D**evelop discrepancy. | |
| 5. **S**upport self-efficacy. | |

| Table 8.16 | **Communication Guidelines to Handle a Patient's Resistance**[75] |
|---|---|
| Reframing | Acknowledging the validity of the patient's perspective and observations and offering a new meaning or interpretation. |
| Emphasizing the patient's personal control | Communicating to the patient that it is his or her own decision as to whether to make a behavioral change. |
| Siding with the patient's negatives about the change | Agreeing with the patient that he or she may not need to change; often the patient may respond by presenting a more positive side of change. |

## THE ROLE OF EMPATHY IN MOTIVATIONAL INTERVIEWING

Expressing empathy during motivational interviewing relies on establishing and maintaining a therapeutic rapport with the patient and using reflective listening. The ability to express and feel empathy is critical. This requires skillful reflective listening to understand a person's feelings without judging, criticizing, or blaming. Accepting the patient's feelings and perspectives helps to facilitate change. Physical and occupational therapists who are judgmental, perceive the patient as lazy or uncooperative, or are impatient are likely to fail in assisting a patient with change. The therapist who sees the patient as someone who is struggling with the process of change and respects the patient and the struggle will be far more successful in helping the patient. The therapist's attitude of acceptance and respect contributes to the development of an effective relationship, enhancing the patient's self-esteem (**Table 8.17**).[89] A vital part of empathy is the process of not labeling the patient; for example, labeling a patient as a "diabetic" or an "alcoholic" confirms their status without identifying the positives and negatives of their behaviors. Patient motivation and adherence should be based on a balance of the patient's good things and less good things related to behavior.

Empathy is a multidimensional quality of the therapist. Empathy entails affective and cognitive factors as well as behavioral components.[89] For physical and occupational therapists, the primary need is for their perceptions to be accurate if shared understanding is to be reached, which highlights the importance of cognitive empathy that is totally different than sympathy. "Feeling sorry" for someone is sympathy, and it is characterized by a generalized or global supportive assessment of patient's problem.[26] On the contrary, empathy has an emotional dimension to it with enough clarity of mind in searching for empathetic understanding of the actual thoughts and feelings of the patient. The therapist's empathetic assessment is facilitated and reinforced by the use of communication skills such as an open question style and checking patient agreement. For the therapist, empathy depends on the ability to

| Table 8.17 | | |
|---|---|---|
| **Forms of Reflecting Listening Skills[89]** | | |
| Simple reflection | Acknowledging the patient's point of view (e.g., "Sometimes it is very difficult to start an exercise program."). | |
| Amplified reflection | Reflecting back what the patient stated in an exaggerated way, but without sarcasm (e.g., "Exercising probably will not work for you at this time."). | |
| Double-sided reflection | Acknowledging both sides of the patient's ambivalence by putting together all the patient's information ("On the one hand you really want to feel better and stronger and exercise, and on the other hand, you really dislike the exercises and do not want to do them."). | |
| Shifting focus | Shifting the patient's attention away from the issue (that the provider may be stuck on); moving on to another issue (e.g., "How is work?"). | |

put oneself in a patient's place and experience the patient's feelings of pain, anger, relief, or happiness.[26] Then, a therapeutic relationship between the patient and the provider can be established.

There are three stages of empathy (**Table 8.18**).[26] The first stage, the cognitive stage, involves getting into the position of the patient.[26] This stage requires listening to the patient and trying to imagine what it must be like for the patient to experience what he or she is describing. The second stage, the crossing over stage, is the most significant because for a moment or so, the therapist has the same feeling as the patient, almost living in his or her world.[26] In the third stage (the coming back to own feelings stage), the therapist feels a special alliance with the patient.[26] Empathy helps the provider to maintain therapeutic subjectivity, but at the same time, to listen to the patient and contribute to his or her healing process.[26]

The therapeutic partnerships formed through empathy can facilitate effective interventions by actively engaging the patient in the therapeutic relationship.[26] In this way the therapist encourages patient motivation and behavioral changes. For example, asking the patient "What does having diabetes mean to you?" helps the rehabilitation provider to determine

| Table 8.18 | **Stages of Empathy[26]** |
|---|---|
| Cognitive. | |
| Crossing over. | |
| Coming back to own feelings. | |

which beliefs are accurate and which need to be corrected. In discussing the good things and less good things, the provider can also ask the patient about what they perceive as barriers and facilitators to treating their illness. All of this gives the provider the opportunity to listen to the patient and demonstrate understanding by empathic responding. Identifying barriers and facilitators of behavior change will also allow the therapist to more accurately determine the patient's stage of readiness to change. Finally, knowing the good things and less good things gives the provider the opportunity to develop discrepancies between old, unwanted behaviors and new, desired behaviors. This is an effective skill for moving patients forward.

## ARGUMENTATION AND DISCREPANCY DURING MOTIVATIONAL INTERVIEWING

Trying to avoid arguing is normal when working with patients. As described in psychology, motivational interviewing is confrontational in order to increase awareness of problems and the need to do something about them.[75] However, this kind of confrontation is different than arguing with the patient, trying to convince patients they have a problem when they are not ready to accept it, or labeling patients (overweight, diabetic, hypertensive, anorexic, uncooperative) in order to promote change. Arguing tends to increase resistance rather than increase motivation to change.[75] This type of "confrontation" is actually discussing pleasantly with the patient his or her problem and trying to make the patient see the discrepancy and reflect on it. As a result, the patient confronts the problem (himself or herself) realizing that he or she needs to change. However, in many situations, ambivalence takes over and the patient could be torn between wanting and not wanting to do something. The task of the physical and occupational therapist is to assist in listing the good things and the not-so-good things and comparing them. The rehabilitation provider's communication style should: (1) avoid provoking the patient; (2) encourage careful attention to the patient's readiness to change; (3) encourage the patient to make his or her own assessments of problems and solutions; (4) enhance the patient's motivation; and, most importantly, (5) not give advice.[75,89]

Developing discrepancy is important when patients are ambivalent about change. The rehabilitation provider should begin to move the patient in the direction of the desired change. Persuasive strategies usually work best in the later stages of change and may fail when patients are in the precontemplation or contemplation stages of change. For this reason, developing discrepancies between a patient's present behavior and the desired behavior is important. Patients are much more highly motivated to change when discrepancies exist between current behaviors and desired personal goals. Motivational interviewing attempts to create these discrepancies without making the patient feel threatened or pressured. Through effective communication and questioning, the interviewer identifies discrepancies that already exist within the patient, rather than imposing external pressures. When the interview is done properly, the patient will come up with the reasons that the change is necessary. Typically, the discrepancy occurs between the patient's most deeply held values and his or her current behavior. It means that the health care provider amplifies the costs of the patient's current behavior against current goals, such as the patient's health or positive image of self. A change in the patient's behavior may be likely to conflict with his or her current personal goals. The provider should draw attention to these discrepancies, demonstrating to the patient that there is a real need for change. For example, for a patient with diabetes who is not convinced of the importance of exercise or activities performance, the therapist can ask: What will happen in the next 3 months if things stay the same? What will happen over the next 3 months if the behavior changes and exercises and activities are introduced?

## SELF-EFFICACY DURING MOTIVATIONAL INTERVIEWING

Supporting self-efficacy is the last part of motivational interviewing (**Table 8.19**) and involves building confidence that change is possible.[75] The patients have to believe that they have the knowledge and skills or abilities to carry out the treatment plan. Self-efficacy is a patient's internal belief in him- or herself being able to carry out and succeed with a specific task. Patients believe that they have some control of the situation and can affect the outcome. The process of self-efficacy extends beyond motivational interviewing into all aspects of a patient's behavioral change, including goal setting, problem solving, and relapse management.[75] Self-efficacy enhances a patient's commitment toward achieving a goal.

## APPLYING MOTIVATIONAL INTERVIEWING TO REHABILITATION

Motivational interviewing can be used in rehabilitation by having the physical and occupational therapist select a target behavior and examine with the patient the positives and negatives of that behavior. Then, the therapist and the patient need to compare the positive and negative things related to the target behavior. Subsequently, the therapist can explore in a systematic way how much of a concern the negatives are for the patient. **Table 8.20** provides motivational interviewing questions to try with a patient's inability to stop smoking.

The next step for the therapist is to highlight the discrepancies between positives and negatives, giving the patient the opportunity to convince him- or herself that there is a need for change. In the past, the therapist had to convince the patient about the need for change and give advice and recommendations on how to change. The current trend with

| Table 8.19 | *Methods to Help Increase a Patient's Self-Efficacy*[75] |
|---|---|
| | Ensure adequate education and information on the particular patient's goal. |
| | Clarify the information. |
| | Offer realistic hope and express confidence in the patient's ability to succeed. |
| | Find role models with whom the patient can identify. |
| | Use persuasive communication and express confirmation that the patient can achieve the goal. |
| | Notice the patient's successful attempts at adherence, even if the attempts are short-lived. |
| | Praise ideas from the patient to solve problems. |
| | Continue to emphasize and support the responsibilities of the patient and provider to improve adherence and outcomes. |

motivational interviewing is to assist the patient to convince the therapist that he or she has a problem and needs help. For example, for a patient who recently had a heart attack and is still smoking, the therapist may ask: "What problems do you think are related to your smoking?" The provider should highlight specific aspects and ask for further details such as: "Give me an example of that"; "Tell me more about it"; "How is that a problem?"; "Does your smoking concern you much?"; or "What do you think are the major problems?"

Typically, there is a difference between acknowledging something is a problem and being concerned enough to do something about it. The same happens when a patient is

| Table 8.20 | *Questions to Explore a Patient's Concerns About Smoking Behavior*[1,75] |
|---|---|
| | How does this inability to stop smoking concern you? |
| | Why does this concern you? |
| | Look to the future. Is the good or not-so-good balance going to change? |

asked about his or her home exercise program (HEP). Asking about a patient's treatment adherence, activity level, and exercises at every visit communicates to the patient that these are important issues for the therapist (**Table 8.21**). As a result, the patient realizes that the HEP should be a concern for him- or herself also. This also shows the patient that his or her behavior will be monitored. The therapist's questions may raise the patient's concern about his or her accountability for the program. The questions can also increase the patient's desire to please the therapist.

The therapist's role is to prompt the patient to reflect back and, where necessary, clarify the nature of the problems that the patient perceives. This conveys to the patient that his or her ambivalence or indecisiveness is a normal part of human nature and not a personality defect. For example, the therapist may ask:

- What are the good things about not doing the exercises?

- What other activities do you like most instead of exercises?

- Are reading, doing crossword puzzles, playing cards, or watching television better activities for you?

- So, to summarize, what you have been saying is that there are other activities you can do at home instead of exercises.

- These activities have some benefits for you such as keeping your mind sharp. These activities are also costly for you because they do not require you to move your legs.

- What do you think the balance between costs and benefits is at the moment?

The therapist should be able to acknowledge the patient's difficulty of giving up a sedentary behavior:

- Yes, it is difficult for you to do the exercises because you have other activities you like.

- What do you think you might do in the next few days about starting a physical activity in your home?

| Table 8.21 | Questions to Raise Patients' Concerns About Their HEP |
| --- | --- |
| | So, there is a problem doing your exercises? Please tell me more about it. |
| | How much does this problem worry you? |
| | Why do you think the HEP is a concern for us? |

The therapist should encourage the patient's future contemplation about walking:

- So, at the moment you may find doing exercises while sitting down helpful, but what about the future? If you continue to sit without any movement, what do you think will happen? If you start walking in your home for 5 minutes daily, what do you think will happen?

- Your inactivity and loss of strength in your legs—are these a problem for you?

- Do you find it a problem that you have to use a walker all the time?

- How do you view yourself now that you cannot leave your house to walk without a walker?

- Do you think your life is working out as you would have hoped?

Patients who are motivated tend to agree with the therapist, accept the diagnosis, express a desire or need for help, and may appear distressed about their condition and follow advice. Patients who are unmotivated disagree with the therapist, refuse to accept the diagnosis, express no desire or need for help, do not appear distressed about their condition, and do not follow advice. In general, during motivational interviewing, the therapist may assume the following: (1) this patient ought to change; (2) this patient wants to change; (3) this patient's health is a prime motivating factor for change; and (4) if the patient does not decide to change, the behavioral change will not occur.[75] Other important factors about change are that patients are either motivated to change or not motivated. Patients are also motivated differently, and sometimes it may not be in the direction the therapist thinks it should be. In the walking exercise situation, the patient is motivated but does not agree with the physical or occupational therapist's goal choice. In this case, the therapist can consider a tough approach to convince the patient that he or she is an expert in the area and that the patient must follow the advice. The main emphasis is that the patient believes that change is possible and that they can make the necessary behavioral changes.

After asking the patient about adherence with intervention and/or disease prevention behaviors and exploring the patient's motivational beliefs, the next step for the therapist is to advise the patient about changes in the treatment program, such as increasing activity level or stopping tobacco use. This should be done in a clear and personalized manner that is appropriate for the patient's SCM stage. If the patient is in the precontemplation or contemplation phase, the therapist's general message would be that the patient should change to prevent present or future negative consequences and preserve current valued activities or exercises. For the previous example, the therapist may say: "As your physical therapist, I want you to know that doing your exercise program is very important for protecting your ability to walk with a walker from your bedroom to your living room or kitchen."

Using positive and negative costs may help tip the patient's motivational balance from inaction to action. The patient must believe that more is to be gained from adherence than nonadherence and from exercises than inactivity.

If the patient is in the preparation or the action stage, it is appropriate for the therapist to indicate the type of intervention, and also the frequency, duration, and intensity. At these stages, it is appropriate for the therapist to assist the patient with developing a plan of care that details how he or she can be more adherent with the HEP or other activities or how to start an activity that is enjoyable, convenient, and realistic for the patient's current physical condition and motivation. Developing the plan with the patient in a patient-centered plan of care will involve problem-solving about barriers to change. The barriers can be elicited by asking the patient to describe how the HEP will be followed and what problems the program might cause. Even if the intervention is not medically optimal, small changes that start with what the patient is comfortable doing now but can be gradually increased are more likely to be achieved. By achieving a small goal, the patient has initiated a positive change. After developing the plan of care with the patient, the patient can be asked to set a start date, to tell family and friends of the plan and solicit their support, and to make the necessary preparation for the intervention (such as buying comfortable shoes or having a friend assist him or her). The three-step process of asking, advising, and assisting the patient at each therapy visit can be effective to increase the patient's motivation and adherence with interventions.[75]

In physical therapy during rehabilitation, many patients lack motivation to continue the program.[65] As a result, they cancel appointments and are not able to meet physical therapy goals. Patient adherence to therapy requires motivation and decreased resistance. For physical and occupational therapists, a powerful method to handle a patient's resistance is *reflection*. The following is an example to counter resistance for a patient who keeps missing appointments in physical therapy:

*Physical therapist:* Tell me some of the reasons why you cancel your appointments frequently. (This is a request for information or elaboration of the reason and an attempt to identify a barrier for keeping appointments.)

*Patient:* Well, don't put it like that. It doesn't happen that frequently, only once or twice these last two weeks. (This minimizes the fact that the patient keeps canceling appointments.)

*Physical therapist:* So you don't feel it is often and that I might have exaggerated or used the wrong words? (This represents reflection and rolling with the resistance.)

*Patient:* Yeah!

*Physical therapist:* At least we agree on something! Maybe this is an area that is more complicated than just missing appointments. Would you like to discuss this another time? (Using humor helps to re-establish rapport, avoid confrontation, and re-establish the plan for treatment.)

It is important for the therapist to express in a succinct way what he or she observes. Reflection to handle resistance demands full attention to words, their meaning, and the emotional content.

Section

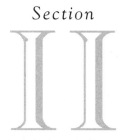

II

# Conclusions

## *Section II Summary*

This section discussed the effects of adherence in interventions and identified adherence barriers and various strategies related to the teaching and learning aspect of rehabilitation interventions. These adherence approaches were related to socioeconomic variables as well as cultural and homelessness factors. Communication issues when delivering patient education were discussed in detail for implementation of effective verbal, nonverbal, and written strategies. Issues and teaching strategies for health literacy and specific communication strategies for older adults with visual and hearing impairments were described. Section II concluded with detailed representations of behavioral modification variables that influence patient teaching and learning and lifestyle modifications in rehabilitation. The significance of the Stages of Change Model and examples of its use in health care and physical therapy also were identified. The value of motivational interviewing for increased patient adherence with rehabilitative interventions also was included.

## *Section II Case Study*

### Patient Education for a Patient with Low Health Literacy

Per the *APTA's Guide to Physical Therapist Practice*, the patient physical therapy diagnostic classification pattern is:[90]

Impaired motor function and sensory integrity associated with acute or chronic polyneuropathies

ICD-9-Cm Codes: 250.6 Diabetes with neurological manifestations

APTA's *Guide to Physical Therapist Practice* recommendations for patient-related instruction:[90]

Instruction, education, and training of patient and caregiver regarding:

- Current condition (pathology/pathophysiology, impairments, functional limitations, or disabilities)

- Enhancement of performance

- Health, wellness, and fitness programs

- Plan of care

- Risk factors (pathology/pathophysiology, impairments, functional limitations, or disabilities)

- Transitions across settings

- Transitions to new roles

## *Patient Description*

Patient is a 43-year-old man with a medical diagnosis of polyneuropathy secondary to diabetes mellitus. He has a 12-year history of impaired glucose tolerance. Medically, he also has HTN. He complains of severe pain and sensations of "pins and needles" in his right ankle and foot. The patient works for a landscape company. Patient is fluent in Spanish and speaks no English. He smokes and uses alcohol regularly. He is more than 50 pounds overweight. He has pain in his right foot and leg and walks holding onto his son's arm. His son is 20 years old and translates for his father. He told the physical therapist that his father cannot go to work anymore, is sad and tired all the time, smokes, and lies in bed all day. Almost 3 weeks ago, he took his father to the emergency room because he was dizzy and vomiting. In the emergency room, the doctor told him his sugar was very high. He was in the hospital for 3 days and sent home with a prescription for medications and physical therapy. The medications have been helping him but not enough to get rid of his pain in his right foot and leg or get rid of tiredness.

The emergency room report described that the patient had double vision, severe pain in the lower back, and pain in the chest and stomach. His blood glucose level was 300 mg/dl. His blood pressure was 190/115. His complete blood count and lipid panel were abnormal. EMG and nerve conduction studies performed in the hospital showed focal neuropathy. During the hospital stay the patient's blood glucose level was stabilized. The neuropathy started to improve but his main problem now is tarsal tunnel entrapment in his right foot. At discharge from the hospital, the patient received information about diabetes and the importance of being physically active.

In physical therapy, the patient presents with a burning type of pain and paresthesia of his right foot and lower leg. He also has bilateral weakness of his lower extremities, but it is worse on the right. He has no open lesions on either foot and has intact protective sensation for both feet. His reflexes are normal and pedal pulses are palpable. He has equinus gait on the right. His blood pressure is 150/95. The patient's son stated his father took his medications in the morning.

*Patient Education Handouts About the Importance of Being Physically Active (Given to This Patient at Discharge from Hospital): English Version*[91]

## BE PHYSICALLY ACTIVE

Physical activity is good for your diabetes. Walking, swimming, dancing, riding a bicycle, playing baseball, and bowling are all good ways to be active. You even can exercise when you clean house or work in your garden. Physical activity is especially good for people with diabetes because it:

- Helps keep weight down

- Helps insulin work better to lower blood glucose

- Is good for your heart and lungs

- Gives you more energy

Before you begin exercising, talk with your doctor. Your doctor may check your heart and your feet to be sure you have no special problems. If you have high blood pressure or eye problems, some exercises like weightlifting may not be safe. Your health care team can help you find safe exercises.

Try to be active almost every day for a total of about 30 minutes. If you haven't been very active lately, begin slowly. Start with 5 to 10 minutes, and then add more time. Exercise for 10 minutes, three times a day.

If your blood glucose is less than 100 to 120, have a snack before you exercise. Being active helps you feel better. When you exercise, carry glucose tablets or a carbohydrate snack with you in case you get hypoglycemia. Wear or carry an identification tag or card saying that you have diabetes.

### ACTION STEPS...if you use insulin:

- See your doctor before starting a physical activity program.

- Check your blood glucose before, during, and after exercising. Don't exercise when your blood glucose is over 240 or if you have ketones in your urine.

- Don't exercise right before you go to sleep because it could cause hypoglycemia during the night.

### ACTION STEPS...if you do not use insulin:

- See your doctor before starting a physical activity program.

*Patient Education Handouts About the Importance of Being Physically Active
(Given to This Patient at Discharge from Hospital): Spanish Version*[91]

## REALICE ACTIVIDAD FÍSICA CON REGULARIDAD

La actividad física es buena para las personas con diabetes. Caminar, nadar, bailar, andar en bicicleta, jugar béisbol y boliche son excelentes formas de realizar actividad física. Usted realiza actividad física incluso cuando limpia la casa o trabaja en el jardín. La actividad física es particularmente beneficiosa para las personas con diabetes porque:

- Ayuda a mantener el peso adecuado (bajo)

- Ayuda a que la insulina funcione para mejor bajar la glucosa en la sangre

- Es buena para el corazón y los pulmones

- Le da más energía

Antes de comenzar a hacer ejercicio, hable con su médico. Es posible que le examine el corazón y los pies para asegurar que usted no tenga problemas especiales. Si usted tiene la presión arterial alta o si tiene problemas de los ojos, algunos ejercicios como levantamiento de pesas pueden ser peligrosos. Su equipo de asistencia médica le ayudará a encontrar ejercicios que no causen peligro.

Trate de realizar actividad física casi todos los días por más o menos 30 minutos. Si últimamente no ha realizado mucha actividad física, comience lentamente. Empiece con 5 a 10 minutos y vaya aumentando el tiempo. Haga ejercicio por 10 minutos tres veces al día.

Si su nivel de glucosa en la sangre es menor de 100 a 120, coma algo ligero antes de hacer ejercicio.

### ACCIONES A SEGUIR...si usa insulina:

- Consulte con su médico antes de comenzar cualquier programa de actividad física.

- Mídase el nivel de glucosa en la sangre antes, durante y después de hacer ejercicio. No haga ejercicio si el nivel es mayor de 240, o si tiene cetonas en la orina. No haga ejercicio inmediatamente antes de irse a dormir porque esto podría causar hipoglucemia durante la noche. La diabetes puede comenzar a cualquier edad.

- Cuando haga ejercicio, lleve tabletas de glucosa o algo ligero con carbohidratos que puede utilizar en caso de que le dé hipoglucemia (nivel bajo de glucosa en la sangre). Lleve siempre una placa o carné de identificación que indique que usted tiene diabetes.

### ACCIONES A SEGUIR...si no usa insulina:

- Consulte con su médico antes de comenzar cualquier programa de actividad física.

*Guidelines for Writing Easy-to-Read Materials About Being Physically Active for the Above Patient*

1. Know your target audience.

2. Determine objectives and outcomes. (What do you want your target audience to learn?)

3. Keep within a range of about a fourth- to sixth-grade reading level.

4. Focus on a few key concepts.

5. Use the "you" attitude. Personalization helps the reader understand what he or she is supposed to do.

6. Structure the material logically. Some users prefer step-by-step instructions. Others may prefer concepts arranged from the general to the specific (because they are easier to understand).

7. Emphasize the benefits of adopting the desired behavior.

8. Do not make assumptions about people who read at a low level. Maintain an adult perspective.

9. Find alternatives for complex words, medical jargon, abbreviations, and acronyms.

10. Keep most sentences short. Use varied sentence length to make them interesting, but keep sentences simple.

11. Use the active voice and vivid verbs.

12. Use colors that are appealing to your target audience. Beware that some people cannot tell red from green.

13. Use pictures and photos with concise captions. Keep captions close to graphics.

14. Avoid graphs and charts unless they actually help understanding.

15. Balance the use of text, graphics, and clear or "white" space.

16. Avoid words or sentences in all capital letters.

17. Avoid italics.

18. Use bolded subheadings to separate and highlight document sections.

19. When possible, use graphics or spell out fractions and percentages.

20. Recommend Web sites with easy-to-read health materials (e.g., Food and Drug Administration, National Institute of Diabetes and Digestive and Kidney Diseases, National Institute on Alcohol Abuse and Alcoholism).

*Section II References*

1. Miller NH, Hill M, Kottke T, et al. The multilevel of compliance challenge: recommendations for a call to action. *Circ.* 1997;95:1085–1090.
2. Falvo DR. *Effective Patient Education: A Guide to Increased Compliance.* Sudbury, MA: Jones and Bartlett; 2004.
3. Marhefka S, Tepper VJ, Farley JJ, et al. Brief report: assessing adherence to pediatric antiretroviral regimens using the 24-hour recall interview. *J Pediatr Psychol.* 2006;31(9):989–994.
4. Delamater AM. Improving patient adherence. *Clin Diabetes.* 2006;24(2):71–77.
5. Chen CY, Neufeld PS, Feely CA, et al. Factors influencing compliance with home exercise programs among patients with upper-extremity impairment. *Am J Occup Ther.* 1999;53: 171–180.
6. Nagy VT, Wolfe GR. Cognitive predictors of compliance in chronic disease patients. *Med Care.* 1984;22:912–921.
7. Swain MA, Steckel SB. Influencing adherence among hypertensives. *Res Nurs Health.* 1981;4:213–222.
8. Fishman T. The 90-Second Intervention: a patient compliance mediated technique to improve and control hypertension. *Public Health Rep.* 1995;110(2):173–178.
9. Tappen RM, Roach KE, Applegate EB, et al. Effect of a combined walking and conversation intervention on functional mobility of nursing home residents with Alzheimer disease. *Alzheimer Dis Assoc Disord.* 2000;14(40):196–201.
10. Whitley HP, Fermo JD, Ragucci K, et al. Assessment of patient knowledge of diabetic goals, self-reported medication adherence, and goal attainment. *Pharm Practice.* 2006;4(4):183–190.
11. Fraser S, Rodgers, WM, Murray TC, et al. The enduring impact of social factors on exercise tolerance in men attending cardiac rehabilitation. *J Cardiopul Rehab Prev.* 2007;27(2):92–96.
12. Beverly EA, Wray LA. The role of collective efficacy in exercise adherence: a qualitative study of spousal support and Type 2 diabetes management. *Health Educ Res.* 2008;23(4):1–32.
13. Shinn M, Weitzman BC, Stojanovic D, et al. Predictors of homelessness among families in New York City: from shelter request to housing stability. *Am J Public Health.* 1998;88(11): 1651–1656.
14. National Coalition for the Homeless. How Many People Experience Homelessness? NCH Fact Sheet #2. Available at: http://www.nationalhomeless.org/publications/facts.html. Accessed November 2008.
15. National Coalition for the Homeless. Who Is Homeless? NCH Fact Sheet #3. Available at: http://www.nationalhomeless.org/publications/facts.html. Accessed November 2008.
16. National Coalition for Homeless Veterans. Facts and Media: Background and Statistics. Available at: http://www.nchv.org/background.cfm. Accessed November 2008.
17. Hwang SW. Homelessness and health. *Can Med Assoc J.* 2001;164(2):229–233.
18. McElroy PD, Southwick KL, Fortenberry ER, et al. Outbreak of tuberculosis among homeless persons coinfected with Human Immunodeficiency Virus. *Clin Infect Dis.* 2003;36:1305–1312.
19. Moss AR, Hahn JA, Perry S, et al. Adherence to highly active antiretroviral therapy in the homeless population in San Francisco: a prospective study. *Clin Infect Dis.* 2004;39:1190–1198.
20. Roter DL, Hall JA, Kern DE, et al. Improving physicians' interviewing skills and reducing patients' emotional distress: a randomized clinical trial. *Arch of Intern Med.* 1995;155: 1877–1884.

21. Spector RE. *Cultural Diversity in Health and Illness*. 8th ed. Upper Saddle River, NJ: Prentice Hall Health; 2000.

22. Osborne H. *Health Literacy from A to Z: Practical Ways to Communicate Your Health Message*. Sudbury, MA: Jones and Bartlett; 2005.

23. Padilla R, Brown K. Culture and patient education: challenges and opportunities. *J Phys Ther Ed*. 1999;13(2):1–14.

24. Maguire, P. Key communication skills and how to acquire them. *BMJ*. 2002; 325:697–700.

25. Stafford L, Canary DJ. Equity and interdependence as predictors of relational maintenance strategies.*J Fam Commun*. 2006;6(4):227–254.

26. Dreeben O. *Introduction to Physical Therapy for Physical Therapist Assistants*. Sudbury, MA: Jones and Bartlett; 2007.

27. Beck RS, Daughtridge R, Sloane PD. Physician-patient communication in the primary care office: a systematic review. *J Am Board Fam Pract*. 2002;15(1):25–38.

28. Hynes P, Kissoon N, Hamielec C, et al. Dealing with aggressive behavior within the health care team: a leadership challenge. *J Crit Care*. 2002;21(2):224–227.

29. Pencheon D. Matching demand and supply fairly and efficiently. *BMJ*. 1998;316:1665–1667.

30. Berlin RE (ed). *Health Communication in Practice: A Case Study Approach*. Erlbaum, NJ: Mahwah; 2005.

31. Office of Disease Prevention and Health Promotion, U.S. Department of Health and Human Services. Healthy People 2010. Available at: http://www.healthypeople.gov. Accessed November 2008.

32. Krueger KP, Felkey BG, Berger BA. Improving adherence and persistence: a review and assessment of interventions and description of steps toward a national adherence initiative. *J Am Pharm Assoc*. 2003;43:668–679.

33. Scott TL, Gazmararian JA, Williams MV, et al. Health literacy and preventive health care use among Medicare enrollees in a managed care organization. *Med Care*. 2003;40(5):395–404.

34. Smith CR, Smith CA. Patient education information: readability of prosthetic publications. *J Prosthet Orthot*. 1994;6(4):113–124. Available at: http://www.oandp.org/jpo/library/1994_04_113.asp. Accessed December 2007.

35. Kessels RPC. Patients' memory for medical information. *J Royal Soc Med*. 2003;96:219–222.

36. Miles SB, Stipek D. Contemporaneous and longitudinal associations between social behavior and literacy achievement in a sample of low income elementary school children. *Child Dev*. 2006;77:103–117.

37. Marcus EN. The silent epidemic: the health effects of illiteracy. *N Engl J Med*. 2006;355(4):339–341.

38. National Assessment of Adult Literacy 2003. A Nationally Representative and Continuing Assessment of English Language Literacy Skills of American Adults. Available at: http://nces.ed.gov/naal/multimedia.asp. Accessed August 2008.

39. Ferguson T. A Guided Tour of Self-Help Cyberspace. *Harvard Medical School*. Available at: http://odphp.osophs.dhhs.gov. Accessed December 2007.

40. Kaplan SH, Greenfield S, Gandek B, et al. Characteristics of physicians with participatory decision-making styles. *Ann Intern Med*. 1996;124:497–504.

41. Runge C, Lecheler J, Horn M, et al. Outcomes of a Web-based patient education program for asthmatic children and adolescents. *Chest*. 2006;129:581–593.

42. Spadero DC. Assessing readability of patient information materials. *Pediatr Nurs*. 1983;9(4):274–278.

43. Hester EJ, Benitez-McCrary M. (2006). Health literacy: research directions for speech-language pathology and audiology. *ASHA Leader*. 2006;11(17):33–34.

44. McLaughlin GH. SMOG grading: a new readability formula. *J Reading*. 1969;12:639–646.

45. Hochhauser M. (2004). Summary of presentation by Mark Hochhauser (appearing via conference call). GLB Interagency Meeting on the ANPR on Privacy Notices—January 29, 2004. Federal Trade Commission. Available at: http://www.ftc.gov. Accessed October 2007.

46. Medline Plus. How to Write Easy-to-Read Health Materials. Available at: http://www.nlm.nih.gov/medlineplus/etr.html. Accessed August 2008.

47. Center for Medicare Education. Writing Easy-to-Read Materials. Available at: http://www.medicareed.org/PublicationFiles/V1N2.pdf. Accessed August 2008.

48. Class Action. Interactive Classroom Materials for Introductory Astronomy. Available at: http://astro.unl.edu/classaction. Accessed August 2008.

49. Reo JA, Mercer VS. Effects of live, videotaped, or written instruction on learning an upper-extremity exercise program. *Phys Ther*. 2004;84(7):622–633.

50. American Foundation for the Blind. Blindness Statistics. Available at: http://www.afb.org. Accessed September 2007.

51. Cienkowski KM. Auditory aging: a look at hearing loss in older adults. *Hearing Loss*. 2003; 24(3):12–15.

52. Gray SL, Mahoney JE, Blough DK. Medication adherence in elderly patients receiving home health services following hospital discharge. *Ann Pharm*. 2001;35(5):539–545.

53. Lorish C. Facilitating behavior change: strategies for education and practice. *J Phys Ther Ed*. 1999;13(2):1–11. Available at: http://findarticles.com. Accessed July 2008.

54. Martin PC, Fell DW. Beyond treatment: patient education for health promotion and disease prevention. *J Phys Ther Ed*. 1999;13(2):1–12.

55. Bassett SF. The assessment of patient adherence to physiotherapy rehabilitation. *NZ J Physiother*. 2003;31(2):60–66.

56. Forkan R, Pumper B, Smyth N, et al. Exercise adherence following physical therapy intervention in older adults with impaired balance. *Phys Ther*. 2006;86(3):401–410.

57. Bassett SF, Prapavessis H. Home-based physical therapy intervention with adherence-enhancing strategies versus clinic-based management for patients with ankle sprains. *Phys Ther*. 2007; 87(9):1–12.

58. Luszczynska A, Sutton S. Physical activity after cardiac rehabilitation: evidence that different types of self-efficacy are important in maintainers and relapsers. *Rehab Psych*. 2006; 51(4): 314–321.

59. Dunbar-Jacob J, Sereika S, Burke LE, et al. Can poor adherence be improved? *Ann Behav Med*. 1995;17:1–2.

60. Poirier P, Turbide G, Bourdages J, et al. Predictors of compliance with medical recommendations regarding pharmacological and nonpharmacological approaches in patient with cardiovascular disease. *Clin Invest Med*. 2006;29(2):1–12.

61. Mayoux-Benhamou MA, Roux C, Perraud A, et al. Predictors of compliance with a home-based exercise program added to usual medical care in preventing postmenopausal osteoporosis: an 18-month prospective study. *Osteoporosis Int*. 2005;16(3):325–331.

62. Mori DL, Sogg S, Guarino P, et al. Predictors of exercise compliance in individuals with Gulf War veterans' illnesses: Department of Veterans Affairs Cooperative Study 470. *Military Med*. 2006;171(9):917–923.

63. Alexandre NMC, Nordin M, Hiebert R, et al. Predictors of compliance with short-term treatment among patients with back pain. *Rev Panam Salud Publica*. 2002;12(2):86–94.

64. Searle A, Norman P, Harrad R, et al. Psychosocial and clinical determinants of compliance with occlusion therapy for amblyopic children. *Eye*. 2002;16(2):150–155.

65. Donohoe G, Owens N, O'Donnell C, et al. Predictors of compliance with neuroleptic medication among inpatients with schizophrenia: a discriminant function analysis. *Eur Psychiatry*. 2001;16(5):293–308.

66. Nielsen B, Nielsen AS, Wraae O. Factors associated with compliance of alcoholics in outpatient treatment. *J Nerv Ment Dis*. 2000;188(2):101–107.

67. Lewthwaite R. Motivational considerations in physical activity involvement. *Phys Ther*. 1990;70(12):808–819.

68. Abella R, Heslin R. Health, locus of control, values, and the behavior of family and friends—an integrated approach to understanding preventive health behavior. *Basic Appl Soc Psychol*. 1984;5:283–294.

69. Kristiansen CM. A 2-value model of preventive health behavior. *Basic Appl Soc Psychol*. 1986;7:173–183.

70. Kripalani S, Yao X, Haynes B. Interventions to enhance medication adherence in chronic medical conditions: a systematic review. *Arch Intern Med*. 2007;167(6):540–549.

71. O'Donohue WT, Byrd MR, Cummings NA, Henderson DA (eds). *Behavioral Integrative Care: Treatments That Work in the Primary Care Setting*. New York: Routledge; 2005.

72. Schneider A, Körner T, Mehring M, et al. Impact of age, health locus of control and psychological co-morbidity on patients' preferences for shared decision making in general practice. *Patient Ed Counsel*. 2006;61(2):292–298.

73. Taplin SH, Barlow WE, Ludman E, et al. Testing reminder and motivational telephone calls to increase screening mammography: a randomized study. *J Natl Cancer Inst*. 2000;92(3):233–242.

74. Maclean N, Pound P, Wolfe C, et al. The concept of patient motivation: a qualitative analysis of stroke professionals' attitudes. *Stroke*. 2002;33:444–448.

75. Miller WH, Rollnick S. *Motivational Interviewing: Preparing People for Change*. 2nd ed. New York: Guilford Press; 2002.

76. Prochaska JO, DiClemente CC, Norcross JC. In search of how people change: applications to addictive behaviors. *Am Psychol*. 1992;47:1102–1114.

77. Prochaska JO, Norcross JC, DiClemente CC. *Changing for Good*. New York: William Morrow; 1994.

78. Maiman LA, Becker MR. The Health Belief Model: origins and correlates in psychological theory. *Health Ed Monogr*. 1974;2:336–353.

79. Bandura A. *Social Foundations of Thought and Action: A Social Cognitive Theory*. Englewood Cliffs, NJ: Prentice Hall; 1986.

80. Shirazi KK, Wallace LM, Niknami S, et al. A home-based, Transtheoretical Change Model designed strength training intervention to increase exercise to prevent osteoporosis in Iranian women aged 40–65 years: a randomized controlled trial. *Health Educ Res*. 2007;22(3):305–317.

81. Gorely T, Bruce DA. 6-month investigation of exercise adoption from the contemplation stage of the transtheoretical model. *Psychol Sport Exerc*. 2000;1:89–101.

82. Plotlikoff RC, Hotz SB, Birkett NJ, et al. Exercise and transtheoretical model: a longitudinal test of a population sample. *Prev Med*. 2001;33:441–452.

83. Jordan PG, Nigg CR, Norman GJ, et al. Does the transtheoretical model need an attitude adjustment? Integrating attitude with decisional balance as predictor of stage of change for exercise. *Psychol Sport Exerc*. 2002;3:65–83.

84. Schreiner LO. Application of the transtheoretical model to clinical exercise prescription. *Cardiopul Phys Ther J.* 2000;12:1–5.

85. Pizzari T, Taylor, NT, McBurney H, et al. Adherence to anterior cruciate ligament rehabilitation: a qualitative analysis. *J Sport Rehabil.* 2002;11(2):90–102.

86. Pearson L, Jones G. Emotional effects of sports injuries: implications for physiotherapists. *Physiother.* 1992;78:762–770.

87. Austin MM. *Yes, You Can! Helping Patients Change Behavior.* American Overseas Dietetic Association Conference—March 23, 2006. Available at: MAustinRD@aol.com. Accessed December 2008.

88. Astolfi H, Evans, M. Motivational interviewing. *GP Drug Alcohol Supp.* 1997;4:1–4.

89. Bassett SF. The assessment of patient adherence to physiotherapy rehabilitation. *NZ J Physiother.* 2003;31(2):60–66.

90. American Physical Therapy Association. *Guide to Physical Therapist Practice.* 2nd ed. Alexandria, VA: APTA; 2001.

91. National Diabetes Information Clearinghouse, National Institute of Diabetes and Digestive and Kidney Diseases, National Institutes of Health. Taking Care of Your Diabetes Every Day: Be Physically Active. Available at: http://diabetes.niddk.nih.gov/dm/pubs/type1and2. Accessed November 2007.

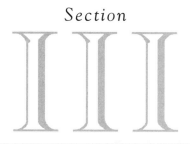

# TEACHING AND LEARNING THEORIES: APPLICATIONS TO PATIENT EDUCATION

Section III of this book, "Teaching and Learning Theories: Applications to Patient Education," describes basic learning theories and their significance in patient teaching and learning. Behaviorism, cognitivism, constructivism, and other related instructional designs and learning preferences are introduced in connection to patient education in physical and occupational rehabilitation. An andragogical model of instruction and elements of adult learning are also presented. Section III concludes with methods for applying educational strategies to an individual's stages of cognitive and psychosocial development. Section III is divided into the following four chapters:

# MAIN TEACHING AND LEARNING THEORIES AND PATIENT EDUCATION

## Objectives

After completing Chapter 9, the reader will be able to:

- Identify the importance of teaching and learning theories in physical and occupational rehabilitation.

- Describe basic teaching and learning principles and their application to rehabilitation.

- Identify motivational strategies and factors that promote learning and reasoning.

- List the significance of the three basic learning theories: behaviorism, cognitivism, and constructivism.

- Discuss examples of learning activities in rehabilitation considering the three basic learning theories.

- Compare and contrast behaviorism and constructivism when related to patient teaching and learning.

- Determine the applications of Social Cognitive Theory (SCT) to patient teaching and learning.

- Determine the applications of Social Learning Theory (SLT) to patient teaching and learning.

# The Significance of Instructional Design in Patient Education

Most physical therapists, occupational therapists, and physical and occupational therapist assistants would agree that when they went to school, they never anticipated becoming teachers in their clinic-based professions and having to know specific instructional designs. However, these health care providers would readily admit that most of their time as clinicians is spent teaching patients rehabilitation skills, information about pathological conditions, and lifestyle changes. Therapists may wonder whether their profession requires them to use instructional design and prescribe a sequence of learning events to help patients reach their rehabilitation goals and outcomes during patient education. The answer is definitely "yes." As rehabilitation providers, physical and occupational therapists must understand the importance of learning theories, learning events and sequences, and methods so they can incorporate them into patients' teaching and learning experiences. Additionally, establishing therapeutic relationships with patients in a patient-centered care approach promotes a relationship for therapists and patients to experience reciprocal teaching and learning. For the most part, effective teaching and learning can take place only through therapists' continuous reflection, scholarship, and development of their instructional abilities.

Patient teaching and learning is a central skill in physical and occupational therapy. The *Guide to Physical Therapist Practice*[1] and the *Occupational Therapy Practice Framework: Domain and Process*[2] strongly emphasize the teaching role of physical and occupational therapists and assistants in areas of patient-related instruction, consultation, education, and patient management. The American Physical Therapy Association (APTA) indicates in the guide that patient-related instruction promotes and optimizes physical therapy services and should be applied by physical therapists in every setting.[1] The American Occupational Therapy Association (AOTA) also incorporates patient and client instruction in each occupational therapy process to communicate goals and objectives, the nature of the disorder or injury, etiology, prognosis and treatment, self-care, and ways to prevent recurrent health problems.[2] In physical therapy rehabilitation, clinical teaching and learning relates to impairments, functional limitations or disabilities, appropriate performance, job or place modifications, risk factors, and needs for health, wellness, and fitness programs. Furthermore, physical and occupational rehabilitation uses teaching and learning to influence behavior and produce changes in patients'/clients' knowledge, attitudes, and skills to improve and maintain health.

Although some health care providers may not consider teaching and learning formal processes, patient education should be a systematic, sequential, logical planned teaching approach.[3] Some providers also equate teaching with establishing only therapeutic relationships with the patient without using formal teaching methods. Furthermore, some clinicians believe that only telling patients what to do means they are teaching them.[3] Physical therapist educators do not agree with this simple concept because patient teaching and learning is a much more complex procedure.[4] When receiving instruction, the expected outcome is for a change to occur in what the patient knows, in how they perform, and in his or her attitudes, beliefs, or behaviors. Behavioral change is the major goal of patient education, and implicitly of teaching and learning. Facilitating patient learning requires an effective approach to teaching characterized by actively involving the learner in the educational process.[5,6]

Patient instruction is a participatory, shared approach of teaching and learning. Incorporating patient-centered care as a collaborative method is considered one of the most important parts of patient education.[7–14] In the patient-centered care approach, the key to effective teaching is to develop an equal partnership that enables patients (as well as families, caregivers, and partners) to self-manage health care problems and make decisions with skill and confidence. Another aspect is to be able to educate patients regarding how to be in command of their health. In patient teaching and learning, the main responsibility of the health care provider is to assist patients in achieving and maintaining health by:

- Sharing knowledge
- Helping them with practical problems of carrying out instructions
- Supporting them as they integrate new knowledge and skills

The first step in teaching and learning is to ensure that the health care instructions are understandable and that the instructions match patients' goals.[14] It is important to remember that patients cannot follow recommendations they do not understand, and they will not follow recommendations they do not agree with. The next step is to make sure patients are included in health teaching as partners rather than simply as passive recipients.[14] By using teaching strategies that are interactive and that allow patients participation as equals, the provider can help promote compliance.

The third step in patient instruction is to view patient teaching as a process that requires a strong interpersonal relationship with the patient and his or her family (partner, caregiver).[14] Effective rehab educators need first to evaluate patient's interventional needs as well as educational needs. After that, a teaching plan must be created including the patient's needs and goals and the intended outcomes.[14] The teaching and learning process in physical and occupational therapy must be based, similar to nursing, on a structured progression that may include the following variables: evaluation of each patient's learning needs, style, and readiness; establishment of a patient-centered teaching plan based on patient's/therapist's goals and anticipated outcomes; utilization of patient-specific instructional methods; and evaluation of the patient's outcomes (**Table 9.1**).[14]

# *Principles of Teaching and Learning Applied to Physical and Occupational Rehabilitation*

When applied to physical and occupational therapy, teaching and learning represent two inseparable processes that work well together. At any given moment, the patient, the

| Table 9.1 | **Variables of Effective Teaching and Learning[14]** |
| --- | --- |
| | Detailed examination and evaluation of the patient's learning needs, readiness to learn, and learning style. |
| | Development of a patient-centered teaching plan of care based on patient's/therapist's goals and anticipated outcomes. |
| | Utilization of specific instructional methods and tools during the teaching process that meet the patient's individual needs. |
| | Evaluation of the patient's outcomes related to interventions as well as changes in the patient's knowledge, attitudes, and skills. |

rehabilitation provider, or the patient's family member can be the learner or the teacher. Typically, three conditions are required for teaching and learning to occur:[3]

1. The therapist should understand the topics very deeply, have passion for the topics, and continually seek new knowledge in order to reflect on new experiences.

2. The therapist should know his or her patients very well in order to be able to effectively capture their curiosity and interest and impart information to them.

3. The therapist should be acquainted with various educational techniques to facilitate learning for diverse groups of patients.

## TEACHING AND LEARNING

Teaching and learning are multifaceted events involving several actions. Teaching can be described as a complex process that includes facilitation of learning and providing direct instruction.[3–6] Teaching also involves a number of procedures (**Table 9.2**) that help the learner to acquire new or improve skills, knowledge, and attitudes. Learning is also a complicated course of action that incorporates cognitive and neural processes of acquiring knowledge, skills, and behaviors (**Table 9.3**).

# Learning and Motivation in Patient and Health Education

In patient and health education, physical and occupational therapists and assistants become teachers of their patients, clients, families, caregivers, and communities. However, being able to teach is totally dependent on being able to motivate the learners. In the classroom

| Table 9.2 |
| --- |

### *Actions During Teaching in Rehabilitation*[3–6]

The therapist must be able to facilitate patient's learning by providing direct and clear instruction.

The therapist must arrange conditions to assist patient's learning (such as planning the lesson, structuring the material, and/or organizing the physical environment for patient's comfort).

The therapist must modify the teaching process based on a given set of conditions (such as for patients with disabilities).

The therapist must use teaching-learning situations that systematically assist the patient to acquire new or improve knowledge, skills, and attitudes.

| Table 9.3 |
| --- |

### *Actions During Learning in Rehabilitation*[3–6,15]

Patient's learning represents a cognitive process of acquiring knowledge and/or skill.

Patient's learning is the acquisition and/or development of specific behaviors.

Patient's learning means a change in the neural function as a result of teaching experience.

Patient's learning requires interpretation of information.

Patient's learning involves permanent changes of cognitive and behavioral functions.

Patient's learning can be related to prior experience(s).

Patient's learning entails practice of knowledge, skill, and/or behavior.

Patient's learning can include the following progression: "motivation, apprehension, acquisition, retention, recall, generalization, performance, and feedback."[15(p.87)] setting, many students seem very excited about learning, but many need or expect their instructors to inspire, challenge, and stimulate them. Students' motivation also depends on the teacher's ability to maintain interest during the learning process. In general, motivating students in the classroom is a difficult task for the teacher. Motivating students in health care and specifically in rehabilitation is even more difficult considering the physiological and psychological challenges experienced by the patient or client. Learning specific motivational strategies applied in the classroom can help rehabilitation providers in patient education.

Many factors affect learners' motivation to be trained and be successful. These factors may include: (1) interest in the subject matter, (2) general desire to learn and accomplish a task, (3) level of self-confidence and self-esteem, (4) the learner's perception of the usefulness of the topic, and (5) the learner's patience and persistence in acquiring the needed information.[6] Strategies used to promote learning and motivation to learn consist of the following: building upon the learner's existing needs or goals, encouraging the learner to become an active participant in learning, and incorporating specific instructional behaviors that motivate the learner.[6] During patient education, therapists can influence patients' teaching and learning behaviors and, as a result, increase patients' enthusiasm for learning. Basic instructional methods could enhance patients' motivation for learning. These methods may include: (1) the therapist holding high but realistic expectations for the patient's learning, (2) the therapist helping the patient set achievable learning goals for him- or herself, (3) the therapist facilitating the patient's abilities to acquire the necessary information, and (4) the therapist being enthusiastic about the subject matter.[6]

## APPLICATION OF MOTIVATIONAL STRATEGIES TO PATIENT TEACHING AND LEARNING

During classroom teaching, teachers must complete the following tasks to help students learn: structure the course to motivate students, respond to students' work by giving them quick feedback (and rewarding success), and avoid demeaning comments. During teaching, the most critical concepts of the subject matter must be emphasized continuously; for example, in patient education in physical and occupational rehabilitation, instructing the learner about safety is a critical concept. Safety is important to successful rehabilitation outcomes. As a practical example, when educating a patient about how to use crutches on stairs, the therapist has to teach him or her not to lean on the crutches and ask the patient to bend the injured limb, allowing the other leg to bear his or her weight. Additionally, critical safety concepts should be reiterated constantly, and every meeting with the patient should include questioning about these concepts. Additionally, the therapist also can use visual aids to explain difficult or abstract concepts. Many students in the classroom and patients in clinical settings are visual learners. Diagrams, flowcharts, and pictures are much more valuable than words written in a text.

Teaching in a logical manner and helping the learner to study and retain new information is another strategy for motivating the patient. Having the learner use deductive reasoning also is helpful. Deductive reasoning, also called critical thinking, encourages the learner to discover the correct answer to a question he or she may not have been anticipating. With patients, this means to apply a general idea to a specific example. Deductive reasoning permits the patient, as the learner, to arrive at the logical answer. For example, using deductions, the patient can reason why he or she should first step with the involved limb instead of the uninvolved limb. This form is more helpful than inductive reasoning, which combines pieces of unrelated information to develop a general idea.

Deduction is a more fundamental thinking skill than induction. Good reasoning is also more important than fallacies or inaccurate ideas. For example, it would be totally wrong to teach a patient how to step incorrectly first, then teach how to step correctly. Teaching a correct method of performing a skill first and then an incorrect one later allows the material to be better understood. An understanding of an accurate solution to a problem will enable patients, in most cases, to recognize faulty answers even if they have never formally learned to identify them.

Another method to increase motivation is to reinforce the newly presented material with hands-on activities. In rehabilitation, most patient teaching takes place using demonstrations and activities. Also, learners need to be encouraged to link the new material with the already learned material. For example, in outpatient settings, the easiest way for the therapist to connect new material with information the patient has already learned is to relate the new exercises/activities with the patient's day-to-day actions and life experiences outside the clinic.

Additionally, the terminology used when instructing the learners is very important, especially in the beginning of the learning process. When introducing a new topic, the teacher should identify new and confusing terms and use alternative terminology if necessary. In rehabilitation, similar to health care, therapists must be careful not to use medical terminology with patients or clients. Layman's terminology is the standard of practice for all health care encounters with the patient, family, and caregivers.

Another element that increases patients' motivation is the relationship between the teacher and the learner. Teachers should always treat learners with respect. Patronizing behaviors or "drill sergeant" strategies do not work well in the classroom and should never be used in clinical settings. Ethical and legal principles of health care require that health care providers show respect and treat patients with dignity. In the classroom, the practice of treating students with dignity produces greater efforts in learning. Learners always need to be held to a high level of performance to be successful in the learning process.

To enhance the learner's motivation, it is important to consider that learning is also an addition of skills and knowledge that results in increased mental activity and behavioral change. As an active process on the part of the learner, learning can be a discovery of meaning and a consequence of experience.[16] As a result, learning is activated and controlled by the learner. For example, in rehabilitation, a patient's sociocultural norms, traditions, and values determine the importance of health topics and his or her preference for specific learning approaches. The therapist's role is to facilitate the learning process by motivating the learner. The learner can also be motivated by environmental factors, motivational praise, internal reinforcement, readiness to learn, and effective organization of the material (**Table 9.4**).

| Table 9.4 | *Motivational Factors Influencing Patient Teaching and Learning*[6,15,17] |
|---|---|

The environment can be used to focus the learner's attention on the topic that needs to be learned. Patient educators who create a warm and accepting atmosphere can promote persistent effort and favorable attitudes toward learning. This strategy applies successfully to adults and children. Visual aids such as booklets, posters, or practice equipment can be used in rehabilitation settings, increasing the patient's motivation, attention, and curiosity.

The use of incentives in teaching and learning (especially in health care) is extremely important because it increases learner satisfaction. An example of incentives includes praise from the instructor. The rehabilitation provider can determine an incentive that is likely to motivate the patient at a particular time. In learning, self-motivation does not work without rewards. The learner must find satisfaction in learning based on understanding that his or her goals will be reached or based (less commonly) on the pure enjoyment of exploring new things.

The learner's internal motivation needs to be repeatedly reinforced by praise or concrete rewards. Internal motivation that comes from within and is based on the patient's values and goals lasts longer than external motivation (that comes from outside sources). However, external rewards can also be exercised, but with caution because they can cause a decline in internal motivation.

Learning is most effective when the patient or client is ready to learn and wants to be involved with rehabilitation goals. Sometimes the patient's readiness to learn comes with time, and the therapist's role is to encourage its development.

The learner's motivation is enhanced by the way in which the instructional material is organized. The best organized learning material makes the information meaningful to the individual. One method of organization is relating new tasks to those already known. Another important method is to determine whether the patient understands the desired final outcome. This also can encourage motivation.

The motivating factors and strategies used in learning should start when the learner enters the learning process. The most important motivational factors when the learner begins the learning process are: (1) the learner's attitudes toward the environment, (2) the teacher, (3) the topic, and (4) the basic needs and goals experienced by the learner. Patients' fundamental needs and goals should receive high consideration in the rehabilitation process. For example, when teaching patients after a cerebral vascular accident, patients' personal goals are highly correlated with their levels of motivation.[18] Patients whose personal goals are independence and self-sufficiency have high levels of motivation to learn, recover, and actively participate in rehabilitation.[18] This indicates that patients' goals have a positive effect on their levels of learning. Patients who establish goals also have high motivation, appreciate the importance of learning, and approach rehabilitation activities in the best possible manner. These patients also understand and perform the exercises and activities better than patients who have no goals and motivation.[18]

Additionally, patients showing high motivation generally meet the desired rehabilitation outcomes.[18] Contrarily, patients who do not have personal goals and needs show no motivation to learn.[18] These patients are totally dependent on caregivers. Patients with low motivation do not understand the exercises and activities and have a decreased desire to participate in the rehabilitation. During the process of learning, motivational strategies are important to increase the learner's confidence and self-esteem and to decrease his or her negative and erroneous beliefs and expectations (**Table 9.5**).

Typically, patients have very little desire to learn when they show signs of decreased enthusiasm for learning. As mentioned previously, patients who have had a stroke who have no personal needs or goals and believe others (caregivers) can do everything for them show low motivation to learn and negative rehabilitation outcomes. These patients require specific motivational approaches to learn, such as: (1) to change the style and content of

| Table 9.5 | *Strategies to Enhance a Patient's Confidence*[18] |
|---|---|
| | The conditions surrounding the topic should be positives (such as in the case of stroke patients with favorable comparisons to other stroke patients and a patient's desire to leave the hospital). |
| | The patient's erroneous beliefs, expectations, and assumptions must be addressed to decrease the effect of a negative attitude toward learning. |
| | Components of learning that lead to failure or fear must be reduced or removed. |
| | The therapist should plan activities to allow the patient to meet self-esteem needs. |

the learning activity; (2) to make learner reaction and involvement essential parts of the learning process using problem solving, role playing, and stimulation; (3) to use the learner's concerns to organize the content and develop themes and teaching procedures; and (4) to use group cooperation goals to maximize learner involvement and sharing.[18] When the learner completes the learning process, the motivational strategies should concentrate on providing consistent feedback about his or her mastery of learning, acknowledgment of the learner's responsibility in having completed the learning task, and constructive reinforcement, especially when the learning was successful.

## The Importance of Learning Theories for Patient Teaching and Learning

There are three main categories of learning theories, divided according to the three dominant paradigms: behaviorism, cognitivism, and constructivism. *Behaviorism* focuses on observed behaviors, attempting to determine ways to shape behaviors by using reinforcements and punishments.[19] Learning is a change in behavior that is dependent on the environmental stimuli. From a behaviorist perspective, the transmission of information from teacher to learner is essentially the transmission of the response appropriate to a certain stimulus. Consequently, the learner needs to be provided the appropriate range of behavioral responses to specific stimuli, and those responses need to be reinforced through an effective reinforcement schedule.[19] Using behaviorism, the role of the educator is to organize the environment in such a way as to be able to elicit a desired response from the learner.[19] In health care, behaviorism becomes significant when using behavioral objectives and when applied to adult learning for skill development and training.

*Cognitivism*, the second large category of learning, tries to understand how information gets processed, stored, and used.[19] Cognitivism uses the learner's internal mental processes to help him or her increase cognitive structuring. The purpose of cognitivism is to help the learner develop better skills. The role of the educator is to structure the content of the learning activity. In health care, cognitivism may be important to help learners, especially older adults, remember the learned information.

The last main category, *constructivism*, believes that knowledge is uniquely constructed by each individual.[19] The community and the individual's interactive observations in a social context are important. The educator is a facilitator of learning. In health care, constructivism could help the learner construct new knowledge by building on prior knowledge and by considering the learner's experiences and social contexts.

Other learning theories have also developed as expansions of or in opposition to behaviorism, cognitivism, and constructivism. Some of these paradigms rejected behaviorism for its ideas of rewards and punishment; for example, the humanistic approach considers that learning should be done only through affective and cognitive abilities. The purpose of education from the humanistic perspective is for the learner to become self-actualized and autonomous. The educator's role is to facilitate the development of the whole person.

Other learning theories expanded and related the three main theories with the experiential learning hypothesis. In addition, theorists such as Bloom and Maslow extended the cognitivism paradigms, trying to understand the hierarchical nature of knowledge or the affective domain and how learners control their own life development.

Not all learning theories are applicable to health care and patient education in rehabilitation. However, all theories described in this section are essential for their contribution to the educational techniques of learning and can be used in combination or alone to help health care providers to organize their educational material, apply the curriculum, and better understand their learners from the motivational and participatory perspectives.

Health care providers' knowledge of learning theories can increase their abilities to provide effective patient education and meet the patients' desired learning outcomes (**Table 9.6**).[20,21] As a whole, physical and occupational therapists and assistants can use teaching and learning theories in patient education to impart better instruction, especially when related to the patient's level of development and their strengths, limitations, and abilities.

In addition, learning theories can help the educator to define his or her teaching philosophy and understand the best educational practice for increasing the patient's or client's knowledge.[20,21] Furthermore, learning theories are important because they explain how people learn and factors that may promote or hinder the learning process.[20,21] The theories promote different educational techniques to help health care providers define their own philosophies as teachers and respect their patients' learning processes. Some consider

| Table 9.6 |
|---|
| ***The Goals of Learning Theories*[20,21]** |
| Increase the ability to better understand the developmental stages and their relation to learning. |
| Increase the ability to value individual differences in regard to learning. |
| Increase the ability to assess the learner's readiness to gain knowledge. |
| Increase the ability to define the learner's philosophy and learning preference(s). |
| Increase the ability to provide instruction appropriate to the learner's level of development. |
| Increase the ability to become aware of the strengths and limitations of the learner at different stages of development. |
| Increase the ability to apply the best educational design to increase the learner's knowledge. |

that the learning theories most relevant to teaching in clinical settings are behaviorism, cognitivism, experiential learning, and humanistic learning. Physical and occupational rehabilitation educators can be guided by each of the educational technologies presented in this section. Some theories will be more helpful than others in particular contexts; however, several teaching and learning principles have emerged from these theories, and they can provide helpful direction for rehabilitation providers as clinicians and educators.

# *Behaviorism and Patient Education*

Behaviorism is a worldview that functions on a principle of the stimulus–response mechanism.[19] All behavior is caused by external stimuli and can be explained without the need to consider internal mental states or consciousness. The most important element in this theory is the environment. If the environment is right, learning occurs as connections are made between a stimulus and response and between response and reinforcement.

In behaviorism, the learning process is very simple. The learner is essentially passive, responding to environmental stimuli. The environmental stimuli can use positive or negative reinforcement. Positive reinforcement involves applying a stimulus in response to an action, whereas negative reinforcement withholds the stimulus.[19] An effective reinforcement schedule requires: (1) consistent repetition of the learned material; (2) a small, progressive sequences of tasks; and (3) continuous positive reinforcement.[19] Without positive reinforcement, learned responses will quickly become extinct because learners will continue to modify their behavior until they receive some positive reinforcement.

## THE BEGINNINGS OF BEHAVIORISM

In behaviorism, there are only two ways to change behavior and encourage learning using two types of conditioning: classical (respondent) and operational. Classical conditioning (also called Pavlovian) has to do with conditioning of behaviors that were elicited from an association between two stimuli.[19] Classical conditioning involves involuntary behaviors. Operational (or operant) conditioning has to do with the use of consequences to modify the behavior.[22] Using stimulus–response conditioning and operating based on the environment, operational conditioning forms an association between the behavior and the consequence.[19] Contrary to classical conditioning, operational conditioning involves voluntary behaviors.

Originators of and contributors to behaviorism include John B. Watson, Ivan Pavlov (classical conditioning), B.F. Skinner (operant conditioning), E.L. Thorndike (connectionism), Albert Bandura, and Edward C. Tolman (moving toward cognitivism). The most used example of behaviorism is Pavlov's classical conditioning theory and its most basic form of learning called *associative learning*. During physiological research studies of salivation and stomach function, Pavlov used the ringing of a bell and meat powder to trigger the salivation response in dogs.[19] He noticed that the dogs salivated shortly before they were given food. When the bell was rung at repeated feedings, the sound of the bell alone as a conditioned stimulus caused the dogs to salivate as a conditioned response.[19] Pavlov's classical conditioning theory included the following steps:[19]

1. Food equals salivation.

2. Food and stimulus equals salivation (conditioned stimulus).

3. Ringing of the bell produces salivation (conditioned response).

In his theory, Pavlov demonstrated how stimulus–response works.[19] Pavlov's findings are considered by some to be the basic blocks of learning. John Watson continued Pavlov's classical conditioning theory, believing that human behavior results from specific stimuli that elicit certain responses. Expanding on Watson's basic stimulus–response model, B.F. Skinner developed a comprehensive view of conditioning called *operant conditioning*. Skinner's theory is based on the premise that satisfying responses are conditioned whereas unsatisfying responses are not.[22] Animals and humans repeat acts that lead to favorable outcomes and suppress acts that produce unfavorable results. For example, if a rat presses a bar and receives a food pellet, the rat will press the bar again. The bar-pressing response is called the operant and the food pellet is called the reinforcement. Skinner's theory states that punishment suppresses a response and decreases the probability that the response will occur in the future.[22] Skinner's hypothesis concentrated on a person's behavior and the reinforcement that occurs after a response. The reinforcement strengthens the probability that the response will take place again under similar circumstances and can be negative or positive. Positive reinforcement increases the probability that a positive response will occur again; negative reinforcement removes or prevents an adverse condition.[22] It also increases the likelihood of a positive behavior because it can remove an unpleasant consequence. Punishment involves presenting a strong stimulus that decreases the frequency of a particular response.

## PROS AND CONS FOR USING BEHAVIORISM IN PATIENT EDUCATION

Skinner's operant conditioning theory can be used in teaching to promote desirable behavior.[22] In the classroom, teachers employ contracts, consequences, reinforcement, extinction, and behavior modification to help students acquire positive learning behaviors. For example, if a student does not complete his or her homework assignments, the teacher and the student design a contract stating that: (1) the student will stay for extra help, (2) the student will ask family member(s) for help, and (3) the student will complete assigned work on time.[22] In rehabilitation, the behavioral learning contracts are especially useful when working with children.

Consequences take place after the target behavior occurs, when either positive or negative reinforcement may be offered. Positive reinforcement in the classroom can be provided by smiling at students, commending students for their work, or praising students' ability to their family. Teachers use negative reinforcement by telling students that submission of assignments on time results in the lowest grade being dropped or that obtaining a score of 80% or higher on the assignments makes the final exam optional. Operant conditioning using extinction decreases the probability of a response by contingent withdrawal of a previously reinforced stimulus.[22] As a classroom example, a student has developed a habit of making squeaky noises every time the teacher asks a question in class. The classmates reinforce the behavior by laughing at his noises. The teacher asks the classmates not to laugh, extinguishing the student's behavior.

In the United States, before the 1960s, behaviorism was used mostly in behavioral psychology and did not have a large impact in educational theory.[19] The impact of behaviorism on American education started with the behavioral objectives movement and continued with other educational systems such as Skinner's programmed instruction method and today's computer-assisted learning.[5] In the late 1950s and early 1960s, many educators realized that a behavioral objective can help the learning process if each learning task is identified as a terminal behavior and is also quantifiable.[22] To develop behavioral objectives, teachers had to break down the learning task through analysis into specific measurable objectives.[22] In this way, the student's learning success was measured by tests developed to consider each objective. The largest contribution to behavioral objective development in education in the United States was provided by Bloom's, Gagne's, and Briggs's taxonomies of learning. (See Section V for more on Bloom.) By the late 1960s, most teachers were writing and using behavioral objectives.

Another impact of the behaviorist school of psychology, particularly Skinner's operant conditioning, was the idea that behavior is a function of its consequences. The learner will repeat the desired behavior if positive reinforcement such as a pleasant consequence follows the behavior.[22] Positive reinforcement can include verbal reinforcement or tangible rewards such as certificates and promotions. Negative reinforcement can also strengthen a behavior in a situation when a negative condition is stopped or avoided as a consequence of the behavior. Reinforcement can be given continuously. New behaviors are learned fastest with continuous reinforcement. Every time the target behavior is performed, the reinforcer can be administered. Reinforcers also can be given intermittently, either at random intervals (unpredictable) or at fixed intervals (such as every third time a behavior occurs). Typically, however, behaviors persist longer when reinforcement is unpredictable.[22]

Punishment weakens a behavior, because a negative condition was introduced or experienced as a consequence of the behavior and teaches the individual not to repeat the behavior that was negatively reinforced. Many educational behaviorists believe that the behaviorist concept of punishment should not be used in education.[22] Others believe that punishment is a necessary everyday notion that should be used in learning repetitive tasks and work skills that require a great deal of practice and in situations where higher order learning skills are necessary.[22]

## APPLICATION OF BEHAVIORISM TO PATIENT TEACHING AND LEARNING

Using aspects of behaviorism, such as the operant conditioning technique, in teaching and learning can be effective, especially when assessing the types of reinforcement needed to decrease or increase a behavior. As an example of behaviorism in physical therapy, the therapist can teach a patient gait training with a walker by doing the following: (1) breaking down the skill into components, (2) giving understandable directions to the patient on how to practice each component, and (3) offering positive reinforcement immediately after the patient performs each component of the skill. In this example (as with any operant conditioning method), the success of conditioning depends largely on the timing of reinforcement. In the beginning of the learning process, patient learning should be reinforced every time it occurs. Typically, positive reinforcement is used frequently in physical and occupational therapy teaching activities and exercises. Patients are reinforced with wholehearted praise for attempting or achieving their tasks and skills. Praising and encouraging the learner's correct performance increases the probability that the same response will occur again. After a response is established, the patient is able to independently perform the gait training skill without reinforcement and backup.

However, not all patients respond well to operant conditioning and reinforcement such as the therapist's smiling after a correct response and commending and praising the patient for his or her achievement. For example, patients in nursing homes and long-term residential facilities, who are typically quiet and not outspoken or who are very reflective, are successful learners using the operant conditioning technique.[10] However, patients who are forthright and insightful may resent behaviorist teaching and learning techniques, being sensitive to the therapist's reinforcement remarks. These patients feel that cognitive reinforcement is demeaning and/or manipulative. In addition, rewards and incentives that are offered in operant conditioning learning are considered narcissistic values and not altruistic perceptions.[23,24] Furthermore, the biggest setback when using operant conditioning for patients' teaching and learning is based on the fact that patients are not usually participating in patient-centered care because they are not actively involved with their goals.

In physical and occupational rehabilitation, behaviorist teaching methods such as a behavioral learning contract may be recommended when working with patients or clients who are children or who have cognitive and perceptual deficits. Simple contracts can be effective in helping children focus on behavior change.[24] The relevant behavior should be identified, and the child and therapist should decide the terms of the contract. Behaviorist instructional methods may also be used with patients with traumatic brain injury, especially when teaching and learning very structured material and/or where the material is easily memorized. For example, after a traumatic brain injury, positive reinforcement using a reward system can improve patient participation with rehabilitation.

In physical and occupational rehabilitation, one drawback to behaviorist instructional methods may be the inability to effectively stimulate a patient's comprehension and analytical abilities, especially when related to the patient's safety. For example, using a walker and conditioning the patient to perform gait training on tiles (an even surface) will not help the patient understand how to perform the same task (gait training) on grass (an uneven surface). In this example, when trying to walk outside on the grass (where the patient was not conditioned), the patient may fall. Nevertheless, using behaviorism for teaching and learning cannot be totally discarded considering the success of behavioral modification therapy. This form of noninvasive therapeutic intervention is based on the interaction of research and clinical studies of physiology, psychiatry, psychology, and physical medicine.[25] Behavior modification therapy can be used by physical and occupational therapists for progressive relaxation and specific behavioral modification education related to hypertension, incontinence, headache, chronic respiratory problems, and chronic pain. Additionally, in psychosocial occupational therapy, therapists can apply behavioral modification instruction for patients with disorders such as schizophrenia.[25] As an example in rehabilitation, positive reinforcement such as smiling and complementing the learner on his or her performance can be offered to affect a patient's teaching and learning of activities of daily living such as shopping, dressing, cooking, and grooming.

# Cognitivism and Patient Education

Cognitive theories consider learning as an internal process that involves higher mental activities such as memory, perception, thinking, problem solving, reasoning, and concept formation. Any previous experience and knowledge may augment the learning process.

## DESCRIPTION OF COGNITIVISM

The cognitivism model essentially argues that the mind is a "black box" that should be opened and understood.[26] The learner is viewed as an information processor, similar to a computer.[26] Information comes in, is processed, and then results in certain outcomes. Any previous experience and knowledge may augment the process of learning.

Cognitive theories were developed in response to behavioral theories and include meaningful learning and discovery learning.[26] Cognitive psychologists believe that learning cannot be described in terms of a change in behavior because behavior is not a factor of learning.[26] Learning occurs regardless of changes in behavior or other noticeable changes in the learner. Cognitive theorists believe that throughout the learning process, instruction is motivated through mental stimulation, not behavioral modification.[26] The cognitivism model believes that an instructor can produce learning by transferring information to the learners and helping them to organize it in such a way that they are able to recall it later. Reinforcement of learning does not need a stimulus (as in behaviorism) but is accomplished through a process of retrieving existing knowledge and presenting new information.

## PIAGET'S STAGES OF DEVELOPMENT AND THEIR APPLICATION TO PATIENT TEACHING AND LEARNING

The best known psychologist who promoted the cognitive development theory was Jean Piaget.[26] He observed children and their process of making sense of the world around them. Piaget developed a four-stage model of how the mind processes new information. He established four stages of learning:[26]

1.  The sensorimotor stage from birth to 2 years old

2.  The preoperational stage from 2 to 4 years old

3.  The concrete operational stage from 7 to 11 years old

4.  The formal operational stage from 11 to 15 years old

In the sensorimotor stage, the infant builds an understanding of him- or herself and reality by interacting with the environment.[26] At this stage the child is only able to differentiate between itself and other objects. The child's outlook is essentially egocentric in the sense that he or she is unable to take into account others' points of view. The learning process takes place through assimilation and accommodation.[26] Assimilation represents organization of information and absorbing it into the existing schema; accommodation happens when an object cannot be assimilated and the schema has to be modified to include the object.[26] The child also recognizes self as an agent of action and begins to act intentionally, such as shaking a rattle to make a noise. In the sensorimotor stage, the child achieves object permanence, realizing that things continue to exist even when they no longer are present to the senses.[26]

In Piaget's preoperational stage, the child is not able to conceptualize abstract ideas, instead requiring concrete physical situations.[26] Objects are classified in simple ways considering their important features. For example, a child can classify objects by a single feature such as grouping together all the red blocks regardless of shape or all the square blocks regardless of color. The child learns to use language and to represent objects by images and words. Thinking is still egocentric, meaning the child has difficulty taking the viewpoint of others.[26] However, the child learns to classify items using different criteria and to manipulate numbers. Linguistic skills increase and open the way for greater socialization of action and communication with others.

In Piaget's concrete operational stage, the child begins to think in the abstract and is able to conceptualize by creating logical interpretations of various physical experiences.[26] The child can think logically about objects and events attaining conservation of number (at age 6), mass (at age 7), and weight (at age 9). The child classifies objects according to several features and can order them in series along a single dimension such as size. From the ages of 7 to 11 years, children begin to develop logic, although they can only perform logical operations on concrete objects and events.[26] In the concrete operational stage of development and learning, the physical experience accumulates and the accommodation process is increased.

In the last stage of Piaget's formal operations, cognition reaches its final form of development.[26] The child is an adolescent now entering the formal operational stage that continues throughout the rest of his or her life. The child can think logically about abstract propositions and test hypotheses systematically.[26] He or she becomes concerned with the hypothetical, the future, and ideological problems. The child no longer requires concrete objects to make rational judgments, but is able to use deductive and hypothetical reasoning in his or her thinking process. In the formal operational stage, children develop the ability to perform abstract intellectual operations and reach affective and intellectual maturity.[26] Most importantly, children build up their capacity to appreciate others' points of view as well as their own. Their ability to use abstract thinking is very similar to that of an adult.[26]

In regard to rehabilitation, especially in pediatric physical and occupational therapy, Piaget's stages of development are important to understand children's perceptions and reasoning in given situations. Patient and family education has to be geared toward the idea that children's thinking is qualitatively different than adults'. Children as patients/clients need to construct or reconstruct knowledge in order to learn. They also need intense opportunities to interact with the physical world and their peers. The predictive nature of

Piaget's stages allows therapists to anticipate which cognitive processes will develop if given adequate environmental support. The relationship between environment and cognition is critical for planning rehabilitative interventions for children with compromised skills. For example, for children with mental disabilities, therapists need to consider simple concrete activities that are demonstrated first and applied passively to the child. For better learning, the activities can be transformed into familiar actions that affect the child's daily life. Environmental distractions and stimuli should be removed to allow the child to concentrate and perform the activity.

Piaget's cognitive development theory is also important for adult learning in cases when adults never reach a formal operational stage of reasoning to think abstractly. For example, during rehabilitation of patients with traumatic brain injury, Piaget's stages can be applied to teach simple and concrete concepts instead of abstract ones. The cognitive development theory of patient education also can be used for older adults who have decreased stages of thinking, especially when influenced by disease, stress, depression, or medication effects. As an effective patient educator, rehabilitation professionals should be able to evaluate the patient's style of cognitive reasoning and apply the best method of teaching and learning.

## THE INFORMATION-PROCESSING APPROACH AND ITS APPLICATION TO PATIENT TEACHING AND LEARNING

Similar to Piaget's cognitive development theory, the information-processing approach believes that the process of reasoning is extremely important because it emphasizes the way information is approached and stored. The information-processing approach studies cognition and cognitive development in relation to the reasoning processes of the mind.[5] These processes are considered similar to a computer.[5] Rather than focusing on simple input and output, psychologists who adhere to this approach place emphasis on the processes of cognitive development. As a result, specific attention is given to the concepts of information processing as they relate to the study of cognition. The information-processing theory began in the mid-20th century and was developed as a reaction to behaviorism.[27] The general definition of the theory is that learning is a change in knowledge that is stored in an individual's memory.[27] Typically, the information-processing approach connects the new learning to prior knowledge.[27] The information-processing theory states that to learn something new, learners must focus their attention on the new information, compare the new information with the old, and create new mental groupings for the new information (**Table 9.7**).

There are four major learning stages in information-processing theory: (1) attention, (2) processing, (3) memory storage, and (4) action. During the first phase, the teacher has to be able to capture the learner's attention.[28] In patient education, the rehabilitation provider has to be able to use stimuli to orient the learner toward the educational material. If the learner cannot be stimulated to become attentive to the rehabilitation provider's stimuli, the learning process cannot take place. The sensory modes of obtaining information for the patient may be reading, looking at pictures or graphs, listening, writing notes, observing and experiencing events and activities, and using kinesthetic awareness such as touching. In the second stage, the processing phase, information is processed by the

| Table 9.7 | **Elements of Information Processing Theory[27]** |
|---|---|

1. Focus attention on the new material.

2. Compare the new material with the old material (that is already stored in long-term memory).

3. Add the new material to the old material or create new mental categories for the new material that does not fit in any established mental category.

learner's different senses. During this phase, the educator has to consider the learner's preference for a learning mode. It can be kinesthetic, visual, auditory, or mixed. The educator must evaluate whether the patient has any sensory and/or motor deficits that may interfere with the learning process and use the learning mode that best fits the patient. In clinical settings, patients with hearing deficits have to receive educational material in a different way than patients with visual impairments. For example, patients with hearing impairments could benefit from visual instruction whereas verbal training could be a learning mode for individuals with visual deficits.

The third major learning stage is called the memory storage phase. During this phase, two important learning processes called encoding and storage take place.[27] Encoding depends upon attaching new information to knowledge that already exists in the brain.[27] First, the educational material is transferred for a short period of time (less than 30 seconds) to the working memory, called the short-term memory.[27] At this point, the information can be either ignored and forgotten or moved and stored in deep memory, called long-term memory.[27] This step of moving the newly learned material from short-term memory to long-term memory is essential. If new material is not added to existing knowledge in long-term memory, it is quickly forgotten. New, fresh information demands attention and "space" in the working memory. For some patients, especially older adults, the storage process may be very slow and demanding, requiring extra effort and a lot of repetition and reinforcement. Information in long-term memory can be stored by using associations such as relating the new information with data that is already in long-term memory or by developing certain images of the new matter. Long-term memory is long-lasting, but the retrieval of information can be difficult.

The last phase of information processing is the action part when the learner recalls the new information.[27] For rehabilitation providers, the recall process must address necessary corrections to emphasize data accuracy, especially when patient safety issues are involved. Also, the learner's cognitive style and methods of processing should be appreciated and respected.

Using the information-processing teaching strategy in the classroom may be a challenge, especially when scientific information has to be encoded and properly stored for retrieval.[27]

Contrary to patients, students are not necessarily affected by physical and emotional difficulties and have the ability to attend to new information, compare it to existing knowledge, and assign the new information to mental categories; however, many students may be awkward and slow at the encoding process.[27] As nonexperts, all the new information looks the same to them. They do not have well-defined categories in their minds, they are not adept at accurately comparing new material with their existing knowledge, and they may not be able to form effective new categories. These students can increase their ability to process information by having the teacher sort and organize the data into categories, give examples and fill in details, and encourage them to practice the new information (**Table 9.8**).

Physical and occupational therapists and assistants need to help patients integrate information into their working memory. Integrative teaching and learning occurs when the information is meaningful to the learner. As a result, linking a patient's prior knowledge or experience to new knowledge is extremely important. As an example, when teaching a patient shoulder exercises for flexion, abduction, or external or internal rotation, connect

| Table 9.8 |
|---|
| ***Methods to Increase Ability to Process Information[27]*** |
| Identifying the key features to be learned. |
| Defining important concepts in their most essential terms. |
| Focusing learners' attention on important concepts by highlighting the main ideas. The teacher has to be selective about the main ideas. Giving too much material will make the situation worse by overloading the short-term memory. |
| Helping learners attach new information to what they already know. |
| Organizing the new information into categories. |
| Filling in details that elaborate on the new concepts. |
| Giving examples. |
| Asking learners to suggest connections among new and old material. |
| Allowing learners to practice using new information. In the classroom, this needs to happen during a lecture as well as in homework. |
| After defining, highlighting, and elaborating on a new concept, asking the learners to do something with the information such as writing a sentence or drawing a picture about it. |

these actions with activities the patient performs daily at home or at work. Additionally, incorporating a patient's personal and cultural backgrounds helps to integrate the topic even more with the patient's everyday life. This allows easier understanding, recognition, and recollection of the new material. Therapists should organize and structure the material by helping patients create their own framework to store the information effectively. This is also dependent on the patient's learning preference; for example, if a patient is a visual learner, he or she can be provided with illustrations to organize the exercises as a visual map.

Structuring the learning environment facilitates patients' physical and emotional well-being, allowing enhanced learning and better data integration. A quiet environment with proper lighting and temperature can assist the learning process. Helping the patient to elaborate on the learned material can further promote storage and retrieval of information. Group teaching can also help expand and connect the information with prior knowledge. Furthermore, especially with movement performances, teaching and learning must include practice and repetition to facilitate the patient's data storage and retrieval of new knowledge.

## SOCIAL COGNITIVE AND SOCIAL LEARNING THEORIES AND THEIR APPLICATIONS TO PATIENT TEACHING AND LEARNING

Social Cognitive Theory is another form of cognitivism that was proposed by Miller and Dollard and expanded by Bandura and Walters.[29,30] Social Cognitive Theory (SCT) stresses the effects of social factors on an individual's thinking, perception, and motivation. It explains how people acquire and maintain certain behavioral patterns, while also providing the basis for intervention strategies.[29] The theory deals with cognitive, emotional, and behavioral aspects for understanding behavioral change and provides methods for behavioral research in health education.[29] Evaluating an individual's behavioral change depends on factors such as the environment, people, and behavior. Environments can be social or physical. Social environments include family members, friends, and colleagues; physical environments include the size of a room, the ambient temperature, or the availability of certain foods.[29] Psychologists who promote SCT believe that the environment and the situation provide the framework for understanding the behavior.[30] The situation refers to the cognitive or mental representations of the environment that may affect an individual's behavior.[30] The situation is a person's perception of the place, time, physical features, and activity. Additionally, SCT states that three factors of environment, people, and behavior are constantly influencing each other.[29,30] Behavior is not only the result of the environment and the person, and environment is not only the result of the person and the behavior. The environment provides models for behavior. In SCT, observational learning occurs when a person watches the actions of another person and the reinforcements that the person receives.[29]

Social Cognitive Theory forms the basis of Bandura's Social Learning Theory (SLT), which explains that people learn by observing other people's behaviors and attitudes, and the outcomes of those behaviors (**Figure 9.1**).[30] SLT promotes observational learning, stating that human behavior is learned observationally through modeling.[29,30] It means that

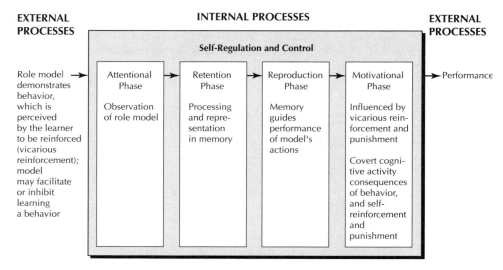

Figure 9.1
### Social Learning Theory[5]

individuals first observe others, then they form ideas of how new behaviors are performed, and finally they use the information as a guide for their actions. SLT describes that people can learn through observation of other people.[29] The theory identifies three types of observational learning: (1) verbal instruction model using verbal explanations of a specific behavior; (2) individual live demonstration model using acting of a specific behavior; and (3) symbolic description model using real or imaginary characters from movies or books of a specific behavior.[29] SLT also explains that the individual's psychological well-being can influence the learning process.[29] For example, internal factors such as pride, satisfaction and internal reward help a person to learn. Additionally, in SLT, learning is not a permanent change in behavior. An individual can learn new information without demonstrating new behaviors.[29] Furthermore, SLT considers that observational learning requires four modeling factors called the learner's attention, retention (storing information), reproduction (performing the learned behavior), and motivation.[29]

Social Learning Theory is relevant for designing patient and health education and health behavior modification programs. This theory also explains how people acquire and maintain certain behavioral patterns. When applied to health care, SLT encourages appreciation of the patient's individuality and diversity.[5] Consequently, the teacher needs to identify the learner's level of cognitive development, goals and expectations, modes of processing information, and social influences affecting the learning process.[5] Then, the teacher can encourage the learner to use new methods to solve problems and achieve his or her goals and expectations.[5] SLT also can be used for providing the basis for compliance with intervention strategies and promoting healthy behaviors using the learner's attention, retention, reproduction, and motivation (**Table 9.9**).[29,30]

Because these four conditions (attention, retention, reproduction, and motivation) vary among individuals, different people will reproduce the same behavior differently. The effects of modeling on behavior are that it: (1) teaches new behaviors, (2) influences the frequency of previously learned behaviors, (3) may encourage previously forbidden behaviors, and (4) increases the frequency of similar behaviors.[5,29] Individuals are more likely to engage in certain behaviors when they believe they are capable of executing those behaviors successfully. This means they will have high self-efficacy, showing self-confidence towards learning. The Social Learning Theory encourages not only observational learning through modeling but also self-efficacy. For an individual, self-efficacy allows him or her to produce the desired effect and succeed in their enterprise. Self-efficacy affects behaviors because individuals choose activities they feel they will be successful in doing and tend to put more effort into

| Table 9.9 | **Four Modeling Factors of Social Learning Theory**[29,30] | |
|---|---|
| Attention | The person must first pay attention to the model. Attention is important for learning to take place. The learner's characteristics such as sensory capacity, arousal, or past reinforcement affect attention. |
| Retention | The observer must be able to remember the behavior that has been observed. Retention also has to do with the learner being able to convey mental images of learned behavior and rehearsing the steps. |
| Reproduction | Actually replicating the behavior. This means the observer has to be able to replicate the action, which could be a problem for a learner who is not ready developmentally to replicate the action. For example, little children have difficulty doing complex physical motions. In physical and occupational rehabilitation, the observer needs the necessary motor skills to be able to reproduce the action. |
| Motivation | Having a good reason to imitate or adopt the behavior. Motivation is the final necessary ingredient for modeling to occur. The learner must want to demonstrate what he or she learned. |

activities and behaviors they consider themselves to be successful in achieving. Learners with high self-efficacy tend to learn better and achieve more.

In classroom learning, students typically have a good sense of their own efficacy in considering what they can and cannot do. In clinical settings, patients have difficulties with self-efficacy because of physiological and psychological impairments and limitations.[5] Other negative factors can be their own previous failures, negative messages received from others, or previous failures of others.[5] Rehabilitation providers need to find methods to encourage patients' self-efficacy. For example, the therapists can link new learning to recent patient-acquired skills as well as help the patient to create and work toward their own personal goals. Increasing self-efficacy will positively influence patients' functional abilities. Some of the methods to increase self-efficacy in physical and occupational therapy may include role modeling, emotional arousal, realistic goal setting, reduction in negative feedback, verbal persuasion and encouragement, individualized care, social support, and a reduction in unpleasant sensations associated with functional activities.[5] To enhance a patient's self-efficacy, the environment must also be considered in addition to the use of humor. Additionally, the patient should be surrounded by a caring, kind, and competent rehabilitation team. The therapist's and family's continuous encouragement and the patient's active participation in his or her rehabilitation including teaching and learning can also positively influence self-efficacy.

Bandura's Social Learning Theory is significant in health care for two important reasons: (1) much of the learning happens through observation of models, and (2) it promotes the concept of self-efficacy. SLT also is applied extensively to understanding of aggression and psychological disorders in the context of behavior modification.[30] The principles of behavioral modification based on SLT require coding modeled behavior in words, labels, and images and adopting the behavior if it has characteristics similar to the patient's personality (**Table 9.10**).[25,30]

| Table 9.10 | **_Three Principles of Behavioral Modification_**[25] |
| --- |
| The highest level of observational learning is achieved by first organizing and rehearsing the modeled behavior symbolically and then enacting it overtly. For this reason, coding modeled behavior into words, labels, or images results in better retention than simply observing the behavior. |
| Patients are more likely to adopt a modeled behavior if it results in outcomes they value. |
| Patients are more likely to adopt a modeled behavior if: (1) the model shows similar characteristics with the observer's personality, (2) the model has a popular status, and (3) the behavior has functional value. |

Bandura's principle of self-efficacy states that the individual's own judgment regarding his or her ability to deal with different situations is central to his or her actions.[30] It means that people's actions are dependent on what they choose to do, how much effort they invested in activities, how long they persist in the situation of adversity, and whether they approach the task anxiously or assuredly. For these reasons, teachers and learners must view anxiety or nervousness in difficult situations as excitement or anticipation. The self-efficacy concept is important in clinical teaching and learning and in health care education for prevention, wellness, and health promotion. For example, therapists must always consider that success can increase a patient's self-efficacy whereas failure can lower it. If failures occur early in the learning process and are not due to lack of effort or difficult situations, they will definitely lower the patient's self-efficacy. For the same reason, when teaching a task in the beginning, it is important for a patient to observe other patients performing the task successfully. This can strengthen the patient's belief that they can perform similar tasks effectively. Verbal persuasion from the therapist as a credible source can also help. Additionally, in physical and occupational therapy, a patient's self-efficacy can be increased by: (1) modeling; (2) setting clear goals; (3) providing knowledge, skills, and practice; and (4) asking the patient to reflect on their learning (**Table 9.11**).[31]

Social Learning Theory also promotes self-regulation, which is a form of self-efficacy that is used for behavioral modifications. Self-regulation takes place when the individual has his or her own ideas about what is appropriate or inappropriate behavior and chooses actions accordingly.[31] In the classroom setting, self-regulation is the process where the student activates and sustains behaviors that are oriented toward the attainment of his or her academic goals.[32] These behaviors may include activities such as concentrating on instruction, rehearsing the information to be remembered, using resources effectively, valuing

| Table 9.11 | **Methods to Increase a Patient's Self-Efficacy[31]** |
| --- | --- |
| Using modeling or demonstrations. |
| Setting a clear goal or image of the desired outcome. |
| Providing the basic knowledge and skills needed to be the foundation of a task. |
| Providing guided practice with constructive feedback. |
| Giving the patient an opportunity to reflect on his or her learning. |
| Interpreting the patient's anxiety or nervousness in difficult situations as anticipation and excitement (and not as a sign of vulnerability). |

learning, and experiencing pride and satisfaction with their efforts.[32] The main aspects of self-regulation are: setting standards and goals, self-observation, self-judgment, and self-reaction.[30] Self-observation is the learner's deliberate attention to aspects of his or her behavior.[32] Learners can regulate their actions if they have goals and set standards to achieve these goals. Self-judgment refers to the learner comparing his or her own present performance with the achievement of his or her goals.[32] The learner's question may be: "How is my performance to achieve my goals?" Self-reaction is the learner's honest response to his or her performance and the learner's plans to correct and improve his or her learning behavior.

When related to behavioral modifications, promoting self-regulation can be an important technique to be used by rehabilitation providers for patient and health education. Self-regulation can play in important role in patients'/clients' teaching and learning in general, especially for prevention and health promotion. For example, in regard to integrating healthier nutrition in American lifestyles, a 2007 research study found that self-regulatory behaviors are extremely important in the healthier food choices of adults.[33] Self-regulatory behaviors helped 712 adults (a majority of whom were overweight or obese) overcome negative outcome expectations and become successful in changing their diets.[33] By increasing these individuals' nutrition-related self-efficacy, the study showed that people can be successful by changing their behavior to buy and eat healthier foods.[33] As a behavioral modification approach, self-regulation also is supported by teaching the patient to reward him- or herself after accomplishing the necessary behavior. As a final point of SLT, through self-regulation patients can give themselves instructions that guide their behavior (**Table 9.12**). Through self-monitoring, they monitor and observe their own behavior, sometimes even scoring the behavior, and through self-reinforcement, they are able to change their behavior.

As previously stated, the Bandura principle of modeling is also known as observational learning.[29] It is used in schools and in clinical situations. The modeling also is the basis for explaining a variety of children's behaviors. Children acquire many favorable and unfavorable responses by observing those around them. For example, in the classroom setting, a student who is always late for class because his friends are late displays the result of an unfavorable response of observational learning. In the clinical setting, modeling can be used for patients to learn and understand various skills. Through observational learning, patients can model (imitate) other patients or the therapists. For example, for a patient who has had a stroke, seeing another patient (who also has had a stroke) taking a few steps at the parallel bars would help to reinforce the patient's desire to try the same activity.

Other instructional strategies related to SLT that promote patients' self-efficacy are brainstorming and briefing (and debriefing).[34] In the clinical settings, these approaches can help patients to process information by activating their prior knowledge.[34] For example, during stair ambulation, the therapist can brainstorm with the patient regarding ideas to enhance his or her safety. This will activate the patient's prior knowledge regarding safe methods to ascend and descend stairs and will provide the necessary framework for the next session of ambulation. Importance should always be given to what the patient already knows.[34] The patient needs help to elaborate on his or her existing knowledge and connect the old to the new information.

| Table 9.12 | **Significance of the Social Learning Theory in Patient Teaching and Learning**[30–32] |
| --- | --- |

Patients as learners often learn a great deal simply by observing other people (observational learning).

Describing the consequences of behavior can effectively increase the appropriate behaviors and decrease inappropriate ones. This can involve discussing with patients the rewards and consequences of various behaviors.

Modeling provides an alternative to shaping for teaching new behaviors. Instead of using shaping (which is operant conditioning), modeling can provide a faster, more efficient means for teaching new behavior. To promote effective modeling the therapist must make sure that the four essential conditions exist: attention, retention, motor reproduction, and motivation.

Therapists as teachers must always model the correct behavior that needs to be learned. This means therapists must demonstrate accurate movements from the beginning of the therapy. Showing the patient certain performance errors can take place only after the patient has modeled the correct behavior.

Therapists as teachers should expose learners to a variety of other models. This technique is especially important to break down traditional stereotypes. If the patient has erroneous beliefs in regard to certain activities, the therapist has to be able to expose the patient to correct ones.

Patients as learners must believe they are capable of accomplishing rehabilitation tasks. This is very important for developing a sense of self-efficacy in all patients. Self-efficacy can be promoted by having patients watch others be successful and also experience success on their own.

Therapists as teachers should help patients set realistic learning expectations for their accomplishments. For example, a patient who is very weak in the legs should not be advised, as a short-term goal, to anticipate ambulating without an assistive device.

Self-regulation techniques provide an effective method for improving a patient's behavior.

After the first learning session, the learner needs debriefing. Debriefing is used to facilitate the cognitive process of learning, promoting discussion and reflection of the information that was learned.[34] The process of debriefing includes the following steps: (1) identifying the impact of experience; (2) identifying and considering the processes that were developed; (3) clarifying the facts, concepts, and principles; and (4) identifying different views of the learner including the emotional aspects.[34] Through debriefing, the therapist as the teacher can provide the patient with increased significance about the learned information. Feedback and discussions can supply opportunities for elaboration of knowledge. Understanding what the patient has learned is important for the therapist to be able to approach the patient's next encounter and also to evaluate the current session. The quality of the resulting new knowledge depends on activating prior known information and the degree of elaboration on the resulting knowledge.[34] The more elaboration on the resulting knowledge, the more easily it will be retrieved by the learner.

# Constructivism and Patient Education

The constructivist approach to teaching and learning is based on a combination of cognitive psychology and operant conditioning theory within behavioral psychology. The basic premise is that learning (cognition) is the result of "mental construction."[35] It means that learners learn by fitting new information together with what they already know.[35] As a result, learners must actively build knowledge and skills.

## THE IMPORTANCE OF CONSTRUCTIVISM TO TEACHING AND LEARNING

According to constructivism, an individual's knowledge is a function of his or her prior experiences, mental structures, and beliefs that are used to interpret objects and events.[35] The learned information exists within built mental constructs and not in the external environment.[35] Learners construct their own knowledge and interpret the information based upon their perceptions of experiences or what they already know.[35] In constructivism, teaching and learning are active processes (not passive). The learner makes judgments about when and how to modify his or her knowledge. Constructivists also believe that much of reality is shared through a progression of social negotiation.[35] All constructivist teaching agrees on the same idea that adaptive behavior is not produced by stimuli but by the individual who processes stimuli from the environment.[35]

Constructivist theories were promoted by prominent psychologists, sociologists, and philosophers, such as Brunner, Piaget, Goodman, Kant, Dewey, Habermas, Vygotsky, and McMahon. Jean Piaget is considered the chief theorist among the cognitive constructivists. Piaget paved the way for the social constructivism of Belarusian psychologist Lev Vygotsky.[36] Piaget's cognitive constructivist theory of learning promotes the idea that knowledge is internalized by learners. Piaget's theory states that individuals use the processes of accommodation and assimilation to "construct" new knowledge from their experiences.[37] When they assimilate the information, they incorporate the new experiences into an already existing framework without changing the framework.[37] This phenomenon occurs when the individuals' experiences are aligned with their internal representations of the world. It also occurs when individuals have a faulty understanding of the information about the world. In contrast, when individuals' experiences contradict their internal representations, they may change their perceptions of the experiences to fit their internal representations.[37,38] In constructivism, Piaget's accommodation is the process of reframing learners' mental representations of the external world to fit new experiences.[38] Accommodation is understood as the mechanism by which failure leads to learning.[37,38] It means that people are able to learn from their experiences, regardless of whether the experiences are positive or negative. Furthermore, the theory indicates that people can learn from successes as well as from failures.[37,38]

In contrast to Piaget, who believed that a child's development necessarily precedes learning, Vygotsky asserted the idea that a child's social learning precedes development.[36] He thought that a child's developmental processes lag behind the learning processes.[36] In his social constructivism theory, Vygotsky felt that every function in a child's cultural development appears twice, first on the social level, between people (interpsychological), and later on the individual level, inside the child (intrapsychological).[36] Other themes of social constructivism promoted by Vygotsky are the more knowledgeable other (MKO) and the zone of proximal development (ZPD).[36] The MKO refers to anyone who has a better understanding or a higher ability level than the learner in regard to a particular task, process, or concept.[36] An MKO can be a teacher, a coach, an older adult, peers, a younger person, or computers.[36] The ZPD is the distance between a student's ability to perform a task under adult guidance and/or with peer collaboration and the student's ability to solve the problem independently.[36] Vygotsky believed that learning occurred in this zone. The MKO and ZPD themes promote the idea that learners can, with help from teachers or peers who have more advanced knowledge, master information that they cannot understand on their own.[36] Learners actively construct knowledge and meaning through participation in activities and challenges. The emphasis is on the interaction between learners and instructors (or facilitators) to be able to arrive at a higher level of truth. Vygotsky's focal point of constructivist teaching was on the connections between people and the sociocultural context in which they act and interact by using speaking and writing to mediate their social environments.[36] Teachers and students collaborate, and many times change their roles from student to teacher and vice versa, in order to facilitate meaningful instruction in students. Learning becomes a reciprocal experience for the student and the teacher.

Brunner, another prominent constructivist who performed research on cognitive development, identified three stages of cognitive growth in childhood development. These are the enactive, iconic, and symbolic stages (**Table 9.13**).[38]

Brunner's constructivist theory advocates active learning, in which the learner is able to construct new ideas or concepts based upon his or her current knowledge.[39] Brunner provided the following principles of constructivistic learning: (1) Instruction must be concerned with learning experiences that promote learner readiness for learning; (2) Instruction must be designed to facilitate extrapolation and/or fill in the gaps, meaning that instruction should have enough information to stimulate cognitive skills and student inquiry; (3) Instruction must be structured in such a way as to be easily grasped by the student.[39] This is called the spiral organization of instruction when the student can easily build on prior knowledge. Brunner stated that instruction should address four important aspects of learning: the learner's predisposition toward learning, modes to structure the knowledge and be readily grasped by the learner, the most effective sequences in which to present the information, and the nature and pacing of rewards and punishments.[39]

Constructivism is important for the educational system of the 21st century.[40] In addition to influencing other contemporary teaching techniques such as discovery-based teaching and problem-based learning, constructivism influences computer programming and computer science learning.[40] Computer programming languages have even been created to support the constructivist theory of Piaget.[40] Some of these computer programming languages produced in the 1980s, 1990s, and more recently in the 21st century are Logo, Etoys, and Scratch. These languages are used to help students in primary and secondary education to create interactive stories and animations for younger students and to help older ones learn math and science.

## APPLYING CONSTRUCTIVISM TO PATIENT TEACHING AND LEARNING

In general, constructivism does not suggest one particular way of teaching or learning. Constructivism describes that learning should happen by promoting active learning or learning by doing. The strength of constructivism is that the learner is able to interpret multiple realities and deal with real-life situations. As generally described, in the constructivist theory, a learner who can problem-solve can also apply his or he existing knowledge to a new situation.

When comparing the behaviorist learning theory and constructivism, the difference is that in the behaviorist inductive manner the instructor will teach the learner a skill step-by-step, whereas in constructivism the instructor will start with the learner's prior

| Table 9.13 | **Brunner's Stages of Cognitive Growth in Children[38]** |
|---|---|
| | 1. The enactive stage is when the child represents and understands the world through action involving motor responses and ways to manipulate the environment. |
| | 2. The iconic stage is when the child represents the world in images that stand for certain events or objects; this stage corresponds to Piaget's preoperational thinking stage. |
| | 3. The symbolic stage is when the child is able to use abstract ideas, symbols, language, and logic to understand and represent the world. |

knowledge and understanding of the skill and fill in the necessary gaps to solve a situation-specific problem. For example, in behaviorism, when teaching an activity of daily living such as brushing hair to a patient who has had a stroke and has hemiparesis of the dominant arm, the therapist will provide the information to the patient step-by-step in a didactic approach without the patient's active participation. In the constructivist mode, the therapist will ask the patient about ways he or she used to brush hair prior to the stroke. Then, after discussing and observing the patient trying to perform the skill, the therapist can facilitate the patient's own ideas for corrective feedback. Another discrepancy between behaviorism and constructivism is the manner in which the curriculum would be introduced to the patient. Behaviorists use a predesigned curriculum whereas constructivists use students' experiences and knowledge base to "construct" more knowledge and expertise.

In social constructivism in patient clinical education as well as health care education, the therapist should view the patient as a unique individual with unique needs and backgrounds. The learner's uniqueness and complexity should be encouraged, used, and rewarded as an integral part of the learning process. The patient as the learner should be supported to arrive at his or her own version of the truth, influenced by his or her background, culture, or worldview. The learner's development, language, logic, and other systems contributing to learning are inherited by the learner as a member of a particular culture and are also learned throughout the learner's life. For these reasons, patient teaching and learning must consider the patient's social interaction with other more knowledgeable members of the family or community that will help them in the learning process. The responsibility for learning should be with the learner. This characteristic of learning encourages patient-centered care, emphasizing the active role of the patient as the learner in understanding, reflecting, and looking for meanings. The learner's feelings of competence and belief in the potential to solve new problems are derived from their first-hand experience of mastery of problems in the past. These can increase the learner's present motivation. This concept specifically links with Vygosky's zone of proximal development, where learners are challenged within close proximity to, yet slightly above their current level of development.[37] By experiencing the successful completion of challenging tasks, learners gain confidence and motivation to start more complex challenges.

Using the social constructivism approach, the therapist (as the instructor) is a facilitator, helping the learner to obtain his or her understanding of the content. The facilitator is not the typical teacher who gives a didactic lecture covering the subject matter by telling and not asking the student.[38] A facilitator is different because he or she supports the learner by continuously providing guidelines and creating the environment for the learner to arrive at his or her own conclusions. The facilitator is in a continuous dialogue with the learner, taking the initiative to steer the learning experience to where the learner wants to create value.[38] The learner and the facilitator are equally involved in learning from each other. The learning experience is objective and subjective, requiring that the facilitator's culture, values, and background also become an essential part of the interplay between learners and tasks in the shaping of meaning.

In physical and occupational therapy, constructivist teaching and learning can engage the patient as a whole. The teaching does not address just the patient's intellect but the entire person. Effective constructivist teaching and learning recognizes that meaning is personal and unique and that the learner's understanding is based on their unique experiences. However, the search for meaning occurs through the patient's already known "patterns" or "schemas."[38] The therapist has to be able to connect the patient's isolated ideas and information with the general concept that needs to be learned. For example, when teaching balance training to a patient the therapist can ask the patient what he or she knows in regard to standing on one leg with his or her eyes open. The patient has to think about it and offer different solutions on how he or she can stand on one leg. From prior experience, the patient may consider various variables that affect being able to stand on one leg, such as vision, the type of surface, having something to hold on to, trying to feel the ground with one leg, moving back and forth to keep equilibrium, or asking someone to hold their hand and help them. Patients' emotions are critical, and learning also is influenced by the environment, culture, and climate. Some patients may remember how they hopped on one leg when they were children. Some patients may cry. Feelings and attitudes are highly involved in constructivist learning.

Patients need time to be able to process what they learned. The teaching and learning climate has to be relaxed but challenging. A threatening environment inhibits learning. Also, the teaching and learning approach is reflective with respect to investigating performance modes. The principal role of the therapist as the teacher is to guide the patient to generate hypotheses, interpret the information, and develop constructs.

Additionally, in physical and occupational therapy, considering the patient-centered care model, the therapist's role is of motivator, facilitator, and manager of the rehabilitative session. The patient's role is to investigate hands-on new and safe methods of skill performance. When teaching techniques that the patient cannot relate to, the learning environment needs to be structured to guide the patient first to practice a certain task. In this way, the patient is acquainted with the activity in order to relate it to prior experience. Then, the patient can integrate the task into the new experiential knowledge. By practicing the novel task, the therapist shapes the environment from an unstructured to a structured one. Consequently, the patient creates a mental pattern or a schema of the task necessary for the learning by doing. Constructivist-learning theorists believe that unstructured environments rely too much on the learner to be able to discover problem solutions.[41] Theorists promote having learners with no prior experiences be taught novice tasks in order to create a well-structured learning environment.

The social constructivism approach to learning is important for physical and occupational rehabilitation because it creates a dynamic interaction among task, instructor, and learner, taking into consideration and blending together the patient's and therapist's beliefs, standards, and values. In addition, the constructivism theory allows the therapist to acquire from the patient information regarding methods of achieving tasks, modifying tasks, cooperation, consideration, and application of various experiences. The assessment process is dynamically linked with learning as a continuous interactive procedure, and the feedback created by the assessment serves as a direct foundation for further development. The therapist needs to engage patients, constantly challenging them with tasks that refer to skills and knowledge just beyond their current level of mastery. This will capture their motivation and build on previous successes to enhance their confidence. Because the learning environment is important, the learner's emotions and the life contexts of everyone involved in the learning process (including the patient's family) must be considered.

Negotiation is another important aspect of constructivism teaching and learning in rehabilitation because it unites the therapist and the patient in a common purpose. In a patient-centered care approach, negotiating means inviting the patient to contribute to and modify his or her interventional goals, including teaching and learning objectives. The process requests patients to invest in their learning needs and the outcomes. As a result, patients will work harder and better toward their physical/occupational therapy goals because they are closely involved in decision making. Furthermore, teaching and learning becomes an interactive process when learning activities promote closer connections and ties between the therapist and the patient.

From the patient's perspective, the down side of constructivism may be that patients as learners need to be ready to change their perceptions and mental conceptualizations when using this approach. Some patients, especially in the context of rehabilitation, may want to be taught and understand better from a didactic approach. This means that therapists need considerable time, energy, and patience to convince patients to apply the concept of constructivist learning. From the therapist's perspective, therapists must also believe that all learners can learn and find their own best way to learn, and that eventually the learning will become meaningful to them. Also, therapists have to demonstrate superior knowledge of the subject matter and excellent communication skills. Additionally, they need to create a strong relationship with the learner, discouraging old ways of medical paternalism and encouraging patient-centered teaching and learning.

# ADDITIONAL TEACHING AND LEARNING THEORIES AND PATIENT EDUCATION

## Objectives

After completing Chapter 10, the reader will be able to:

- Describe humanistic theory and its role in patient instruction.
- Explain the role of experiential learning in patient teaching.
- Discuss multiple intelligences and their application to patient teaching and learning.
- Recognize the role of visual-auditory-kinesthetic teaching and learning in rehabilitation.
- Identify Bloom's taxonomy of learning and its role in patient education.

## Humanism and Patient Education

In the 1970s and 1980s, a great deal of theoretical writing about teaching and learning in the United States concentrated on humanistic psychology. In education designs, a strong linkage exists between constructivist theories of learning and humanistic psychology.[42] The humanistic trend of teaching came about as a reaction against scientific reductionism, which explained everything on the basis of science. An individual affective and subjective world had to be reaffirmed. Also, personal freedom, choice, motivation, and feelings needed attention. For these reasons, the American psychologist Abraham Maslow proposed the *hierarchy of needs* to explain motivation (**Figure 10.1**).[5]

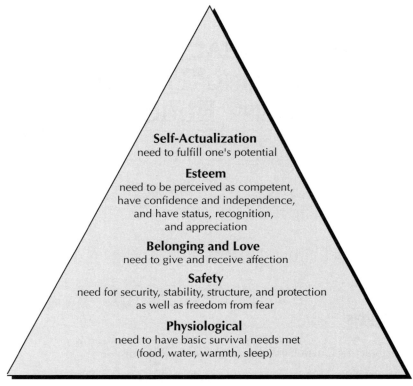

Figure 10.1
**Maslow's Hierarchy of Needs[5]**

## MASLOW'S HIERARCHY OF NEEDS

Abraham Maslow believed that learning is not an end in itself. Learning is the means to progress towards self-development, which he called *self-actualization*. At the lowest level of Maslow's hierarchy are physiological needs.[42] Only when the lower needs are met is it possible for an individual to fully move on to the next level. A motive at the lower level is always stronger than those at higher levels. At level one, the physiological needs include hunger, thirst, sex, sleep, relaxation, and bodily integrity.[5] These must be satisfied before the next level comes into play. At level two, the safety needs call for a predictable and orderly world. If these are not satisfied, individuals will look to organize their world to provide for the greatest degree of safety and security.[5] If satisfied, they will come under the force of level three, belonging and love, in which individuals seek warm and friendly relationships.

At level four, esteem, they desire strength, achievement, adequacy, mastery, and competence.[5] They also want confidence, independence, reputation, and prestige.[5] The last level is five, self-actualization, representing the full use and expression of talents, capacities, and potentialities.[5] In self-actualization, learners are able to submit to social regulation without losing their own integrity or personal independence. Achieving this level means developing to the full stature of which they are capable. Learning can be seen as a form of self-actualization, contributing to a person's psychological health. However, although self-actualization may be seen as the primary goal, other goals also exist. These include a sense of accomplishment and the controlling of impulses.

Maslow's theory received much criticism, mostly in regard to its reliability. Many issues were brought up, such as whether a person's lower needs really have to be satisfied before higher ones come into play.[42] Also, many psychologists felt that individuals may well put physiological needs to one side to satisfy the need for love. However, Maslow's idea of a hierarchy of needs, identifying different needs, and the notion of self-actualization maintained a powerful hold over adult education theorists such as Malcolm Knowles.[42] Humanistic psychology's positive view of people and their ability to control their own destiny, and the seemingly unlimited possibilities for individual development, provided hope for educators.[42]

In patient education, Maslow's theory is important because it establishes a patient's priorities before applying teaching and learning. Physical and occupational therapists must be aware of patients' priorities. Many obstacles can hinder patient education such as illness, communication barriers, educational background, age, impairments and functional limitations, and others. For example, the patient's physiological needs must always be met before trying to teach the patient. If the patient has pain or discomfort, it will be impossible to teach him or her exercises or activities. At the same time, the theory of self-actualization emphasizes a patient's self-government and self-regulation toward autonomy, moving away from didactic instruction and toward a patient-centered learning approach. Self-actualization may also explain the humanistic principles of instruction that emphasize a patient's motivation toward learning.

## CARL ROGERS'S HUMANISTIC VIEW OF LEARNING

The most persuasive exploration of a humanistic orientation to learning came from another American psychologist, Carl Rogers.[43] In educational psychology, special attention is given to Carl Rogers's contribution to the humanistic view of learning. Rogers believed that education must engage the whole person and their experiences because learning combines the logical and intuitive, and the intellect and feelings.[43] He felt that an individual learns with all their capacities, physical and psychological. Rogers's humanistic approach to learning is similar in many ways to constructivism (discussed in Chapter 9) because it promotes personal change and growth and facilitates learning if the learner participates completely in the learning process. Rogers's concept is also primarily based upon direct confrontation with practical, social, personal, or research problems.[43] Further, the learner's self-evaluation is the principal method of assessing progress or success (**Table 10.1**).

| Table 10.1 | **Carl Rogers's Learning Concepts[43]** |
|---|---|
| | Learning has a quality of personal involvement of the whole person (including feelings and cognitive aspects). |
| | Learning is self-initiated. Even when the impetus or stimulus comes from the outside, the sense of discovery, and grasping and comprehending the material, comes from within. |
| | Learning is all-encompassing. It affects the behavior, the attitudes, and the personality of the learner. |
| | Learning is continuously evaluated by the learner. The learner knows whether it is meeting his or her need or whether it leads toward what he or she wants to know. The locus of evaluation is found definitely with the learner. |
| | The essence of learning is in its meaning. When learning takes place, the element of meaning to the learner is built into the whole experience. |

## HUMANISM APPLIED TO PATIENT TEACHING AND LEARNING

The biggest benefit of the humanistic learning theory in teaching and learning is its motivational characteristic. The educator is a facilitator of learning, encouraging the learner's curiosity, questions, creativity, and positive self-concepts.[42] The educator does not use traditional didacticism but is very concerned about the learner's emotional needs. In humanism, the learner's feeling and thinking are interlinked. Feeling positive about oneself facilitates the learning process. Similar in many ways to constructivism, humanistic teaching and learning facilitates patient-centered learning.

The physical or occupational therapist is a facilitator using participatory and discovery methods to help the patient learn. Humanistic learning helps the patient and the therapist define the problem, propose solutions, and jointly implement rehabilitation goals. The patient is able to strive for self-actualization by moving towards self-regulation and autonomy and by taking responsibility for his or her own learning. The patient's behavior is within the context of his or her own personal realities, and open communication is necessary for the rehabilitation provider to understand the patient's point of view. In humanistic learning, the patient becomes self-responsible, flexible, and creative. Working in groups allow patients as learners to express their feelings more openly and explore new programs. Additionally, in the humanistic approach to patient education the emphasis is on the patient's personal values facilitating development of self-identity and self-actualization. Humanistic learning is the foundation of health education that promotes prevention and wellness programs in rehabilitation. However, the biggest criticism of humanistic learning is that it promotes self-centered learners who cannot compromise or take criticism.[5]

## CARL ROGERS'S EXPERIENTIAL LEARNING THEORY

Experiential learning theory (ELT) is a form of education that occurs as a result of direct participation in life events. Experiential learning theory also was created as an offshoot of constructivism, stating that knowledge must be "constructed" by the learner and cannot be supplied by the teacher.[43] Thus, the construction of knowledge is a dynamic process that requires the active engagement of the learner. All learners are responsible for their own learning and the teacher is responsible for creating an effective active learning environment. The knowledge is directly experienced, constructed, acted upon, tested, or revised by the learner. Experiential learning theory builds on the work of renowned psychologists such as John Dewey, Carl Jung, and David Kolb. The theory provides a framework for understanding the cyclical nature of experiential learning and individual learning tendencies or styles. In regard to patient education, experiential learning theory is embraced in clinical teaching and learning as well as in health care education.[43,44] This form of learning involves a direct encounter with the phenomenon being studied.

Carl Rogers suggested that experiential learning is equivalent to personal change and growth.[43] Rogers felt that all human beings have a natural propensity to learn, and the role of the teacher is to facilitate such learning. He proposed that learning should include the following characteristics: (1) setting a positive climate for learning, (2) clarifying the learner's purposes, (3) organizing and making available learning resources, (4) sharing feelings and thoughts with learners (but not dominating them), and (5) balancing intellectual and emotional components of learning.[43]

According to Carl Rogers, learning is facilitated by students' direct participation in the learning process (**Table 10.2**).

| Table 10.2 | ***Carl Rogers's Ideas Regarding Student Participation in Teaching and Learning***[43] |
| --- | --- |
| The student participates completely in the teaching and learning process and has control over its nature and direction. | |
| Learning is primarily based upon the student's direct confrontation with practical, social, personal, or research problems. | |
| The student's self-evaluation is the principal method of assessing progress or success. | |

# *Additional Learning Styles and Patient Teaching and Learning*

Successful patient education occurs when health care providers affirm the presence and validity of diverse learning styles and maximize the conditions for using instructional designs that best fit the patient's learning style(s). These teaching and learning designs should be taken into consideration as a way to increase the possibilities of success for all learners. Although people learn continuously, they have a preference about how they learn. This means that everyone has a learning style. Effective teaching and learning cannot be limited to just delivering the information; learners must be actively involved in the learning process. Recognizing each patient's learning style is part of effective patient instruction. Trying to teach exclusively in a manner that favors the patient's preferred learning style(s) can influence their ability to learn. Usually, patients respond better to new information when it is provided using a learning style with which they are most comfortable. Additionally, the therapist must know his or her own personal learning style because when teaching, individuals tend to teach by predominantly using their personal learning style(s).

## DAVID KOLB'S MODEL AND ITS APPLICATION TO PATIENT TEACHING AND LEARNING

David Kolb also contributed to experiential learning theory by providing the Cycle of Learning model, which states that learning is a continuous process.[45–47] Kolb's learning model sets out four distinct learning styles or preferences, which are based on four learning cycles: concrete experience, reflective observation, abstract conceptualization, and active experimentation.[5] Kolb conceptualizes learning styles as dynamic states resulting from the learner's preferences. Consistent with the experiential learning theory, Kolb considers that every learner approaches a topic based on past experiences and the demands of the environment.[45] Kolb's Cycle of Learning model also states that each learning style preference is actually the product of two pairs of variables, or two separate choices.[45] These learning preferences are related to two variables: (1) the way the learner approaches a task, called the processing continuum, and (2) the learner's emotional response (or how the learner feels about it), called the perception continuum.[45] Processing includes two opposite orientations to learning, watching (reflective observation, or RO), and doing (active experimentation, or AE) (**Table 10.3**).[46,47] Individuals characterized as RO learners may prefer to learn by watching and listening to others and relying on objectivity, careful judgment, and personal thoughts and feelings.[47] Individuals characterized as AE learners learn best by actively being involved with tasks, experimenting with tasks, and trying to change situations.

Perception also includes two opposite perspectives to learning, thinking (abstract conceptualization, or AC) and feeling (concrete experience, or CE). Individuals characterized as having CE viewpoints rely more on feelings than on thinking when dealing with tasks, situations, and conditions.[47] They benefit from group learning experiences and being able to relate to others. Contrarily, individuals with AC perspectives rely more on logic and ideas than feelings when tasks, situations, and conditions arise.[47] They learn best by thinking and analyzing.

In Kolb's theory, the learner cannot grasp an experience by simultaneously doing and watching.[46] Also, the learner cannot transform the experience by simultaneously feeling and thinking.[46] The learner has to pick one choice for each approach. For example, the learner approaches the task by opting to: (1) watch others involved in the experience and reflect on what happens (RO) or (2) jump in and just do it (AE).[46] At the same time, emotionally, the learner can transform the experience into something meaningful and useful by opting to: (1) gain new information by thinking, analyzing, or planning (AC) or (2) experience the concrete, tangible, felt qualities of the world (CE).[46]

According to Kolb, the ideal form of learning is for the learner to be able to integrate all four cycles of learning.[45,46] The result of this integration means truly transforming the experience into knowledge. This forms the basis of Kolb's definition of learning: the production of knowledge through the transformation of experience.[45] Additionally, in Kolb's view, the process of learning may begin anywhere in the Cycle of Learning. Furthermore, Kolb's theory requires that the learner gives full consideration to each stage because the outcomes of one stage would nourish the next stage of the model to the point where the cycle was started.[45] Going through each cycle means important activity and function that are essential for the final learning achievement.[45] When learners are able to approach all four learning cycles, they are experiencing the full cycle of learning. These learning stages show how experience is translated through reflection into concepts. These, in turn, are used as guides for active experimentation and the choice of new experiences.[45] Kolb's theory suggests that learning is a complex and adaptive process integrating a range of mental

| Table 10.3 | **Kolb's Experiential Learning Cycles[46,47]** |
|---|---|
| Concrete experience (CE) | Feeling |
| Reflective observation (RO) | Watching |
| Abstract conceptualization (AC) | Thinking |
| Active experimentation (AE) | Doing |

processes, and that experiential learning is a process created through the transformation of experience.[45] When combining all four experiential learning cycles, the learner demonstrates four types of learning styles, called accommodator, converger, diverger, and assimilator (**Table 10.4**).[45,46]

Experiential learning involves thoughts, feelings, and cognitive processes. It is a process and not an outcome, requires an individual to resolve dialectically opposed modes of adaptation, derives from experience, is a holistic integrative process, requires interplay between a person and the environment, and results in the creation of knowledge.[45] The concept of learning through experience is fundamental in development training and academic programs such as those in physical and occupational therapy. The learners learn by selectively reflecting on their experience in a critical way. It means that the experience is essential for the learning to take place. In physical and occupational rehabilitation, experiential learning is intensively used in all academic programs. In patient education, experiential learning, and especially Kolb's Cycle of Learning, can be used when teaching patients different skills, taking into consideration each patient's preferred learning style(s).

| Table 10.4 | Kolb's Learning Styles and Patient Teaching[45,46] | |
|---|---|
| **Learning Styles and Teaching Strategies** | **Characteristics** |
| "Accommodator" Learning Style | This type of learner combines concrete experience (CE) with active experimentation (AE). He or she typically completes hands-on tasks and enjoys experiencing new and challenging situations. The learner acts on intuition dealing with his or her feelings. The learner needs to determine his or her own criteria for relevance of materials or techniques. The accommodator's strengths lie in doing things and being involved in new experiences. He or she excels in adapting to specific immediate circumstances and tends to solve problems intuitively, relying on others for information. The accommodator is at ease with people, but is sometimes seen as impatient and pushy. |

*(continues)*

| Table 10.4 | *Kolb's Learning Styles and Patient Teaching*[45,46] *(continued)* |
| --- | --- |

| Learning Styles and Teaching Strategies | Characteristics |
| --- | --- |
| "Accommodator" Teaching Strategies | The teacher should model specific teaching and "hands-on" techniques. The best techniques for the accommodator are role playing, skill practicing, problem solving, small group discussions, and peer feedback. When working with patients with this learning style, the therapist should observe and guard them carefully for safety reasons. Because they are happy to explore new interventions, they may be willing to take risks and get hurt. Also, including the family and the caregiver in the rehabilitation session (and in patient education) can be helpful. Patients with this learning style prefer to work as a team to complete the task, sometimes trying different methods to achieve their goals. |
| "Converger" Learning Style | This type of learner combines abstract conceptualization (AC) with active experimentation (AE). The learner likes to think about the subject. He or she finds practical applications for ideas and theories and can use deductive reasoning for problem solving. Factual information takes precedence over social and interpersonal issues. The converger is a pragmatist. The greatest strength of this learning style is the practical application of ideas. The learner tends to be relatively unemotional. The converger prefers to deal with things rather than people. He or she tends to have a few technical interests and quite often chooses to specialize in the physical sciences. |

*(continues)*

| Table 10.4 | Kolb's Learning Styles and Patient Teaching[45,46] (continued) | |
| --- | --- |
| **Learning Styles and Teaching Strategies** | **Characteristics** |
| "Converger" Teaching Strategies | The best teaching and learning approaches for patients with this learning style are peer feedback and activities that apply skills and tasks. The rehabilitation provider's role as a teacher for these learners is not very complicated because they prefer a self-directed, autonomous type of teaching and learning. The therapist mostly is a coach and facilitator. However, sometimes these patients may spend too much time solving the wrong problem and may make hasty decisions. |
| "Diverger" Learning Style | This type of learner combines concrete experience (CE) with reflective observation (RO). The learner is able to look at the information from different perspectives. The diverger prefers to watch rather than perform tasks, also gathering information and using imagination to solve problems. The learner is best at viewing concrete situations from several different viewpoints. The diverger solves problems the best when brainstorming. Also, the learner has an active imagination and is emotional. |

(continues)

| Table 10.4 | *Kolb's Learning Styles and Patient Teaching*[45,46] *(continued)* |
|---|---|
| **Learning Styles and Teaching Strategies** | **Characteristics** |
| "Diverger" Teaching Strategies | These learners need plenty of reflection time. The teacher should provide expert interpretation and judge the learner's performance by external criteria. Patients with this learning style tend to be interested in people and also can be very sensitive to feelings. Rehabilitation providers should involve the patients in group rehabilitation. Additionally, connecting the tasks with familiar experiences is very important. |
| "Assimilator" Learning Style | This type of learner combines abstract conceptualization (AC) with reflective observation (RO). The learner prefers to use a concise and logical approach to learning. The learning focus is on abstract ideas and concepts. The logical soundness of the theory is more important than its practical value. Patients with the "assimilator" learning style are best at understanding a wide range of information and organizing it in a concise and logical form. They do not like to work with other people and prefer to reflect on the information prior to its application. |
| "Assimilator" Teaching Strategies | Rehabilitation providers should work with patients one-on-one, allowing them enough time to read the information and apply it in a methodical fashion. The information should be organized and presented in a logical order, making sure that the theory fits the factual interventions. |

The therapist's responsibility in experiential learning is to structure and organize a series of experiences that positively influences the patient's goals and outcomes. Patients are able to learn from direct experiences. Good or positive experiences can motivate and encourage patients to accept more valuable learning experiences. Poor or unsuccessful experiences tend to lead patients to turn away and not to trust the teacher. Although experiential learning involves a semi-structured approach of learning (giving the learner the freedom to perform and "experience" an activity), planning is still important to facilitate cognitive thinking about the experience. Physical and occupational therapists and assistants have to be careful in situations when experiential learning may lead to miseducative experiences if the learning process is wrongly applied or unstructured.

## GARDNER'S MULTIPLE INTELLIGENCES AND ITS APPLICATION TO PATIENT TEACHING AND LEARNING

Multiple intelligences is an educational theory developed by psychologist Howard Gardner (**Table 10.5**).[48] It describes an array of different kinds of "intelligences" exhibited by human beings. Gardner suggested that an individual manifests varying levels of different intelligences.[48] This gives each individual a unique cognitive profile. According to Gardner, the implication of the theory is that teaching and learning should focus on the particular intelligences of each person.[48] For example, if an individual has a strong musical intelligence, the individual should be encouraged to develop his or her musical abilities. Gardner's concept argues that traditional intelligences do not encompass the wide variety of abilities an individual can display.[48] For example, a child who easily masters the multiplication table is not necessarily more intelligent overall than a child who struggles to do that. The second child may be stronger in another type of intelligence, and therefore may best learn the given material through a different approach. It is also possible that the second child may be looking at the multiplication learning process through a deeper level than memorizing the concept. Gardner's multiple intelligences theory suggests schools should offer student-centered education, with curricula tailored to the needs of each child.[48] This includes the idea that educators should help students develop the intelligences in which they are weaker.

Gardner identified seven core intelligences: (1) bodily-kinesthetic, (2) interpersonal, (3) intrapersonal, (4) spatial, (5) linguistic, (6) logical-mathematical, and (7) musical. In 1999 he added an eighth, the naturalistic intelligence, and indicated that investigation continues on whether there is an existential intelligence.[48] Gardner based his classification of intelligences on various criteria from different domains: case studies of individuals exhibiting unusual talents in a given field (such as child prodigies or autistic savants), neurological evidence for areas of the brain that are specialized for particular capacities, the evolutionary relevance of the various capacities, psychometric studies, and the existence of symbolic notation (such as written language or musical notation).[48]

Gardner's *bodily-kinesthetic intelligence* is related to physical movement and the knowledge of the body. This type of intelligence has various capacities such as control of voluntary and preprogrammed movements, expanding awareness through the body, mimetic abilities, a

| Table 10.5 | |
|---|---|
| ***Gardner's Main Principles of Multiple Intelligences[48]*** | |
| Individuals should be encouraged to use their preferred intelligences in learning. | |
| Instructional activities should appeal to different forms of intelligence. | |
| Assessment of learning should measure multiple forms of intelligence. | |

stronger mind and body connection, and improved body functioning.[48] Individuals in this category are adept at physical activities such as sports or dance and often prefer activities that utilize movement.[48] They may enjoy acting and performing, and also may be good at building and making things. Those with strong bodily-kinesthetic intelligence seem to use what might be termed *muscle memory*.[48] This means they can remember things through their body rather than through words or images. Bodily-kinesthetic intelligence includes the skills and dexterity for fine motor movements such as those required for dancing, athletics, surgery, craftmaking, and computer engineering.

In physical and occupational therapy, the therapist should be aware that patients with bodily-kinesthetic intelligence like to move, dance, walk, wiggle their bodies, and swim. They have good fine motor skills. They like to take things apart and put them back together. Bodily-kinesthetic learners tend to increase their learning potential when they are given the opportunity to do something for themselves. Patients' knowledge can be enhanced through touching when talking, moving around, and using body language. For patient education, the therapists can use demonstrations and body movements to help patients learn. Using gestures while making a point is important. Additionally, the sensory neurological technique of tracing letters on the hand or on the patient's back (graphesthesia) could increase the patient's ability to remember a specific exercise. Taking a walk with the patient while discussing an activity or exercise for home use also can increase the patient's ability to apply the technique at home. Asking the patient to write letters and words in the air or to handle a ball enhances the individual's intelligence and helps with patient education. As learning strategies, patients could be trained to use exercise equipment in physical therapy and perform manipulative activities in occupational therapy. Examples of instructional strategies are: build it, touch it, act it out, get a "gut feeling" of it, or dance it.[49]

Gardner's *interpersonal intelligence* has to do with the ability to interact with others.[48] Individuals in this category are typically extroverts. They are characterized by their sensitivity to other peoples' feelings, temperaments, and motivations, and their ability to cooperate with each other and work as a group.[48] Individuals with interpersonal intelligence communicate effectively, empathize easily with others, and may be either leaders or follow-ers. They typically learn best by working with others and also enjoy discussions and debates.[49] This type of learner likes to be part of group activities. In patient education, patients with interpersonal intelligence have strong social skills and like to develop ideas and learn from other people.[49] They like to have lots of friends, talk to people, and join groups. Interpersonal learners are good at understanding people, leading others, organizing, and communicating.[49] In rehabilitation, therapists could encourage interpersonal learners to work with others by participating in group discussions, reading dialogues, or doing team learning/investigating projects. Also, when the family is involved in patient education, the therapist can ask the patient to set up interview questions in regard to the learned material and interview the family. Writing notes in regard to the content of new material can help the patient commit the information to long-term memory. Patients with this learning style learn best by sharing, comparing, relating, cooperating, and interviewing. Role play, community involvement, simulations, cooperative learning, peer tutoring, and social gatherings should be encouraged. Examples of instructional strategies are: teach it, collaborate on it, and interact with it.[49]

In contrast to interpersonal, Gardner's *intrapersonal intelligence* has to do with an individual's introspective and self-reflective capacities.[48] Individuals with this type of intelligence are typically introverts and prefer to work alone. They are usually highly self-aware and capable of understanding their own emotions, goals, and motivations.[48] Their affinity is for thought-based pursuits such as philosophy. They learn best when allowed to concentrate on the subject by themselves.[49] Many times, there is a high level of perfectionism associated with this intelligence.[49] Philosophers, theologians, writers, psychologists, and scientists are the best careers for someone with intrapersonal intelligence.[49]

In patient education, patients with intrapersonal intelligence are strong in self-intelligence and like the rhythm and sound of language. They like poems, songs, and jingles. They enjoy humming or singing along with music. Patients who are intrapersonal learners have the ability to reflect upon many different ideas, issues, and perspectives. Independence in learning enhances the patient's personality. It also allows the patient to set goals and work towards them. Physical and occupational therapists should encourage the patient to work alone on individual projects such as to write a daily journal of exercise performance at home. When learning a new technique, the patient needs time to reflect on new information. Breathing techniques are perfect for relaxation. The therapist should help the patient increase his or her self-esteem and allow self-paced instructions. Also, patients need to have their own space for learning. Examples of instructional strategies are: connect it to your personal life, or make choices with regard to it.[49]

Gardner's *visual-spatial intelligence* has to do with vision and spatial judgment.[48] These individuals have a very strong visual memory and can visualize and mentally manipulate objects.[48] People with this form of intelligence typically have a good sense of direction, excellent hand-eye coordination, an active imagination, and skill at image manipulation and graphic representation.[48] Careers that best suit this intelligence include artists, engineers, and architects.[49]

In regard to patient education, visual-spatial learners benefit from ocular stimulation. Extensive use of color in the treatment room would increase their learning capacity. Patients who are strong in spatial intelligence can remember things visually, including exact sizes and shapes of objects. They like posters, charts, and graphics. They prefer to learn using visual cues and drawing.[49] The therapist can use posters, charts, and graphics to stimulate the acquisition of new information. Patients should be encouraged to take the information and create diagrams or graphs. Words should be color-coded so that syllables have different colors.[49] Montages illustrating activities work best for these spatial intelligence learners because they stimulate their reading abilities.[49] Home exercise programs (HEPs) should be presented in an array of colors or as crossword puzzles. At the same time, therapists should be aware that visual-spatial learners are sensitive to visual distractions and are often involved in daydreaming. Examples of instructional strategies are: draw it, visualize it, highlight important information, or use visual aids.[49]

Gardner's *verbal-linguistic intelligence* has to do with words, spoken or written.[48] People with this type of intelligence have the ability to use words and learn languages, have excellent reading and writing skills, are able to tell stories, and also can memorize words and dates.[48] Individuals with verbal-linguistic intelligence tend to learn best by taking notes, reading, listening to lectures, and taking part in discussions and debates.[49] Careers best suited for verbal-linguistic intelligence are writers, lawyers, politicians, philosophers, and teachers.[49]

In patient education, individuals with verbal-linguistic intelligence enjoy saying, hearing, and seeing words. These patients like telling stories and are motivated by books, records, and opportunities for writing. The therapist could work with them by asking patients to read the information out loud or write a story about it. Patients should keep a journal of his or her HEP or use a tape recorder for daily activities. New information can be retrieved easily by asking the patient to read it out loud to a member of the family (or to the therapist). Then, the patient could explain what they read. Patients also should be asked to use emotional tones or viewpoints when reading or to connect the material to various life events. An example would be to teach an older patient who had a stroke to comb her hair and asking her to tell you how she combed her hair when she was a young girl. Stimulating the love for and the meaning of words can increase these patients' capacity for learning. Verbal-linguistic learners can also memorize names, dates, places, and trivia.[49] Examples of instructional strategies are: read about it, write about it, talk about it, or listen to it.[49]

Gardner's *logical-mathematical intelligence* often is called scientific thinking.[48] It has to do with logic, abstractions, inductive and deductive reasoning, and numbers.[48] These individuals with this intelligence have strong reasoning capabilities and excel in abstract pattern recognition, scientific thinking and investigation, and complex calculations.[49] Although many associate this type of intelligence with mathematics and computer programming, the research shows that the logical capacity is strongly correlated with verbal rather than mathematical abilities.[49] Careers that suit this intelligence best include scientists, mathematicians, doctors, engineers, and economists.[49]

In physical and occupational rehabilitation, patients who are strong in the logical-mathematical intelligence enjoy exploring how things are related. They also like to understand how things work. They like mathematical concepts.[49] These patients are good at critical thinking. For patient education, the therapist should arrange the material in a logical sequence. Everything that needs to be learned should be sorted, categorized, and characterized.[49] Patients like to play word games that require critical thinking. For example, when teaching a patient gait training and why he or she needs a clear path for locomotion, pick a word such as *chair* and ask the patient why it should not be there. When writing the HEP, the therapist should write the directions for completing the exercises in the most logical order and label the most important parts. Ask the patients to look for patterns in words. For example, ask a patient who has been a diabetic for 10 years to tell you the relationship between overeating, overweight, and obesity. Or ask a patient who just had a lumbar laminectomy and needs to protect the surgical area to tell you the relationship between bending, rotating, and lifting. Examples of instructional strategies are: quantify it, conceptualize it, or think critically about it.[49]

Gardner's *musical/rhythmic intelligence* is based on the recognition of tonal patterns, including various environmental sounds, and hearing.[48] Another capacity is the individual's sensitivity to rhythm and beats.[48] Individuals excelling in musical/rhythmic intelligence appreciate the structure of music; recognize, create, and easily reproduce melody and rhythm; sense the quality of musical tone; and show sensitivity to sounds.[48] Learners with musical/rhythmic intelligence learn best via lectures and can use songs or rhythm to learn and memorize information.[49] They also work best with music playing in the background. Careers best suited for musical/rhythmic intelligence are musicians, singers, conductors, and composers.[49]

In physical and occupational rehabilitation, patients in this category learn best when humming or singing the information. Familiar songs or tunes can be used to teach or to remember important skills. The therapist can create a simple song for learning tasks emphasizing certain pitches, rhythm, or beats. When teaching gait training, use marching music, especially for patients with Parkinson's disease (or Alzheimer's disease). The material can be remembered when using music in the background or when reading together (choral reading). Examples of instructional strategies are: sing it, listen to it, or rap it.[49]

Gardner's eighth intelligence, *naturalistic intelligence*, was discovered in 1999.[48] This type of intelligence deals with sensing patterns and making connections to elements in nature.[48] Individuals possessing naturalistic intelligence are interested in the environment, the earth, and other species.[48] They have a strong affinity to the outside world or to animals and enjoy stories or shows that deal with animals or natural phenomena.[49] They also exhibit an unusual interest in subjects such as biology, zoology, botany, geology, meteorology, paleontology, or astronomy.[49] Naturalistic intelligence individuals are intensely aware of their surroundings and changes in their environments, even if these changes are at minute or subtle levels.[49] Often this is due to their highly developed levels of sensory perception. They can also categorize or catalogue things easily. Frequently, they may notice things that others might not be aware of. In addition, people with naturalistic intelligence show a heightened awareness of and concern about the environment and for endangered species.[49] Examples of notable people who had a naturalistic intelligence are John Muir, Rachel Carson, and Charles Darwin.[49] Examples of cultural groups possessing and valuing this form of intelligence are many Native American tribes and aboriginal peoples.[49]

In regard to patient education in physical and occupational therapy, the therapist should be aware that individuals with naturalistic intelligence enjoy interacting with the outside world. They can notice patterns in nature and easily distinguish between different species of flora and fauna. The best place to conduct physical or occupational therapy would be outside or on a large terrace. Spending time outside with the patient and relating information to nature such as observing patterns in nature could enhance the rehabilitation.

## VISUAL-AUDITORY-KINESTHETIC LEARNING STYLES AND THEIR APPLICATION TO PATIENT TEACHING AND LEARNING

Gardner's eight intelligences can be further illustrated by evaluating another classical intelligence and learning style model, known simply as the *visual-auditory-kinesthetic (VAK)* learning style (also referred to as visual-auditory-physical or visual-auditory-tactile/kinesthetic). The VAK theories originally dealt with the teaching of children with dyslexia and other learners.[50] They were developed around the 1920s by psychologists and teaching specialists such as Fernald, Keller, Orthon, Gillingham, and Stillman and Montessori.[50] The early VAK specialists recognized that because people learn in different ways, children who cannot easily learn words and letters visually (by reading) might learn them more easily in a kinesthetic way (by tracing letter shapes with their finger).[50] The VAK learning model does not overlay Gardner's multiple intelligences but provides a different perspective for understanding and explaining an individual's preferred or dominant thinking and learning styles and strengths.[45,50]

According to the VAK model, most individuals possess a dominant learning style.[50] However, some people have a mixed and evenly balanced blend of the three styles.[50] The visual learning style includes the use of seen or observed things such as pictures, diagrams, demonstrations, displays, handouts, films, or flip-charts.[50] The auditory learner transfers information through listening and speaking.[50] The auditory learner also prefers listening to the spoken word (their own or others), and to sounds and noises. The kinesthetic learning style has to do with the physical experience of touching, feeling, holding, doing, and practical hands-on experiences.[50] The learner prefers kinesthetic stimulation for learning to occur.

In physical and occupational therapy, when working with patients with a visual learning style, the therapist should give them written instructions or use a notepad for them to write questions for the therapist. Highlighting the most important information helps, as does using graphs, diagrams, and charts to demonstrate the key points. Other learning tips for visual learners are organizing information as acronyms, mind maps, or mnemonics. Using CD-ROMs or other computer software, videotapes, photographs, illustrations, and visual metaphors, and encouraging patients to visualize the scene and words, can also help visual learners remember the material.

When working with patients with an auditory learning style, the therapist should encourage them to read the explanations aloud and describe the material verbally in their own words. When the patient learns something new, the information must be stated out loud immediately, and all important facts must be verbally reviewed. Sequences of steps have to be written out by the therapist in a sentence form and be narrated by the patient. Videotapes of the information are also helpful in addition to mnemonics, word links, learning together with a spouse (or friend/partner or in a group), and many discussions of the material. Saying words in syllables and repeating rhymes to remember facts are also useful for auditory learners.[50]

Patients who are kinesthetic learners gain knowledge when they receive tactile and physical stimulation to understand the tasks. They need demonstrations and presentations of the material with gestures and hands-on feedback. The sequences need to become automatic. Videotapes and audiotapes for home use need to be played during the skill performance. The learning process can be reinforced by using gestures or certain movements.

# Bloom's Taxonomy and Patient Education

Bloom's taxonomy of learning domains is a design and evaluation tool for training and learning. Bloom's Taxonomy of Educational Objectives was initially partially published in 1956.[51] The taxonomy's role was to develop a system of categories of learning behaviors to assist in design and assessment of educational learning in the United States.[51] Over the years, the taxonomy was expanded by many contributors such as Anderson and Krathwhol.

## DESCRIPTION OF BLOOM'S TAXONOMY AND ITS APPLICATION TO PATIENT TEACHING AND LEARNING

Bloom's taxonomy is a useful template for developing appropriate types of learning experiences considering the cognitive, psychomotor, and affective domains of learning.[51] These three domains of learning (also referred to as knowledge, skills, and attitude [KSA]) overlap.[51] They are typically utilized as goals of any teaching and learning process. In patient education, the taxonomy can be used for explanation and application of learning objectives, methods to teach and train the patient, and measurement of learning outcomes. The taxonomy can also be implemented as a sort of checklist to ensure that patient education is planned to deliver all the necessary development.

The *cognitive domain* involves knowledge and the development of intellectual skills. This includes the recall or recognition of specific facts, procedures, and concepts that serve in the development of the learner's intellectual abilities and skills.[52] The cognitive domain has six categories. The *psychomotor* and *affective* domains include five categories each. Bloom's psychomotor domain includes physical movement, coordination, and use of the motor skill areas.[52] Development of these skills requires practice and is measured in terms of speed, precision, distance, procedures, or techniques in execution. Bloom's affective domain includes the development of the learner's emotions, feelings, and attitudes.[52] It provides a framework for teaching and training, assessing, and evaluating the effectiveness of training and lesson design and delivery, and also the retention and its effect on the learner.[52] The educational objectives of the affective domain take into consideration the learner's values, appreciation, and enthusiasm.[52]

**Table 10.6** represents a modification of Bloom's cognitive domain to be applied to educational objectives in patient education. **Table 10.7** and **Table 10.8** also are modifications of Bloom's psychomotor and affective domains for objectives that can be used in patient teaching and learning. All three tables consist of categories, descriptions of behaviors, and examples of activities or demonstrations. All categories are listed starting from the simplest behavior to the most complex. These categories can be considered degrees of difficulty. The first category must be mastered before proceeding to the second or third one. In patient education, some patients may remain at the first or second behavioral category, depending on the patient's degree of impairment, functional limitation, and disability.

Bloom's taxonomy is important for the therapist to consider when planning the instructional objectives and educational outcomes with the patient (family/caregiver). Typically, in the cognitive domain, the patient as the learner receives knowledge and understanding of a certain topic. He or she can recall the data or the information. For example, in physical and occupational therapy, the therapist may teach a patient about the purpose and the necessary steps for performing a task or skill. Then, the patient is able to recite the reason and the needed steps to complete the activity. In addition to cognitive knowledge, the patient always needs to receive information regarding the physical skills necessary to implement the learned procedure. These skills are part of the psychomotor domain. Cognitive and psychomotor skills always complement each other. The development of psychomotor skills requires practice and feedback. The patient has to use sensory cues to guide his or her motor activity. In the early stages of learning, a complex skill needs imitation and trial and error for tasks to be adequately performed. Toward the end of the psychomotor stage, the patient's proficiency may be indicated by a quick, accurate, and highly coordinated routine requiring a minimum amount of energy. Some patients may not be able to advance to the adaptation and naturalization categories of psychomotor learning, where the skills are perfectly developed and the individual is able to modify movement patterns or create new patterns to fit a particular situation. These actions are dependent on the patient's recovery process, especially with patients who are older or who have neurological impairments and functional limitations.

The affective domain will help patients' motivation and self-efficacy. Patients may have the knowledge of how to perform the necessary skills but may not be motivated enough or able enough to synthesize the knowledge to fit new situations and behaviors. Additionally, a person's set of values is difficult to predict because values are based on a variety of variables such as society, culture, family, friends, health, or illness. Many times, values can also be related to particular objects, phenomena, or behaviors. As a result, emotionally, an individual can simply accept a behavior or, from a more complex perspective, make a commitment to it. The affective domain of learning, especially the fourth and fifth stages

Table 10.6

## Cognitive Domain: Educational Objectives for Development of Patient Knowledge[51,52]

| Category | Behavior | Examples of Activities and Demonstrations and Their Measurements | Examples of Verbs Used to Describe and Measure the Activity |
|---|---|---|---|
| Knowledge | The learner's ability to recall or recognize information | Recounting facts; recalling a process or tasks or skills; repeating the steps of a task. | Arrange, define, describe, label, list, memorize, recognize, relate, reproduce, select, or state. |
| Comprehension | The learner's ability to understand the meaning; restate the information in their own words; interpret the information; translate the information in their own words. | Interpreting the meaning of the learned tasks; interpreting the scenario describing the behavior; suggesting solutions for the problem. | Classify, critique, discuss, estimate, example, explain, illustrate, interpret, paraphrase, reference, reiterate, reword, rewrite, summarize, theorize, or translate. |
| Application | The learner's ability to use or apply the knowledge of the information; take the theory and explain it into practice; use the knowledge of information in response to real circumstances. | Take the theory and include it in a practical example; demonstrate the theory; solve the problem; manage the activity. | Apply, change, conduct, construct, discover, execute, implement, manage, perform, react, respond, or role-play. |

| | | | |
|---|---|---|---|
| Analysis | The learner's ability to interpret elements of information; to interpret organizational principles and structure of information; to interpret the quality of individual components of information. | Identify constituent parts and functions of the process or concept; deconstruct the process or the methodology; make a qualitative assessment of the elements, relationships, effects, and values; measure requirements or needs. | Analyze, break down, compare, catalogue information, diagram, divide, examine, experiment, create a graph, quantify, relate, plot, or value. |
| Synthesis (creating and building) | The learner's ability to develop new plans or unique structures, systems, models, ideas, and approaches of the learned information; the ability to build creative thinking in regard to the information. | Develop plans and procedures; design solutions; integrate methods, resources, ideas, and parts; create new approaches. | Develop, plan, design, revise, organize, formulate, assemble, integrate, rearrange, or modify. |
| Evaluation | The learner's ability to assess the effectiveness of the whole concept in regard to its value, efficacy, and viability; critical thinking about this information; strategic comparison and review of information. | Reviewing strategic options or plans in regard to efficacy or practicability of the information; calculating the effects of a plan or strategy and making recommendations. | Justify, assess, defend, appraise, direct, argue, or manage the project. |

Table 10.7

## Psychomotor Domain: Educational Objectives for Development of Patient Skills[51,52]

| Category | Behavior | Examples of Activities and Demonstrations and Their Measurements | Examples of Verbs Used to Describe and Measure the Activity |
|---|---|---|---|
| Imitation | The learner's ability to copy the action of task or behavior from the therapist; to observe and replicate the task or behavior. | Watch the therapist and repeat the action, process, or activity. | Adhere, copy, follow, replicate, or repeat. |
| Manipulation | The learner's ability to reproduce the activity from the instruction or from memory. | Reproducing tasks or behaviors from written, verbal, or videotaped instruction. | Recreate, build, perform, execute, or implement. |
| Precision | The learner's ability to execute the skill consistently and without help. | Perform a skill or procedure with high quality, proficiency, and independence (from instruction or assistance); demonstrate the activity or task to the therapist or family (caregiver). | Demonstrate, complete, show, control, or achieve. |
| Articulation | The learner's ability to adapt the skill and integrate expertise into it to higher levels than regular standards. | Relate and combine associated skills or tasks to develop new and varied methods of performance. | Construct, solve, combine, coordinate, integrate, adapt, develop, formulate, modify, or master. |
| Naturalization | The learner's ability to automatically and routinely show mastery of the skill and also related skills at the highest level of performance. | Identify methods to approach and the necessary strategy to meet the highest level of performance. | Design, specify, manage, invent, or create. |

# Table 10.8

## Affective Domain: Educational Objectives for Development of Patient Attitude[51,52]

| Category | Behavior | Examples of Activities and Demonstrations and Their Measurements | Examples of Verbs Used to Describe and Measure the Activity |
|---|---|---|---|
| Accept (Receive) | The learner is open to the learning experience and willing to receive it. | Listens to the instructor (therapist); takes interest in the learning session; makes time for the learning experience; shows up for the therapy session; takes part in the therapy session. | Ask, listen, attend, discuss, acknowledge, follow, read, do, feel, or hear. |
| Respond | The learner actively participates and reacts to the learning experience. | Participates in group discussion; demonstrates active participation in learning activities; shows interest in outcomes; shows enthusiasm for tasks; questions ideas; suggests interpretation. | React, respond, seek, clarify, provide examples, contribute, perform, question, or cite. |
| Value | The learner attaches values to learning and expresses personal opinions. | Decides on relevance of ideas and experiences; accepts or commits to a particular task or skill. | Dispute, challenge, confront, critique, justify, or persuade. |
| Organize or conceptualize values | The learner resolves internal conflicts and develops a value system in regard to the learning experience. | Quantifies and qualifies personal views; states personal position and reasons; states beliefs. | Build, develop, formulate, defend, modify, relate, prioritize, reconcile, contrast, or compare. |
| Internalize or characterize values | The learner adopts the belief system and philosophy of the learning experience. | Self-reliant; behavior is consistent with personal value set. | Act, display, influence, solve, or practice. |

225

(conceptualizing and internalizing), may become impossible to accomplish in patient teaching. Internalizing the values is generally a long process and difficult to attain for everyone. When a person internalizes a learned behavior, he or she is able to add to his or her personal morals a new set of beliefs, attitudes, and values. Psychomotor internalization is easier to accomplish, because after the person has learned the skill, he or she will make use of it from then on. For affective internalization to occur, the individual has to show self-reliance, cooperate in group activities, use an objective approach in problem solving, and revise changes to behavior in light of new evidence of learning.

In classroom teaching, measurable student outcomes that require higher levels of expertise also require more sophisticated teaching and assessment techniques.[52] Nevertheless, for patient education, Bloom's taxonomy is a convenient way to describe the degree to which therapists want their patients to understand and use concepts, to demonstrate particular skills, and to have their values, attitudes, and interests affected. Basic knowledge of the taxonomy may prove helpful in rehabilitative interventions for better patient teaching and learning. Furthermore, the main goal of Bloom's taxonomy is to motivate therapists to focus their teaching on all three domains and as a result create a more holistic form of patient education.

# ADULT LEARNING AND PATIENT EDUCATION

## Objectives

After completing Chapter 11, the reader will be able to:

- Compare and contrast pedagogy and andragogy models of instruction.
- Implement learning activities in rehabilitation using principles of andragogy.
- Identify all elements of adult learning including the four critical variables of motivation, reinforcement, retention, and transference.
- List the characteristics of the brain-dominance theory of learning preference.
- Discuss elements of active and reflective learning in adults.

## Andragogy and Patient Education

The word *pedagogy* derives from the Latin word for education. Generally, the word *pedagogy* refers to the science or theory of educating, including the actual instructional operations. However, when discussing educational theories, the term *pedagogy* specifically refers to instructional methods for children.[53] The contemporary educational system uses the terms *andragogy* or *critical pedagogy* to describe adult education. Pedagogy flourished during the Middle Ages, whereas andragogy started in the 1800s and expanded in the 20th century. Pedagogical instruction began in the monastic schools of Europe, when young boys were sent to the monasteries to learn from the monks.[53] The Middle-Ages pedagogical model required these children to become obedient, faithful, and efficient servants of the church.[53] Later the tradition of pedagogy spread to the secular schools of Europe and the United States.

In the pedagogical model, the teacher has full responsibility for making decisions about what will be learned, how it will be learned, when it will be learned, and whether the material has been learned.[53] Pedagogy is a teacher-centered style of teaching, placing the student in a submissive role requiring obedience to the teacher's instructions. It is based on the assumption that learners need to know only what the teacher teaches them. The result is a teaching and learning situation that promotes dependency on the instructor.[53] In pedagogy, the mode of transmitting knowledge is through description of facts. This is called fact-based lecturing.[53,54] Additionally, learning is compulsory and tends to disappear shortly after instruction. In the past, in the United States, the pedagogical model of learning was applied equally to children and adults. However, educators realized that as adults mature, they become increasingly independent and responsible for their own actions.[54] Adults resent pedagogy because they are motivated to learn by a sincere desire to solve immediate problems in their lives.[54] Furthermore, adults have an increasing need to be self-directing in their teaching and learning approach.[54]

## DESCRIPTION OF KNOWLES'S ANDRAGOGY

Andragogy first appeared as an educational term in Germany in the 1800s.[53] In the United States, andragogy was defined as the art and science of helping adults learn; however, the meaning of the term enlarged due to Malcolm Knowles's writings (**Table 11.1**).[53,54] Currently, in the 21st century, the term defines an alternative to pedagogy and refers to learner-focused education for people of all ages. Knowles himself stated that four of andragogy's five key assumptions apply equally to adults and children.[53] Knowles's adult learning theory includes four significant hypotheses regarding andragogical teaching: (1) informing the learner why the information is important to learn, (2) showing the learner how to self-direct through the information, (3) relating the topic to the learner's experience, and (4) taking into consideration the fact that people will not learn until they are ready and motivated to learn.[53,54] Knowles's fifth assumption is also important for adult learning because it requires the teacher to help the learner overcome behaviors, beliefs, and inhibitions about the learning process.[53,54]

Knowles's andragogy model of learning is learner-centered. The focus of learning is on application of knowledge and the development of competency in skills needed at that time.[54] The role of the teacher is as a facilitator of learning and a resource to the learner. The adult learner takes total responsibility for his or her education. Each style of teaching is effective in andragogy.[54] At times, the instructor should take control of the learning situation and work to ensure that the learner has a solid base of knowledge for future use. At other times, learners are encouraged and allowed to assess their needs and direct or redirect their learning.

| Table 11.1 | |
|---|---|
| **Summary of Knowles's Adult Learning Theory[53,54]** | |
| Adult learners are independent and self-directed in the learning process. For this reason, the role of the instructor is to engage the learner in a process of inquiry, decision making, and analysis. | |
| Adult learners have a great deal of experience that helps them to learn. Considering the adult's vast experience, the role of the instructor is to plan active participation practices such as discussions and active problem-solving exercises. | |
| Adult learners appreciate learning that incorporates the demands of their daily life. Any previous experience, including life experiences, augment the process of learning. Training activities should be based on information that can easily relate to their daily life. | |
| Adult learners are interested mostly in immediate problem-centered approaches as compared to subject-centered approaches. Life- or work-related situations are more appropriate for learning than theoretical approaches. | |
| Adult learners are motivated to learn more by internal drives than by external ones. They are ready to immediately correct problems related to their determination based on their intrinsic motivation to learn. | |

# Adult Teaching and Learning Applied to Physical and Occupational Rehabilitation

Adults pursue learning throughout their life. There are varied reasons for adults' lifelong desire to learn, as discussed in the next section.

## REASONS ADULTS LEARN

Basically, three categories describe the general orientation of adults toward continuing education or lifelong learning. The first category is the *goal-oriented adult learner*. These learners engage in educational endeavors to accomplish clear and identifiable objectives.[55] Continuing education for the goal-oriented learner is episodic and occurs as a recurring pattern throughout their lives as they realize the need to expand their knowledge and skills.[56] Adults who attend night courses or professional workshops do so to build their expertise in a particular subject or for advancement in their professional or personal lives.

The second category is the *activity-oriented adult learner*. These learners select educational activities primarily to meet social needs.[55] The learning of content is secondary to their need for human contact. The activity-oriented learner has a desire to be around other people and communicate with them regarding similar circumstances such as parenting, divorce, retirement, or widowhood.[55] As a result, the learner may choose to participate in support groups, special-interest groups, or self-help groups, or attend academic classes because of an interest in a particular topic being offered. The learner's drive is typically to alleviate social isolation or loneliness.

The third and last category is the *learning-oriented adult learner*. These learners view themselves as perpetual students who seek knowledge because of their intrinsic need for more knowledge.[55] Learning-oriented learners are active learners all of their lives and tend to join groups, classes, or organizations with the anticipation that the experience will be educational and personally rewarding.[56]

In most cases, all three categories of learners initiate the learning experience for themselves.[55] As a result, when planning educational activities for adults, it is important to determine their main reasons for being involved in the learning process. It is beneficial for the therapist as the educator to understand the purpose and expectations of the individuals who participate in the educational programs in the clinical settings or health education. In that way, the therapist can best serve learners in the role as facilitator for referral or resource information.

The goal-oriented and activity-oriented learners are likely to engage in the learning process mostly during life-changing events such as a new job, marriage, divorce, promotion, losing a loved one, moving to a new city, or being ill.[56] The more life change events an adult learner encounters, the more likely they will seek out learning and become motivated. From that perspective, in health care, patients will seek (many times on their own) to learn everything that triggered their illness as a life-changing event. They are particularly willing to engage in learning experiences if the knowledge will help them cope with the transition. Rehabilitation providers and professionals, as educators, should be aware of this process, understanding that their patients' learning becomes a means to an end, and not an end in itself. For the learning-oriented adult learner, other motivators to engage in learning experiences are to increase or maintain self-esteem and also for enjoyment.

## CRITICAL ELEMENTS OF THE ADULT TEACHING AND LEARNING PROCESS

Adults bring to a learning situation a background of experience that is a rich resource for themselves and for others.[55] As a result, using various teaching and learning techniques such as discussions, case studies, problem solving, or life experiences can provide learners with knowledge from which they can learn by analyzing them. The instructional approach must expand and refine prior knowledge of the adult learner by connecting it with the new information and making the instruction relevant to important tasks in the adult's life.[55] Therapists should know that adult learning is a continuous process throughout an individual's life. Learning results from stimulation of the senses. In some individuals, one sense is used more than others to learn or recall information. Consequently, educators should present materials that stimulate as many senses as possible to increase their teaching success. The critical elements of teaching and learning for adults include motivation, feedback and reinforcement, retention, and transference of knowledge (**Table 11.2**).[55]

In addition to the critical elements of the teaching and learning process, there are other important variables in adult education: (1) curriculum design, (2) learning environment, and (3) assessment of learning. Motivation is essential to help the learner recognize the need for the information.[55] To increase the learner's motivation, the educator must establish a rapport with the learner and prepare him or her for learning. This can be done by using a friendly and open atmosphere, showing sincere concern for the learner, and setting an appropriate level of difficulty to challenge the learner but not so high that they become frustrated by information overload.

In physical and occupational rehabilitation, the majority of patients are autonomous and self-directed adult learners. They need to be free to direct themselves. Therapists must actively engage them in the learning process and serve as facilitators. Andragogical principles are important for patient education because the patients as learners accumulate a foundation of life experiences and knowledge that need to be connected to the new learning.[55] For this reason, the therapist as the facilitator should draw out the patient's experience and knowledge of a particular relevant health care and rehabilitation topic. The therapist must relate rehabilitation concepts to the patient's life events and recognize the value of experience in the teaching and learning process. The therapist should use a patient-centered care approach and allow the patient to assume responsibility for his or her own learning goals. Because adults are goal oriented, the therapist needs, together with the patient, to clearly define and organize educational goals related to the rehabilitation plan of care. The therapist's teaching role is to provide information guiding and facilitating the patient's active learning and involvement toward the goals. Additionally, the therapist must show the patient how the information will help them attain his or her goals. This process must take place in the initial examination and evaluation of the patient.

| Table 11.2 | |
|---|---|
| ***Critical Elements of Adult Teaching and Learning*[55]** | |
| Learner motivation. | |
| Feedback and reinforcement of learning. | |
| Retention of information. | |
| Transference of knowledge. | |

## SOURCES OF MOTIVATION FOR ADULT TEACHING AND LEARNING

The main barrier in adult patient education is the teacher's ability to motivate the learner. Understanding the sources of motivation can increase the teacher's ability to help enhance the student's incentive to learn. Many factors serve as a source of motivation for the adult learner; however, six of these factors seem to be particularly important in relation to patient teaching and learning. The six elements that can increase the adult's learning interest are social relationships, external expectations, social welfare, personal advancement, escape or stimulation, and cognitive interest.[56]

As a motivating factor, *social relationships* have to do with making new friends and meeting the need for associations and friendships.[56] The patient as the learner needs to feel that the therapist is a new friend or associate who could help them to achieve better health. In physical and occupational therapy, this can be accomplished by establishing a therapeutic partnership with the patient, helping the patient actively engage in the teaching and learning process to achieve his or her therapeutic goals.

*External expectations* for the learner involve complying with instructions to fulfill the expectations or recommendations from someone with authority.[56] Health care providers and professionals are considered experts in their field, asking patients as learners to comply with their recommendations or instructions. The therapist as the teacher needs to demonstrate expertise not only in applying physical and occupational therapy interventions, but also in effectively using instructional methods during patient teaching and learning.

*Social welfare*, as a source of motivation for learning, can improve a patient's ability to participate in community activities or go back to work.[56] In physical and occupational therapy, many adult patients want to be able to return to their work or their hobbies as soon as possible. The therapist needs to be able to refer the patients to organizations that provide social support. In addition, patient teaching must include prevention and health promotion topics to ensure the patient's well-being in the community.

Motivation to increase a patient's *personal advancement* to a higher status may apply to patient education of adults who want to return to activities or tasks. In physical and occupational therapy, these individuals, especially athletes, make a great effort to achieve the same high performance of activities or tasks as before hospitalization or surgery. As an example, when working with athletes recovering from orthopedic surgeries, the therapist should use patient education materials regarding safety instructions for caution with rehabilitative interventions. For personal advancement, these patients might actually injure themselves trying to return to playing sports sooner than required.

As another form of motivation, *escape or stimulation* also may affect rehabilitation interventions. Some individuals may find learning an exercise program stimulating. Also, in acute care rehabilitation, a patient may be encouraged to learn skills and "escape" by leaving the hospital sooner and going home to family and friends. Generally patients are strongly motivated to leave the hospital and return to their prior activities. Patients may also be motivated to learn by *cognitive interest*, seeking to understand certain rehabilitation interventions and reasoning beyond them. Therapists as educators should always explain to the patient the rationale of their teaching.

## FEEDBACK AND REINFORCEMENT IN ADULT TEACHING AND LEARNING

Adult patients learn at different rates and degrees of involvement.[55] Many patients are nervous and anxious during the learning process because they are faced with a new learning situation. In clinical settings, adult learners may show extreme anxiety and hesitation when dealing with new information considering their impairments, functional limitations, disabilities, age, cognitive level, education, and other variables. Positive reinforcement by the therapist as the instructor can enhance learning, as can proper timing of the instruction.

Feedback and reinforcement are two important concepts in adult teaching and learning. Feedback is providing learners with information about their responses.[55] Reinforcement means to be able to cause a specific response again.[55] The learner always needs specific knowledge of their learning results (feedback) and reward for their learning. The feedback must be specific and not general. In classroom teaching, feedback is considered to be external whereas reinforcement can be internally generated by the learner or externally generated by the teacher.[55,56] External reinforcement is motivational.[55] The reward for learning has to be directly related to the learner's interest in the subject or topic. Adults want to understand the benefits of learning in order to encourage themselves even more to learn the subject. Reinforcement is necessary in the teaching and learning process to correct modes of behavior and performance.[55,56] It should be used on a frequent and regular basis early in the learning process to help learners retain what they have learned.[55,56] Positive reinforcement is typically used when teaching new skills because it reinforces good or positive behavior.[56] Negative reinforcement also is normally used by the teacher when teaching new skills or information.[56] The result of negative reinforcement is extinction.[56] The instructor uses negative reinforcement until the undesirable behavior disappears or it becomes extinct. After the student has learned the necessary material, the reinforcement should be used only to maintain consistent, positive behavior.[56]

## RETENTION AND TRANSFERENCE IN ADULT TEACHING AND LEARNING

The amount of retention in the learning process is affected by the degree of original learning.[56] If the student did not initially learn the material well, he or she will not retain it well either. Retention by the participants is also directly affected by their amount of practice during the learning process.[56] Retention and application of the learned material should be emphasized by the instructor. After the learner demonstrates correct performance, he or she should be urged to immediately practice to maintain the desired (correct) performance.[56] Distributed practice is similar to intermittent reinforcement. Distributed practice takes place when the student distributes his or her efforts and studies the material immediately after each lecture to keep up with the new information; this is opposite to "cramming," when the student waits until one day prior to the exam to study all the material that was taught over the preceding weeks.

Transfer of learning is the learner's ability to use the information taught in the course in a new setting.[56] Transference of information, similar to reinforcement, can be positive and negative. Positive transference occurs when the learner uses the behavior taught during the educational process.[56] Negative transference occurs when the learner conforms to the teacher's instructions and does not use adverse behavior (such as those recommended for prevention).[56] This results in a positive outcome. During transference, four factors are responsible for the learner successfully transferring the information: association, similarity, degree of original learning, and critical attribute element (**Table 11.3**).[56]

## CURRICULUM DESIGN FOR ADULT TEACHING AND LEARNING

When designing a curriculum for adult learning, the therapist should consider that learners prefer single concept or single theory classes that focus on the application of information to relevant problems.[56] They generally do not like survey classes that consist of summaries of very broad topics.[56] As they become older, adults need to be able to integrate new ideas or concepts with the material they already know. Information in conflict with already known data will be integrated more slowly. Also, concepts that have little theoretical overlap (and are too abstract) in regard to what learners already know are acquired slowly. The best curriculum will integrate new learning with previously learned concepts.[56]

| Table 11.3 | *Learning Factors During Transference*[56] | |
|---|---|
| Association | When participants associate the new information with material that they already know. As a result, patient teaching and learning must relate to daily activities/exercises and other information they already know. |
| Similarity | When the information is similar to material the learner already knew. Similarity helps the learner revisit a logical framework. As a result, patient teaching and learning must connect the information with similar material the patient knows so that the patient can place the information in a logical framework. |
| Degree of original learning | When the learner's degree of original learning is high and accurate. The more accurate the original learning, the better the transference. As a result, attention must be given to the accuracy of information communicated to the patient the first time. |
| Critical attribute element | When the information learned contains elements that are critical or beneficial to the learner to perform a task. As a result, patient teaching and learning must always connect the information to the patient's gains. |

Additionally, adult learners tend to compensate for being slower in some psychomotor tasks by being more accurate and making fewer trial-and-error ventures. They will have the propensity to take errors personally, which can negatively affect their self-esteem.[56] For this reason, adults will apply tried-and-true solutions and take fewer risks.[56] The therapist should understand this aspect of learning and not rush patients to complete a task.

Another curriculum issue to consider is that new information may be in concert or in conflict with the adult learner.[56] In many situations, particularly in health care, patient teaching and learning may be designed to effect a change in the patient's behavior as well as in their belief and value systems. Such a concept needs to be explained to the patient from different perspectives in order to appeal to him or her for future use. For example, teaching an adult who recently had a heart attack to stop smoking (when they have smoked for 30 years) may require an educational curriculum that is explained and justified from a variety of viewpoints. Media such as books, programmed instruction and television, and Internet information also can be helpful in the teaching curriculum. For example, with programmed instruction, the health care provider (as the teacher) gives the patient (as the learner) self-teaching materials to about behavioral modifications (such as to stop smoking). This instruction can be a textbook, a video, or other form of data that presents the information in a logical, step-by-step sequence. Programmed instruction allows the patient to learn the information at home and to answer questions at his or her own rate. Also, the patient can check his or her own answers to see if they are correct or not. When returning to the health care provider, the patient will be given a question to test his or her understanding. If the patient's answer is correct, the patient can progress to another step in the behavioral modification program. If the answer is incorrect, the health care provider must provide the patient with additional information.

In addition, straightforward how-to information is the preferred content orientation for adults. Adults' primary motivation for beginning a learning project is their need for being able to apply the information and how-to material.[53] Furthermore, adults showing self-direction does not mean they are isolated; for example, self-directed projects for adults may involve 10 other individuals as resources, guides, and encouragers. Even for the self-professed, self-directed learner, lectures and short seminars get positive ratings, primarily when these educational events are offered face-to-face or through one-on-one expert instruction.

## THE LEARNING ENVIRONMENT FOR ADULT TEACHING AND LEARNING

The learning environment must be physically and psychologically comfortable for learners, especially for adult learners (**Table 11.4**).[56] Long lectures and long periods of sitting without practice opportunities cause frustration and boredom. Also, in classroom situations, adults experienced self-esteem and ego problems when asked to try a new behavior in front of peers and cohorts.[57] For this reason, many patients may learn better when using a one-on-one practice of new skills or tasks.[57] Dialogues with the instructor and peers are considered the best method of learning for adults.[57] The therapist as the educator should be a facilitator concentrating on open-ended questions to draw on relevant patient

| Table 11.4 | ***Summary of Teaching and Learning Concepts for Adults[55–57]*** |
|---|---|

Adults have experience and a large and varied supply of information. The teacher needs to tap into their experience and provide opportunities for dialogue. The learner can become a teaching and learning resource for the instructor.

Adults have established values, beliefs, and opinions. The teacher needs to show respect for differing beliefs, religions, value systems, and lifestyles.

Adults have different styles and paces of learning. The teacher should employ a variety of teaching strategies using auditory, visual, tactile, and participatory teaching methods.

Adults relate new knowledge and information to previously learned information and experiences. The teacher should use single concepts and focus on application of concepts to relevant practical situations. Frequent summarizing increases retention and recall of information.

Adults have pride and a deep need for self-direction. The teacher should support the learners as individuals, allowing them to admit confusion, ignorance, biases, fears, and different opinions. For self-direction, engage learners in a process of mutual inquiry.

Adults tend to have a problem-centered orientation to learning. The teacher, especially in health care, should emphasize problem-centered learning by applying the new information to current problems and situations. Because adults bring preconceived thoughts and feelings to the learning experience, assessing the level of these traits and the student's readiness to learn must be included in each educational session.

knowledge and experience. The patient must be actively participating in the learning process, depending on the therapist's feedback for skill practices. The therapist is also dependent on the patient's feedback in regard to curriculum and in-class performance.

In regard to teaching and learning designs and styles, skill training tasks for adults are best taught using behavioral approaches whereas personal-growth subjects may benefit from humanistic concepts.[55,56] Also, an eclectic approach rather than a single theory of learning is recommended when matching instruction to learning tasks.[55]

The adult learner always needs to define the relationship between old and new information.[55] This aspect of learning can be achieved only through discussions and reflection. For example, the therapist as the instructor can use small group discussions with the patient and the patient's family (or caregiver). This will increase and deepen the learning process, involving long-term memory practices for permanent learning to occur. Practicing and remembering the information soon after it is processed increases learning retention.[57] Therefore, it is important to provide opportunities for review and remembering by means of activities, discussions, and practice. For example, over a period of 3 days, learning retention is characterized as the following: 10% of what the learner read, 20% of what the learner heard, 30% of what the learner saw, 50% of what the learner saw and heard, 70% of what the learner said (repeating the information), and 90% of what the learner said and did (repeating orally the information and also working out the problem or practicing the information either by discussions, applications, or writings).[5]

Health care providers involved in educating adults need to convey a desire to connect with the learner. They should provide challenges to the learner without causing frustration. Also, feedback and positive reinforcement must be offered at all times. For example, in women's health, the physical therapist may encounter patients who have urinary incontinence. If the patient is concerned about how urinary incontinence is affecting her lifestyle she may be motivated to learn to use the necessary exercises to correct it. Because the learner's past education experiences and information are important, the therapist may ask the patient whether her family or friends have encountered continence problems and if they did any exercises for them. Past educational experience may positively affect or cause bias in a patient's perception about how education will occur. At this time, the therapist can address any erroneous or preconceived ideas and emphasize new beliefs. Physical and occupational therapy support patient-centered care and also patient-centered education that first considers each patient's needs and perspectives of learning. For this learner to completely participate in the learning process and have control over the type of learning and its direction, the therapist must assess the patient's learning needs such as her understanding of urinary incontinence, her expectations for interventions, and her level of motivation to learn and practice the home exercise program.

As another example, when evaluating the learning needs of older adult patients with chronic obstructive pulmonary disease (COPD), most patients prefer learning new information directly from the health care provider by talking to "someone who knows."[58(p.5)] Also, the first learning preference seems to be the auditory, interactive method of learning, indicating that older adult patients learn in an environment that allows them to interact with the educator.[58] The second learning preference is watching a videotape.[58] This is visual learning that could be also considered interaction with the instructor that is supplemented by use of a video or other visual resource.

In regard to patient teaching and learning in acute care, some health care providers may wrongly assume that acutely ill patients do not want education or are unable to identify their learning needs. However, acutely ill patients are actually able to prioritize and are very interested to learn, considering their learning preferences. When teaching patients with COPD, the majority of patients and health care providers identify survival skills as patients' learning needs.[58] These survival skills are related to topics such as methods to improve taking medications, learning emergency signals to be able to ask for help, and ways to avoid or manage shortness of breath.[58] Generally, in physical and occupational rehabilitation, patients' main learning needs may be related to their safety and methods to manage their diseases/ disorders. It is important that rehabilitation providers as educators always assess each patient's unique learning needs prior to initiating patient education.

## ASSESSMENT OF ADULT TEACHING AND LEARNING

Another aspect of adult patient education is to assess the patient's progress or success at the completion of learning. One of the preferred adult evaluation methods is self-evaluation.[57] For patient self-evaluation, the therapist as the educator can provide frequent patient self-checks and practice training. During assessment of patient teaching and learning, the therapist and the patient need to be open-minded and assign enough time for appraisal. This engages the learner in the assessment and also facilitates better transfer of knowledge. Additionally, learners respond more enthusiastically to teachers who demonstrate a genuine interest and concern for them. The patient as the learner needs the opportunity to perform the skill with as little interference from the teacher as possible while also considering his or her safety during the performance. As learning progresses, the patient needs as little assistance as possible, giving him or her the opportunity to perform the skill independently. The patient's progression from one step to another depends on the patient's self-evaluation and comfort level. Nevertheless, a patient reporting comfort with performing a new skill may need closer monitoring to assure that his or her confidence is backed up by appropriate skill.

In addition, patient education for adult learners should consider the learner's level of concentration. Usually, people can consciously think about only one item at a time. Especially with adult teaching and learning, the therapist must provide an environment that helps learners concentrate on their learning tasks.[57] The content, format, and sequence of teaching and learning experiences must be able to compete with challenging environmental interferences.[57] Also, the learner needs to define the relationship between old and new information.[57] This can increase and deepen the learning process, involving long-term memory practices that allow permanent learning to occur.[57] Practicing remembering the information soon after it is processed increases learning retention.

# *Teaching and Learning Preferences for Adults*

All the learning theories discussed in this section are trying to positively influence various learning styles. When learning theories are applied to teaching and learning, the teacher must try to consider students' learning styles or preferences during the educational experiences. This classroom concept is important in patient teaching and learning. Usually, learning is more productive when teachers take different learning styles into account.[59] In classroom teaching, matching instruction to every learner's style and needs is very difficult in terms of administrative matters such as having a different teacher for each learning style or acquiring various classrooms to accommodate each student's learning preference. However, in clinical settings, when working with one patient or a small group of patients, accommodating different learning styles may not be a major problem. Even in the classroom, educators are encouraged to provide a variety of learning experiences to accommodate the various learning styles. In this way, all students will have at least some activities that appeal to them based on their learning styles and preferences.

## VISUAL-AUDITORY-KINESTHETIC ADULT LEARNING PREFERENCE

In educational settings, the visual-auditory-kinesthetic (VAK) learning theory seems to be the main educational tool used in the classroom.[59] The reason for utilizing the VAK most often may be its practical mode of assessing it by asking the learner about ways they receive information the most. These can be through visual (such as sights, pictures, or diagrams), auditory (such as sounds or words), or kinesthetic (such as touch, taste, or smell). As mentioned in Chapter 10 regarding the VAK, visual learners, who constitute the highest percentage of American learners, prefer mostly visual learning resources.[59] The visual learning materials that enhance the adult teaching and learning process may include posters, a chalkboard, drawings, pictures, graphs, diagrams, films, transparencies, digital video discs (DVDs) or videotapes, and computer programs if available. Visual learners also prefer to have written assignments and have the teacher use as many visual information materials as possible.[59]

Auditory learners need lectures, discussions, small group talks, compact discs (CDs), and audiotapes. The teacher should give precise oral directions and explanations. This includes orally setting tasks, giving assignments, discussing resources, reviewing progress, and any other activity requiring auditory comprehension and processing.[59]

Kinesthetic learners prefer to learn from hands-on experience. Teachers should have manipulative and three-dimensional materials that are touchable and moveable and should provide real models and factual, hands-on experiences.[59] Learners must be encouraged to plan, demonstrate, report, and evaluate.

## BRAIN-DOMINANCE THEORY OF ADULT LEARNING PREFERENCE

The brain-dominance theory explains that individuals use different sides of the brain to process different kinds of information.[60] As a whole, people use both sides of their brains, but most individuals tend to prefer learning strategies associated with one side or the other.[60] Such individuals are considered to be left-brain dominant or right-brain dominant, although no person is totally left-brain or right-brain dominant. Some people have about even preferences and are considered to have bilateral dominance. Brain preferences develop early in life and become more pronounced as people grow older. There is no intellectual status or stigma associated with using the right or the left side of the brain.[60] The differences remain related to the different functions of the hemispheres. The degree of specialization varies according to task, and each person has a range for each set of functions. In addition, individuals have culturally conditioned preferences for certain cognitive strategies.

The left side of the brain processes verbal, abstract, analytical information in a linear, sequential manner.[60] It also evaluates differences and contrasts of information, is able to see small signs that represent the whole, and concerns itself with reasoning abilities such as mathematics and language. The left-hemisphere adult learner is often called the linear or analytical learner.[60] The characteristics of the left hemisphere of the brain are verbal, rational, and realistic thought processes. For linear learning, the learner prefers to process information line by line or in a sequence, whereas for analytical learning, the preference is to evaluate details and facts logically.[60] The left-hemisphere learner is usually more logical, organized, and disciplined. Learners want to have a plan for learning, look at details, and make decisions based on facts. For individuals using mostly the left brain, theoretical details are interesting and important.[60] These learners can apply new information quickly and prefer to work alone. In addition, they tend to be more time-oriented and competitive. For patients using mostly the left hemisphere for learning, patient education can emphasize the discovery approach, encouraging learners to find methods to solve problems. New concepts and procedures could be taught by logical explanation and analytical exploration.

In physical and occupational therapy for left-hemisphere learning preference, the therapist can use charts, graphs, tables, handouts, and transparencies to help the learning process. The learning can take place in a functional, organized, and tidy task-oriented environment.[60] The therapist as the educator is expected to have a formal (business-like) relationship with the patient. The patient as the learner must consider the therapist an authority in the rehabilitation area to accept their teaching and learning concepts. The left-hemisphere learner needs recognition of his or her learning achievement, emphasizing the fact that the student excelled at the task.[60]

An adult patient using mostly the left hemisphere for learning will try to always be on time for his or her therapy session and even arrive much earlier than scheduled.[60] The patient will not be very animated, using a few gestures and not much voice fluctuation. When learning something, the left-hemisphere-dominant individual would prefer to sit up and study.[60] He or she will also like to discuss the material with the therapist and ask questions. The new information will be processed from part to whole. To draw conclusions, the patient needs to take the pieces of information, line them up, and arrange them in a logical order. The therapist as the educator needs to explain to the patient each portion of information, allowing the patient to draw the logical conclusion.

In contrast, the right side of the brain handles nonverbal, concrete, and spatial information.[60] The right hemisphere is characterized by recognizing sequencing of symbols, objects, and events; appreciating music; and being responsible for the nonverbal, emotional, empathetic, witty, and humorous side of an individual.[60] The learner using mostly the right side of the brain looks at similarities in patterns forming a whole picture. The information is processed from whole to parts. The learner sees the whole picture first before the details. Right-hemisphere-dominant learners concern themselves with artistic abilities such as music and graphics.[60] They prefer learning to be informal, spontaneous, and creative. The learner makes learning decisions based on feelings and intuition. They need longer to assimilate the material and prefer to work with others. The right-hemisphere learner finds the theory behind the information interesting only after he or she has learned how to apply the new material.[60]

The physical and occupational therapist as the educator is expected to clearly state all concepts, principles, and procedures early during the teaching session, and make the new information very clear and understandable. The adult patient would select the learning steps without any obvious sequence, but instead based on what comes to mind at that moment. The patient decides things on the spur of the moment. The right-brain-dominant patient can be very emotional and have difficulty expressing him- or herself in words. The therapist should encourage the patient to write down and draw what his or her feelings and needs may be. When learning new information, it can also be retained easily if it is written down. The therapist needs to use creative and interesting ways to deliver the information. The role of the therapist is to guide the learner in how to problem-solve in a clear uncomplicated way, and step-by-step. The therapist may use simple graphs or charts and include plenty of explanations. The teaching and learning atmosphere must be friendly and relaxed without tension or pressure. Teaching should take place in a comfortable and attractive environment.

Patients using mostly right-brain dominance will not arrive on time for the therapy session if it is not important to them; however, they may arrive earlier to a theater performance or a choir recital because it is something they really enjoy.[60] The patients in this group will talk using many gestures. Their facial expression and voice may be very animated and entertaining. Adult learners with a right-hemisphere learning preference expect strong personal relationships with the teacher and recognition of their achievements.[60] This can include the therapist's personal expression of enjoyment.

## ACTIVE AND REFLECTIVE ADULT LEARNING PREFERENCES

Learners can have both active and reflective learning styles.[61] Active and reflective learning involves two complex mental processes called active experimentation and reflective observation.[61] Active experimentation is taking new information and discussing it with others or testing it as an experiment. Reflective observation is examining and manipulating new information introspectively.[61] Additionally, individuals who prefer active learning are considered extraverts while reflective learners are introverts.

Learners with an active learning style tend to retain and understand information best by acting on it.[61] In the classroom setting, active learners would not just listen and watch the teacher but question, argue, or brainstorm the material. Active learners prefer to work in groups and resent listening to lectures without doing something physical.[61] It is difficult for active learners to take notes during lectures because they want to jump in and experiment with the information. When teaching an active learner it is important to discuss and try to problem-solve the new information with the learner before allowing him or her to act on it.[61] The therapist as the educator should try to involve active learners in discussions and guide them to work in groups explaining and talking about the information with others. Also, the therapist can give the patients in a group a question to answer facilitating deliberations and practical solutions. Demonstrations and practices are effective with active learners, especially when family or friends are involved, which gives them the opportunity to interact with others.

Reflective learners prefer to work alone.[61] They like to think about the information quietly first, and only after that do they apply it. Reflective learners need time to think about the new material just learned.[61] When the information is abundant, the reflective learner compensates by memorizing the data without review and application. The therapist as the instructor needs to allow them to periodically read, think about the new material, formulate questions, and evaluate possible applications. Writing short summaries of the new information is also helpful for the learner to retain the material more effectively. Open-ended problems that call for analysis of a situation are also indicated.

Learners can express active and reflective learning style preferences in mild, moderate, and strong ways.[61] Every adult learner can be an active learner at one time and a reflective learner at another time.[61] Individual learners who always act before reflecting can throw themselves into untrained circumstances and cause themselves problems. Conversely, learners who spend too much time reflecting have difficulty completing tasks.[61] Usually a balance of the two is desirable.

## SEQUENTIAL AND GLOBAL ADULT LEARNING PREFERENCES

Other learning preferences in adults can be sequential and global. In classroom teaching, sequential learners understand the material in a linear way by following the information step-by-step in a logical sequence.[61] They may not fully understand the information as a whole, but are able to put the pieces together. In rehabilitation, the therapist should know that sequential learners "learn best when the material is presented in a steady progression of complexity and difficulty."[61(p.679)] The therapist should not jump around from topic to topic or skip steps in a procedure. Patients who are sequential learners can follow the material from simple to complex. For example, post lumbar surgery, teaching a patient to transfer from supine (face up) position to sitting following a sequence is the best solution for either sequential or global learner. The therapist should explain to the patient all necessary steps how to move from supine to side-lying and then to sitting taking into account surgical precautions. The sequential learner would readily follow the steps but may have difficulty understanding the procedure in its entirety.

Global learners prefer to learn in large jumps, by understanding the topics randomly and without any connections between them.[61] In the classroom setting, global learners need to see the "big picture" first before mastering the details. Many global learners, although being very creative, are aware of the drawbacks of their learning style.[61] They need help to understand how their learning process works to become more comfortable with it and less critical of themselves.[61]

Global learners need to be encouraged for their unique abilities and also shown how to reshape their learning experiences for better efficiency.[61] In rehabilitation, the therapist may need first to provide a global learner an overview of the entire procedure before explaining the necessary steps to perform such a course of action. With global learners, it is easier to reach them by first, establishing their main rehabilitation goals, and only after that, relate the goals with their prior experiences. As a result, the patient could have the opportunity to devise his or her own method to achieve the goals. For example, teaching a supine to sit transfer after lumbar surgery to a global learner, the patient will want to skip steps and get up immediately without taking safety requirements into consideration. However, the therapist as the teacher must applaud even if incorrect patient's "large-scale" solution and explain to the patient the necessary sequential steps to achieve the correct transfer.

# COGNITIVE/PSYCHOSOCIAL STAGES OF DEVELOPMENT AND PATIENT EDUCATION

## *Objectives*

After completing Chapter 12, the reader will be able to:

- Relate Piaget's and Erikson's stages of development to patient teaching and learning.
- Discuss the significance of teaching strategies to pediatric rehabilitation.
- Apply teaching and learning strategies to adolescents.
- Identify ageism as a barrier to the health care of older adults.
- List the differences between andragogy and gerogogy.
- Describe teaching and learning barriers related to visual and hearing impairments.
- Explain the role of independence and self-sufficiency in older adults' learning.
- Describe the importance of goal setting in patient education for older adults.

## *Stages of Development and the Importance of Patient Education*

Most learners have developed a preference for learning that is embedded in their childhood learning patterns. To understand and address teaching and learning, it is important to recognize the differences in the cognitive and psychosocial developments of an individual.

Two developmental theories identify the individual developmental stages and the necessary processes to progress through the stages. These theories are Jean Piaget's Stages of Cognitive Development and Erik Erikson's Stages of Psychosocial Development.[26,62,63] Piaget's cognitive theory of learning, discussed earlier in this section, is related to a child's development of the cognitive structures necessary for learning. Piaget's stages of sensorimotor, preoperational, concrete operational, and formal operational demonstrate that a child's cognitive structures increase in complexity with development, advancing from innate reflexes such as crying to highly complex mental activities such as analysis, synthesis, and evaluation.[26] Additionally, Piaget's learning hypothesis establishes that children learn best with other children because they are motivated by peer relationships and communication with the teacher and other members of the learning group.[26] The environment, physical setting, emotional atmosphere, and social norms also contribute to the child's learning. Erik Erikson believed the same as Piaget that children develop in a predetermined order; however, instead of focusing on cognitive development, Erikson was interested in a child's socialization and its effects on personality.[63]

## ERIKSON'S STAGES OF DEVELOPMENT

Erik Erikson, a German-born American psychoanalyst, was influenced by Sigmund Freud, the Austrian neurologist and psychiatrist who founded the psychoanalytic school of psychology.[62,63] Erikson explored three aspects of identity from birth to death, the ego (self), the personal, and the social/cultural. Erikson's theory has eight distinct stages of development, each with two possible outcomes. Positive completion of each stage in a timely manner results in a healthy personality and successful learning and interaction in society.[62] Disappointment and dissatisfaction in completion of each stage can result in a reduced ability to advance to further stages, and an unhealthy personality that influences the individual's integration in society. Nevertheless, Erikson's stages can successfully be resolved at a later time. Erik Erikson's psychosocial theory of development also considers the impact of external factors, parents, and society on personality development from childhood to adulthood.[62] According to Erikson, every person must pass through eight interrelated stages representing an individual's entire life cycle (**Table 12.1**).[62,63]

Erikson's first stage is the period from birth through 18 months of age.[62] The psychosocial crisis at this time is basic trust versus mistrust.[62] Developing trust is the first task of the child's personality. The child will become anxious when the mother or father is not present. The child needs to be nurtured and loved to develop trust, security, and optimism. When the child is handled improperly, she or he will become insecure and mistrustful.[62] Psychologically, the balance of trust with mistrust depends mostly on the quality of the maternal relationship.[63] Erikson proposed that the concept of trust versus mistrust is present throughout an individual's entire life.[62] When the concept is not addressed properly at its introduction, during infancy, the individual may be negatively affected and never fully immerse him- or herself in the world.[62] As an example, the individual will not be able to form a long-lasting relationship with other people. If the individual learned, understood, or improperly

| Table 12.1 | |
| --- | --- |
| **Erikson's Eight Stages of Development[62,63]** | |
| Infant | Basic trust versus mistrust. |
| Toddler | Autonomy versus shame. |
| Preschooler | Initiative versus guilt. |
| School-age child | Industry versus inferiority. |
| Adolescent | Identity versus role confusion. |
| Young adult | Intimacy versus isolation. |
| Middle-age adult | Generativity versus stagnation. |
| Older adult | Integrity versus despair. |

used the concept of trust versus mistrust, he or she will not be able to learn and mature into a fully developed person.

Erikson's second stage of development starts around 18 months and lasts until 3 years of age.[62] The psychosocial crisis at this time is the child developing autonomy versus shame.[62] During this age, the child as a toddler discovers that he or she is a separate individual and not attached anymore to the primary caregiver. The child wants autonomy to form his or her own identity.[62] The child has the determination to become independent. This can cause a power struggle between the parents and the child. When handled properly, given reasonable choices and appropriate guidance, the child emerges from this stage happy, confident, and proud. When denied independence, the child will desire to manipulate and discriminate.[63]

Erikson's third stage of development is the period from 3 years old to 6 years old.[62] The psychosocial crisis of this stage is initiative versus guilt.[62] The child is learning to master the world around him or her, planning and initiating tasks. During this stage of taking initiatives, the child learns by imagining, broadening his or her skills through fantasy play, cooperating with others, and leading or following others. The child, as a preschooler, prepares for leadership and goal achievement. Because the child can be aggressive and take risks, the parents need to allow some guilt to keep a healthy balance between self-control and independence.[63] If too much guilt is involved, however, the child will become fearful, restricted in imagination, and continually dependent on adults.[63] At this stage, the importance of responsibility is dominant in the child's relationship with her or his parents.

Providing chores and tasks for the child will strengthen the preschooler's independence, self-efficacy, and confidence.

Erikson's fourth developmental stage starts around 7 years of age and lasts until 12 years of age.[62] The psychosocial crisis of the fourth stage is industry versus inferiority.[62] In this period, the child learns to master more formal skills of life such as relating with peers according to certain rules, progressing to more elaborate teamwork such as playing sports, and learning reading, arithmetic, and social studies. The child must be encouraged to be productive in his or her tasks and be able to realize that good work requires responsibility, sharing, and cooperation with others. Some children will express their independence by being disobedient and rebellious. The parents need to promote the child's successful achievements by teaching self-esteem and resilience.[63] A balance must be kept between too little and too much success. Too little success will develop a sense of inferiority and too much success will lead to narrow skills or talents, rushing the child into adulthood.

The fifth developmental stage created by Erikson starts chronologically from around adolescence until about 18 years old.[62] During this period, the child struggles to define and find her or his own identity. In this phase, the psychosocial crisis is characterized by identity versus role confusion.[62] The adolescent makes great efforts to fit in with peers and to develop a sense of morality and right and wrong. At this stage, some adolescents attempt to delay entrance to adulthood and withdraw from responsibilities.[63] Those who are not successful finding affiliation and devotion to ideals, causes, and friends tend to experience role confusion and upheaval.

The sixth period of development in Erikson's developmental stages represents the young adult stage.[62] It starts around 19 and terminates around 35 years of age. The psychosocial crisis described by Erikson is intimacy versus isolation.[62] At this young adult stage, the role confusion period is ending, and individuals tend to seek companionship and love. Young adults are in search of a close personal relationship and start to prepare themselves for intimacy. The individuals need to learn that a balance between intimacy and isolation allows love to happen. Young adults' personalities need to be prepared for rejection and not to culminate in despair and isolation.[63] Satisfying relationships end up in marriage and family. For the young adults in this developmental phase, the most significant roles are as marital partners and friends.

The last two stages described by Erikson as the middle-aged adult and the older adult represent psychosocial crises of generativity versus stagnation and integrity versus despair, respectively.[62] The middle-aged adult starts around 35 years of age and culminates at approximately 55 to 65 years of age.[62] Career, work, and family are the most important proceedings at this time. At this phase, individuals take greater responsibility and control, attempting to produce or generate something meaningful for society, and especially for the next generation. Usually socially valued work and disciplines are expressions of generativity.[63] Major life changes such as children leaving the household or career moves may occur. Some people struggle to find more noteworthy functions in their personal lives, such as being affiliated with a religious organization or helping in the community.

During the older adult stage, from approximately 55 to 65 years old until the end of life, the individual needs to reflect on their whole life.[62] The development of the person continues in terms of evaluating his or her own mortality, making mistakes and asking forgiveness, having integrity and readiness, and dealing with whatever the remaining life events bring.[62] A positive outcome of this psychosocial crisis is achieved if the individual gains a sense of fulfillment about life and a sense of unity within him- or herself and others.[62] After reflection, the older adult can accept death with a sense of integrity and accomplishment. A negative outcome of the older adult crisis will cause the individual despair and fear of death.

In physical and occupational therapy, Erikson's developmental stages are important for patient teaching and learning because they can influence a person's ability to learn. As described earlier, learning is a permanent change in an individual's behavior. As a result, people's psychosocial crises of growth and development must be taken into consideration by the therapist to be able to effectively apply teaching and learning methods. Constructive patient education techniques can make a difference in a patient's beliefs, cooperation, and performance. Teaching and learning has the ability to temporarily or permanently effect changes in behavior and implicitly increase the patient's learning achievements.

## Teaching and Learning for the Infancy and Toddler Stages of Development

Infancy and toddler stages include children from birth to approximately 3 years of age. In these early childhood stages, the infant's and toddler's growth and development include very multifaceted processes of physical, cognitive, and psychosocial transformations. Piaget describes that the primary modes of learning for the infant and the toddler are sensorimotor.[26] Because the infant is dependent on mother and father, the main focus of instruction is on parents and caregivers. The infant's thoughts derive from sensation and movement. Teaching should be geared toward the sensorimotor system, learning through integration of sensory stimulation activities with motor development.[63] Erikson feels that in infancy, the child must be able to trust the mother or caregiver in order to gain confidence in the future.[63] For this reason, the major emphasis is on the parents' nurturing ability, their care for the child, and their ability to guide and protect them. The infant's knowledge of the environment is limited but increasing because it is based on physical interactions and experiences. At approximately 7 months (or earlier), children acquire awareness of having objects around them even when the objects cannot be seen (called *object permanence*).[63] This is the beginning of memory for the infant. The most significant relationship for the child is with the maternal parent or the most significant caregiver. An infant who is properly cared for and handled will acquire optimism, hope, confidence, and security. The infant's physical development allows mobility and growth of new intellectual abilities.

At the end of the infancy stage and the beginning of the toddler stage, there is an expansion of language abilities.[63] Parents should be encouraged to listen and talk to their children and facilitate their language skills. Between the ages of 1 and 3, children begin to assert their independence by walking away from the parent or making choices about food, toys, or what to wear. In this toddler stage, children should be encouraged and supported in their increased independence to become confident in their ability to survive in the world.[63] Parents need to not criticize or overly control the child. Parents or caregivers must give the toddler the opportunity to assert him- or herself in order to increase self-esteem and self-assurance.

Physical and occupational therapists working in pediatrics must consider all aspects of the child's development and teach parents and caregivers about the expected gross motor skills and developmental milestones. Several screening tests can assess effectively the infant's competence and behaviors and also educate parents about these behaviors. Patient education for parents or caregivers of infants can focus on gross motor status, integration of primitive reflexes, emergence of purposeful movement, language, and personal and social skills. Additionally, health promotion, disease prevention, and safety are considered priorities of instructional activities for parents or caregivers. When the infant or toddler is ill, the main concern is, the same as in nursing, to assess the parents' (caregivers') and child's level of anxiety and offer coping techniques.[5] The therapist needs to consider the child's and parents' separation anxiety and apprehension, especially in situations of acute illness when there is a need for hospitalization or frequent visits with other health care providers. Unfamiliar environments and health care interventions constitute major problems for children as well as parents or caregivers. In such events, teaching activities to cope with stress and anxiety can be directed at the child, as well as parents or caregivers.

Physical and occupational therapists and assistants should consider teaching parents or caregivers how to use the home environment and toys to work toward the child's developmental goals. For example, for infants the toys should be set up close at hand to encourage rolling or propping on forearms.[64] For toddlers, the toys could be set up close enough to promote cruising or put up on tables for standing and kneeling activities. The entire family is involved in physical or occupational therapy. For infants, the parents can be instructed about the importance of stimulation for proper development, concentrating on specific inhibitory or excitatory techniques to achieve the developmental milestone. Simple and playful exercises such as rolling, kicking, and throwing a ball are important for the child's mental and physical growth.[64] Swimming also is considered an excellent activity for muscular and cardiopulmonary development. The child's safety should always be a teaching and learning priority.

For infants who are chronically ill, patient education should concentrate on family-centered care, recognizing the needs of the family and the child.[5] The therapists and the entire health care team must address the impact of illness or injury on the entire family. The therapists' role is to help decrease parents' anxiety and also assist them with decision making. All the rehabilitation activities must involve direct participation of the parents or caregivers. The family should be able to direct the services and support needed for the child even after the professional health care is no longer necessary or involved. Parents or caregivers must be continuously encouraged to take an active role in their child's development and health.[17] In addition to the parents, especially in cases of children with disabilities, instruction is also directed to other members of the family such as grandparents or even to nontraditional family, such as babysitters, neighbors, or stepfamilies. Help and support from the extended group of individuals can make a great difference in the child's life.

Family education for individuals who care for a child with a disability can facilitate constructive interactions between the child and the family.[17] In many situations, parents or the family are not fully aware of the child's capabilities and are not able to put emphasis on specific stimuli and skills. The family needs teaching to support and facilitate the child's performance.[64] Additionally, motivational behaviors encouraging the child to achieve the skill by allowing extra time or modifying the task for enhanced execution could be valuable methods to teach parents and families.

Pediatric physical and occupational therapists must work in partnership with the family to evaluate, plan, and deliver interventions for the child. Physical therapy and occupational therapy in pediatrics include goals written for families as well as for the individual child.[17] For infants, the teaching should concentrate on parents promoting the children's use of gross motor abilities by stimulating the auditory, visual, and kinesthetic (tactile) senses. For toddlers, the teaching sessions are directed at the child. The educational sessions for the toddler must be short but frequent to reinforce the learned material. Explanations must be clear and presented in simple and uncomplicated terms.[17] The teaching can be individualized according to the child's attention level and reaction to material. For example, for infants with Down syndrome, physical and occupational therapists can teach parents activities to help in the development of the child's gross motor skills by increasing the strength of the neck, arms, stomach, and legs musculature. At the same time, parents need to learn about safety measures to avoid injuries to the child's neck if there is vertebral instability of the cervical spine.[17] For children with Down syndrome, rehabilitation interventions are recommended as early as possible, at approximately 1 or 2 months of age. These early interventions can help the child develop the major milestones including walking, running, and stair climbing. Parent or caregiver education and training is typically provided prior to the child starting rehabilitation as well as during the therapy. The parents or caregivers learn about the disorder, interventions, and how to make decisions for the plan of care. The child's positioning and feeding are important tasks for the parents.[17] For the infant, the instruction teaches methods to carry and position the child to practice head control. For the toddler, the teaching involves use of orthoses to support feet and ankles and helping the child stand in a standing frame while playing with the parents.[17] The parents are included in the rehabilitation team working together with other professionals. The child and the family are the most important members of the rehabilitation team and are continuously involved in the instructional process and rehabilitation training.[17]

# *Teaching and Learning for the Preschooler Stage of Development*

This stage includes children from 3 years to approximately 6 years old. Piaget describes this stage as preoperational, when the child's knowledge of language helps him or her to start using symbols to represent objects and personify things.[29] The child is oriented to the present and has difficulty conceptualizing time.[29] The thinking is influenced by fantasy. For this reason, teaching must account for the preschooler's vivid fantasies and undeveloped sense of time. The child's active role in learning can be emphasized using neutral words and equipment for playing or increasing motor skills. At this stage, Erikson indicates that children are able to assert themselves and begin to plan activities or games.[62] Preschoolers develop a sense of initiative and feel secure in their ability to lead others and make decisions. The child's self-initiative should be encouraged and developed during instruction. The skills from toddlerhood continue to expand and new behaviors are learned, allowing the child to acquire more independence and care for him- or herself. The preschooler demonstrates fine and gross motor skills and coordination for independent activities of daily living.[64] Parents and caregivers need instruction for child supervision and injury prevention considering the child's inability to think logically and their curiosity in explorations. For preschoolers, fantasy and reality are not well differentiated. They can mix facts with fiction and develop imaginary playmates. At the same time, they have the knowledge of requiring help when facing the outside environment.

In the preschool stage, children mimic others' behavior.[62] Learning must involve modeling of appropriate behaviors. Also, recognizing and dealing with children's feelings is a vitally important step in handling children's behavior. Parents, caregivers, and health care providers should be able to interpret nonverbal clues, understand feelings, and help the child understand methods to cope with actions and attitudes.[64] For example, preschoolers need to know that physical violence is not an acceptable behavior. Also, taking responsibility for one's actions is important as well as being able to keep a promise and admit mistakes. Children need to be taught respect by modeling and using deferential tones and words. Children in the preschool age are sensitive to nonverbal communication such as facial expressions, voices, and body gestures and movements. Eye contact must be maintained with the child when talking. It reinforces the message telling the child that they are important. When talking to the child, the person must kneel next to or beside him or her in order to be at the same eye level and not to appear in a threatening posture.[64] Closed postures with crossed arms and legs can indicate resistance and hostility.[17] The tone of voice is also a powerful tool when communicating with the child, especially when trying to improve social behaviors. Keeping the voice calm, soothing, and soft helps children feel safe and able to express themselves in return. Showing affection by smiling or tucking a child into bed conveys caring, love, and understanding. For preschoolers, health is a difficult concept to understand. Health means the ability to play with others and participate in daily activities. Illness may be considered a punishment for doing something wrong.

Physical and occupational therapists and assistants interact with preschoolers when they are in need of rehabilitation due to trauma or other chronic disorders/diseases. At this stage, play is an important component of rehabilitation. Vygotsky believed that play contributed to the child's development by helping to increase the level of thinking.[36] The constructivist psychology approach believes that during play, the child uses complex intellectual behaviors.[36] These activities then become a foundation for abstract concepts, typically found in adults. In rehabilitation, the therapist uses play to help increase the imaginative skills of the child while also developing gross and fine motor skills.[64] Additionally, the imaginative tasks can be included in the child's activities of daily living such as dressing, eating, or cleaning.

Family is always involved in physical and occupational therapy of the child as significant members of the rehabilitation team. Siblings and other members of the family can play with the child and incorporate familiar games into the therapy session. A family member can be an asset to meeting the therapy goals by practicing with the child the necessary tasks as well as providing motivation and encouragement. Other disciplines that are part of the rehab team can improve the rehabilitation goals in the areas of communication skills and development of social and cognitive abilities. The rehabilitative teaching sessions for the preschooler include closely planned group activities, imaginative games and computer games, art projects that the child can take home, and exploration of the environment.[64]

For the preschooler with disability, physical and occupational therapy needs to adapt the environment and activities while the child is in school or kindergarten. For example, a child who wears a prosthetic knee needs to be able to navigate using a walker in the classroom. The teacher also learns from the therapist how to assist the child in donning and doffing the prosthesis and adapting the tables or desks for the child's walking and playing. In addition, the parents or caregivers can help the child when in school, especially when the teacher is reluctant to assist.

When teaching the preschooler, the teaching sessions must be kept short and scheduled sequentially at close intervals for continuity and reinforcement of information.[5] The learned material must relate to activities and experiences that are usual for the child. The child needs to participate in the selection of activities to meet the desired goals. Group sessions involving parents, siblings, and friends (if possible) can increase the interaction and be more enjoyable for the child. Verbal and nonverbal communication using praises and rewards are important incentives for learning. For long-term learning and continuity of care, parents can continue the therapy sessions at home and reinforce the learned information and the child's permanent attainment of specific skills.[64]

# Teaching and Learning for the School-Age Stage of Development

This stage includes children from 6 years to approximately 12 years of age. In Piaget's cognitive development theory, the school-age phase represents the concrete operational period.[29] At this developmental stage, children are capable of logical thought. They still learn through their senses but no longer rely only on them for teaching. The school-age child develops the ability to think abstractly and make rational judgments about concrete or observable phenomena. Teaching gives the child the opportunity to ask questions and explain the learned information. In Erikson's psychosocial stages, the school-age child begins to develop a sense of pride in their accomplishments.[62] School-age children initiate and complete projects, being proud of the results of their activities. Teachers and peers play an important role in the school-age child's development. Parents or caregivers are important but no longer represent authority figures as in the earlier stages of development. School-age children approach learning with enthusiasm. They become motivated to learn because of their need to better understand the world and themselves.[5]

Physical growth and development of school-age children includes mature patterns of movement such as throwing, jumping, and running. Competitiveness increases, allowing boys and girls to participate and enjoy sports and games. They exhibit improved coordination, balance, and endurance and can be involved in various curricular and extracurricular activities at school or after school. The prepubescent bodily changes contribute to their physical and psychosocial developments. Children think more objectively, listen to others, and use syllogism as a form of deductive reasoning that explains a notion from the general to the specific. They also develop skills for memory, decision making, and problem solving. In addition, young schoolchildren are able to concentrate for an extended period of time and can independently perform all activities of daily living. They understand the meaning of time and can pursue subjects and activities that will increase their talents in certain areas. Cognitively, the child can make decisions and act accordingly; however, they still have difficulty understanding the consequences or the seriousness of their choices.[5] For this reason, in terms of behavior, young schoolchildren need to understand certain boundaries. Setting limits gives them a feeling of safety and security. The children learn to develop their own limits. The role of the parents is to talk to their child about boundaries and explain how to set them. In this way, parents can help the child and encourage him or her to become more self-disciplined and self-sufficient. Usually, children who have developed a strong sense of self-discipline and internal motivation can better deal with peer pressure and difficulties in life.[65] This allows them to be more independent. Additionally, parents can help children achieve this sense of self-discipline and motivation by giving them coping mechanisms for dealing with disappointments.[65]

Although young school children are involved more with school and peers than home life, the roles of the parents do not diminish. Children need encouragement at every developmental stage. Encouragement is described as the most basic parenting inclination.[66] Through encouragement, children can develop healthy emotions.[66] Parents need to know that encouragement has far more potential to help develop emotionally healthy children than punitive measures.

Physical and occupational therapists teaching parents and healthy school-age children must emphasize education for health promotion and injury prevention. Usually, the instruction occurs in the school system through the school therapist or at community centers, outpatient rehabilitation clinics, and hospitals.[64] Parents and caregivers also must be informed about the content of information. Health education may also be promoted by teachers and health care providers and include topics such as the importance of exercises, nutrition, and sleep; avoidance of alcohol, tobacco, and drugs; and prevention of injuries.[67] For children who have an illness, disorder, or disability, patient education must consider the child's specific learning style and readiness to learn.[67] Together with the parents (caregivers), the children are actively involved early in the planning process including short- and long-term goals of rehabilitation. The therapist has to explain in simple and logical terms the illness/disorder and the necessary interventions. The children can follow directions and receive feedback on their performance.

For children from 6 to 9 years old, symbolic play and imaginative games are still choices for play interventions.[64] For boys, toy guns, adventure fantasy play, and video games are typical for playing. Girls tend to choose dolls, household objects, and fantasy games with familiar roles. School-age children from 10 to 12 prefer interventions that involve playing with video games and computer games and model building. Educational types of games such as Monopoly or LeapFrog Leapster also can be used. Organized athletic activities, group exercise classes, and community programs such as swimming and aerobics classes can be used as continuity of care interventions, especially for musculoskeletal and neuromuscular rehabilitation.[64]

School-age children can follow directions and comply with interventions, but they can easily become bored with routines and repetitions. Occupational and physical therapy should be fun for them. Motivational strategies such as a group exercise program, using kinetic exercise machines, or singing or playing instruments can be employed to make the therapy enjoyable. From the emotional and social perspectives, children with chronic disorder and disability can also benefit from activities involving community integration and support. These measures can help to meet the therapeutic goals.[64]

The teaching sessions for school-age children should be approximately 30 minutes per session.[64] The instruction must be spread out to provide ample opportunity to practice. Depending on the individual child's learning style, diagrams, pictures, videotapes, printed materials, and games including computer games can be used. Layman's terminology is the choice for communicating scientific information.[17] Simple analogies can clarify the material. Teaching sessions that involve important concepts should be individualized, but also include the parents or caregivers if possible. Rehabilitation interventions, especially ones involving playing and other dynamic activities, can be taught in a group. Audiovisual and printed materials must show peers performing the same tasks. Sufficient time should be provided for the child to discuss the learned information and ask questions for clarification. The child needs positive feedback, praise, and rewards for his or her correct performance of tasks.[17] These can motivate and reinforce the learning process.

For injury or illness prevention, the instruction should begin in the early stages of the child's development.[67] The child's early life experiences and environments set the stage for future developments and achievements. Research indicates that at least half of the eventual educational achievement gaps among children exist at kindergarten entry.[67] Regrettably, these gaps widen rather than diminish as children mature and move through the educational system.[67] Usually, lifelong patterns of health and well-being are established early in life. Therefore, young children and their families must have access to resources and services that can promote early health and development in order to pay large dividends over the life course. Additionally, teaching and learning in physical and occupational rehabilitation should be directed at assisting children to incorporate positive health measures into their daily lives. Group activities are effective behavioral teaching techniques because of the importance of peer influence.

# Teaching and Learning for the Adolescent Stage of Development

This stage includes adolescents from 12 years to approximately 18 years old. This stage is represented by Piaget as the formal operational period, when the child no longer requires concrete objects to make rational judgments.[29] Piaget's writings assert that the adolescent is able to think abstractly.[29] Adolescents are also able to reflect, hypothesize, and theorize. In Erikson's developmental stages, the teenager must establish his or her own identity and individuality.[62,63] For the adolescent, identity and role confusion cause struggle and difficulties, especially when developing morality and differentiating right from wrong. During the transition from childhood to adulthood, many adolescents experience uncertainty, insecurity, aggression, and other destructive behaviors that can lead to health issues.[63] The teen tries to integrate many roles into his or her self-image, taking into consideration other adults and adolescents.

The period of adolescence is not an easy one. It is a time of adolescents' resistance against parents and teachers in order to distinguish themselves as unique individuals. Establishing identity is crucial. Consequently, risk taking can be very dangerous, leading to morbidity and mortality. The statistics concerning adolescents' risky behaviors are frightening. In the United States in 2005, one third of adolescents ages 12 to 17 drank alcohol, one fifth used illicit drugs, and one sixth smoked cigarettes;[68] that translates to 8 million teens drinking alcohol, 5 million using illicit drugs, and more than 4 million smoking cigarettes.[68] In 2005, in only one day, 7,970 adolescents between 12 and 17 drank alcohol for the first time, 4,348 used an illicit drug for the first time, 4,082 smoked cigarettes for the first time, and 2,517 used pain relievers nonmedically for the first time.[68] Additionally in 2005, 47% of high school students had sexual intercourse and 14% had four or more sex partners.[68] That same year, 34% of sexually active high school students did not use a condom during their most recent sexual intercourse.[68] Risky sexual behaviors during adolescence account for more than 25% of American teenagers having sexually transmitted diseases (STDs).[68] Each year, there are approximately 19 million new STD infections, and almost half of them are among youth ages 15 to 24.[68] In 2000, 13% of all pregnancies, or about 831,000, occurred among adolescents ages 15 to 19.[68] Approximately every minute one adolescent in the United States has a baby.[68] These statistics should alert health care providers to try to understand the behavioral characteristics of adolescents and apply effective education for teens and their parents. Disease prevention education must be developed by providers with the active involvement of parents and teachers. Additionally, the education should be locally determined and consistent with school and community values.

In regard to health and illness, adolescents are able to understand several concepts, especially the ones related to the causes of diseases and also education for disease prevention. Parents, teachers, and health care providers are considered the most common sources of health information including prevention. The educational needs of adolescents are extensive, including a variety of health care topics ranging from sexual adjustment to drinking and substance abuse,[69] nutrition, and accident prevention. Because teenagers are reluctant to visit health care providers, many times the teenagers' education can be directed by the parents. The best preventive policy is for parents and teachers to educate teens about the growing health problems in this age group. Teenagers' rights need to be respected and they must be given the opportunity to make decisions, choices, and even mistakes.[69] They can learn from experience and understand very early at around 11 or 12 years of age that it is better to be safe than sorry. Parents and family play a big part in this process, but friends do too. Most teenagers want to fit in or belong, and sometimes new ideas learned from friends do not match their parents' views. Most conflict between parents and teenagers is about minor things such as dress and activities. At this time, what their friends think is often more important than their parents' beliefs. Conflict can be reduced by respecting the adolescent's right to have different views and by teaching them to respect all views, including those of the family. Teenagers can be helped by their parents knowing that independence can be risky and that family is there, ready to help them.[69] Reinforcing parental views, values, and concerns can be important to encourage teens to discuss any problem honestly without embarrassment and humiliation.[69] Enlightening a teenager is the best preventive policy to tackle the growing health problems in this age group. For example, relative to drinking, health care providers can educate parents to discuss drinking openly with teenagers.[69] Parents can reinforce the fact that children who begin drinking alcohol before the age of 15 are five times more likely to develop alcohol problems than those who start after the age of 21. Education must include details about the effects of alcohol on the teenage brain, including causing problems with motor coordination and the ability to drive, impulse control by lowering a person's inhibitions, memory by impairing recollection of information, and judgment and decision-making capability by engaging in risky behaviors that result in illness, injury, and even death.[70]

Alcohol use among teenagers is a major problem all over the world. In the United States, alcohol use among teens is strongly correlated with violence, risky sexual behaviors, poor academic performance, and other harmful activities.[71] A survey of high school students found that 18% of females and 39% percent of males feel that is acceptable for a boy to force sex if the girl is high or drunk.[71]

It is known that the relationship between teenagers and their parents is based on conflict, toleration, or alienation. Teenagers tend to rebel against authority and recommendations from their parents. However, in regard to drinking, it seems that the key reason adolescents choose not to drink is parental disapproval of underage drinking.[69,70] The reality is that parents have more influence over their children than they realize. When parents are involved in their children's lives, the adolescents are less likely to drink, smoke, or use illicit drugs.[71] Therefore, health care providers can educate parents and teenagers to be involved in their child's life and openly talk to their child on a daily basis. The parents must be sincere, however, and admit their own oversights. Teenagers are very cognizant of deception and pretense. Open talk will allow the teen to open up and discuss their activities. At the same time, the parents can also share their interests and values with the child. Additionally, family beliefs and history concerning drinking can create an environment of trust and understanding. Parents who drink must explain to the child that moderation is important because women should have only one drink per day, while men can have no more than two drinks per day.[71] Parents who do not drink must explain their reasons for not drinking, whether they are religious, health related, or due to family history.[71] The teen must be encouraged to ask questions, especially when explaining to them that they should not drink until they are 21 years old, and even then, they should drink in moderation. Adolescents must know that drinking is forbidden in the following situations: (1) when they are children and teenagers, (2) when women are trying to conceive or are pregnant, (3) when individuals of any age group cannot restrict their drinking to moderate levels (especially recovering alcoholics and people whose family members have alcohol problems), (4) when people plan to drive or take part in activities requiring attention or skill, and (5) when people use prescription and over-the-counter medications.[71]

When someone in the family has a history of alcoholism, the teenager needs to know that he or she is at a greater risk for problem drinking.[71] The teenager need to clearly understand that some people are unable to drink alcohol at all without drinking to excess, and that alcoholism is a progressive disease combining physical addiction and mental obsession with drinking. Abstaining from alcohol for as long as possible is extremely important for teenagers because the older a person is when starting to drink, the lower the chances he or she will have problems with alcohol.[71] Also, providing information about treatment options for people who drink and develop problems with alcohol can help the teen recognize the parents' honest interest in them.

The adolescent has to know that parents are listening to them and that the teen is important to them. Specificity and consistency are essential when talking to the teen. Being reasonable, not using unrealistic threats, and setting clear and sensible rules can protect the child's physical safety and mental well-being. Because drinking and driving is the biggest killer of adolescents, parents must be persistent and clear about rules concerning drinking and driving.[70,71] The parents have the right to insist that the teenager does not drive after drinking or does not ride with a driver who has been drinking. These same rules should apply to drugs. Parental rule must insist that the teen will call the parent in situations of drinking and driving or riding with an intoxicated driver.[70,71] The parent must assure the teen that they will be helped without questioning, punishment, or lecturing. The lines of communication between the teen and the parents must be kept open at all times and be used without condemnation or reprimand.

Another vital issue in parental and school education of the adolescent is sex education. It is advisable that teenagers receive the correct information from teachers, parents, or health care providers instead of from misleading sources such as friends, magazines, or Web sites. During adolescence, not only do hormones work overtime but also there are physical changes taking place in the body structure and the sex organs. These changes cause curiosity and exploration for teens to be able to understand sexual physiological phenomena. Additionally, the adolescent has the impulse to try something that is considered prohibited. Parents, teachers, and health care providers must understand the benefits of sex education. These are: (1) It can prevent teenage pregnancies; (2) It can stress the role of abstinence and contraceptive methods, including the use of condoms; (3) It can explain to teenagers that pregnancy is a health hazard because adolescents are mentally unprepared to handle pregnancy, childbirth, and parenthood; (4) It can help teenagers become better equipped to understand the repercussions of teenage pregnancy on their health as well as that of the fetus; and (5) It can assist the teenager to recognize the importance of predelivery care and the consequences of hiding the pregnancy.[72] Other benefits of sex education include helping teenagers appreciate the negative impact of teenage pregnancy on their education, and consequently on their future, and also assisting them to understand and prevent STDs such as the human papillomavirus (HPV), which causes over 70% of cervical cancers; gonorrhea; pelvic inflammatory disease; or syphilis.[72]

Sex education, as with other types of education, needs to be repetitive; for example, adolescents whose parental communication in regard to sex education involved more repetition of the same topic felt closer to their parents.[73] Additionally, the teen was able to better communicate in general and specifically about sex and perceived that the discussions had openness.[73] Health care providers must advise parents about the value of discussing sexual topics repeatedly because they can provide reinforcement and the opportunity for the child to ask questions. For many parents, sex education is an uncomfortable conversation; however, it is an important topic to discuss because it builds trust between the parent and the child.[73] The teen should never be penalized for telling the truth about sex (or drugs or drinking). The parent must allow the child to talk to, confide in, and trust the adult parent. The parent needs to become an ally of the teenage child. Plain facts and data about pregnancy or STDs are not considered enough information to allow for discussion and dialogue. The parent must follow the child's lead in conversation, and express their values without lecturing them. Points to stress for the parent may include that sexual involvement must be by mutual consent and that sexuality is a natural part of adolescence but it is not the beginning of sexual activity.[73] Teenagers also must know about birth control, how it is used, and where they can go to obtain it.[74] The adolescent child may need direct support in the form of birth control and information and supplies to practice safer sex.[74] Parents should be instructed that when birth control is discussed in a caring manner, and provided as prevention rather than encouragement, the knowledge and materials will not cause the child to have sex.[74] Similar to preventive education for drunk driving, parents must stress their involvement, concern for the child's safety, and the assurance that they will help the teen in any needed situation.

In physical and occupational therapy, adolescents are physically developing strength and changes in their balance, coordination, and endurance. Therapists need to consider that adolescent patients are typically interested in athletics, academics, jobs, or recreation. Therefore, rehabilitation interventions need to include activities such as athletic practices or games, video games, social activities, or skill-building activities. The plan of care must incorporate the teen's priorities that are relevant to their lifestyle.[64] In orthopedic rehabilitation of athletic injuries, many teens are very motivated to return to their sport activities. As a result they will diligently work toward the rehabilitation goals. Motivational strategies for adolescents may include integrating the adolescent's goals into the therapy, giving the teen a sense of success, and/or developing a system of rewards for home programs.

When teaching adolescents in physical and occupational therapy, the greatest challenge is being able to develop a trusting and mutually respectful relationship with the teen. The important factors in teen patient education are the availability and flexibility of the therapist, the quality of the information, confidentiality, and coordination with other health care providers, schools, and services. For adolescents who have chronic illness or disabilities, the therapist must be able to directly communicate with them without having the parent speak for the child. The therapist speaking directly to the adolescent and asking about his or her needs and preferences shows respect and concern for the teen.[64] As a result, the teen will have the opportunity to assume some personal responsibility for his or her health and wellness. Additionally, as adolescents grow, therapists need to check their perceptions of their disability or chronic illness from time to time. Then, they should help them fill in the gaps in regard to their understanding of their health care needs.[75] Patient education must include condition-specific information and self-management including social and emotional support.[75] Optimal care may depend on the adolescent's level of development.[75] The information can be reviewed several times and may include videotapes and interactive media as well as printed material. The data should also have information on support groups. Additionally, the therapist must supply resource lists, referral sources, and opportunities to learn about alternatives. For teens with disabilities or chronic conditions, it is important to transition to age-appropriate adult care.[75] The process of transition is gradual and occurs together with the adolescent and their family.

The process of parents gradually letting go of the care of their children is critical to the adolescent years. These teens, who will be young adults, will take charge of their own lives including their health.

Adolescents with disabilities face the developmental tasks that any adolescent faces, but their struggle is intensified by their disability. Physical and occupational therapists should realize that the process of transition from adolescent to adult is more difficult for the teen with chronic illness or disability and their families. A subject such as sexuality often is ignored by parents and professionals when disability is involved. However, with an adolescent patient, the subject cannot be overlooked. The therapist should provide families with peer counseling and other families as resources for health promotion and disease prevention. Families must be encouraged to develop a positive attitude about impairments and functional limitations of the teen with disability. Establishing goals together with the teen and the family will help the transition period. For example, a goal for the adolescent with Down syndrome will be the ability to independently take the bus going from school to their job and from the job to their residence. The therapist will need to teach the child which bus to take and where to go in addition to ascending and descending bus stairs independently. The therapist and the parents (if necessary) should take bus rides with the teen and help him or her figure out how to negotiate steps. The route must be practiced with the adolescent, allowing him or her to independently commute from school to the job and back home.

In regard to healthy teens, physical and occupational therapy can promote health and educate adolescents in regard to prevention. Patient education should concentrate on topics such as avoidance of smoking and alcohol or illicit drug use, and sex education. Specific teaching strategies for adolescents may include individualized instruction especially for situations when there is a need for confidentiality of sensitive information. Teens can benefit from peer group discussions by listening to other peers' experiences. For teaching, the rehabilitation provider can use models, diagrams, written materials, role-playing, computer group discussions, and gaming. Having teens meet with other teens and discuss their experiences via computer technology can be very effective, especially when working with teen behavioral changes. Additional teaching materials should include audiotapes, videotapes, simulated games, and other computer-interactive material. Layman's terms should be used instead of scientific or medical terminology.[17] Similar to adults, adolescents should be included in the teaching plans, goals, and teaching strategies.[17] Providing the rationale for the presented information is helpful to promote discussions and choices for action. Therapists should use respect, confidentiality, tact, and flexibility and should not be discouraged by the teen's negative responses or behaviors. Confrontations must be avoided and decision making must be encouraged.

Including parents, families, and siblings in patient education for disease prevention can also be helpful. The therapist as the educator can give guidance and support to families, helping them to better understand adolescent behavior. Parents need education to learn how to sensibly set limits and also promote the adolescent's independence. The therapist must consider the learning needs of the adolescent as well as his or her parents.

# Teaching and Learning for the Young and Middle-Aged Adult Stages of Development

The adult stages of development start around 18 years old and last until the end of adult life, signified by the person's death. Erikson divided the adult stages into three developmental phases: the young adult, from 18 to 35; the middle-aged adult, from 35 to approximately 55 or 65; and the late adult, from 55 or 65 to the end of life.[62,63] The psychosocial development of the *young adult stage* is described as the adult seeking companionship and love.[62] The individual is trying to find a mutually satisfying relationship that will end up in marriage and the beginning of a family. For the young adult, the relationship has to involve a deep level of intimacy to be considered satisfying and successful. From a social perspective, young adults are striving to maintain skills from their teens involving independence and self-sufficiency. Cognitively, Piaget describes the young adult period as a continuation of the formal operational stage of cognitive development.[29] As a result, these adults can tap into their formal and informal experiences to improve their critical thinking and problem-solving capabilities. Additionally, their physical abilities are excellent, allowing a great deal of psychomotor skills.

Generally, the learning interests of young adults are directed toward immediate application of information to enhance their daily activities and tasks. In physical and occupational therapy, teaching strategies for young adults are similar to the ones used for the middle-aged adult population. For example, young adults may be treated for various orthopedic injuries such as sprains, strains, or fractures. Some of the injuries can be caused by trauma or falls during sporting events. Other overuse injuries can be caused by repetitive stresses such as running and throwing. They can occur because of muscular fatigue and poor body mechanics. Therapists have to rehabilitate the individual and teach prevention of future injuries.

In regard to teaching approaches, young adults need to establish their goals and outcomes with the therapist using a patient-centered care approach. The rehabilitation goals are to fulfill the expressed needs of the learner. With the young adult learner, the therapist can use a combination of teaching techniques combining the adolescent style with adult learning. Subject-oriented teaching techniques from adolescence can be combined with the patient-oriented learning used most often in adulthood. The learner can get the necessary knowledge or skills after the therapist explains the subject. Then, in patient-oriented learning, the therapist acts as a facilitator or resource person supporting the patient's own ideas and encouraging the young adult's creativity. The learning should not be a challenging situation. Family members must be included in the teaching sessions. Also, application of learning should take place immediately after teaching each concept. Additionally, the patient should be encouraged to evaluate his or her actions and make changes as necessary. The patient's past experiences can be used as a learning resource to connect them with the new information.

In the area of health promotion and prevention, young adults do not regularly benefit from patient education. The reason for not using health care services often is lack of insurance coverage.[76] In the United States, young adults have the highest uninsurance rates of any age group.[77] They are ineligible for their parents' health coverage and the public insurance that covers adolescents. The risk of being uninsured is greater among certain groups of young adults including the poor, Hispanics, and non–full-time students.[77] Males are more likely to lack insurance than females.[77] This difference may be due in part to Medicaid coverage of poor families, which are disproportionately headed by young single women with children.[77] Because they are not insured, young adult males are not able to receive health care, fill prescriptions, or discuss their health problems with a health care professional. Young adult females use health care services at a greater rate than young males, largely due to their reproductive health needs.

The biggest health care problems for young males and females are obesity and overweight concerns. Substance abuse is also reported to be very high among young adult men, especially whites and American Indians/Alaskan Natives.[77] Additionally, a sizeable portion of young men and women face mental health problems.[77] Other health consideration for the young adult population relate to risk factors such as high cholesterol, smoking, and high blood pressure.[77] Young adults, both insured and uninsured, who do visit health care professionals report difficulties paying medical bills.[77] These include making payments or significantly changing their way of life in order to pay the medical debt. Government initiatives are needed to allow young adults to be covered by their parents' insurance plans at least until they are 25 years of age. The individual states could also ensure that all colleges and universities require full-time and part-time students to have health insurance, and that these educational institutions offer health insurance coverage to both. The school coverage plans can be added to tuition cost along with other required fees. Additionally, increased preventative measures must be instituted to avoid homicide, unintentional injuries, and substance abuse among young men in late adolescence and early adulthood.

The young adult's motivation to learn is dependent on the need for self-esteem, better quality of life, job satisfaction, financial growth, and increased time for recreational activities.[78] When young adults are faced with acute or chronic illnesses, they are motivated to gain the necessary knowledge to be able to maintain their independence and return to their normal lives.[78] In rehabilitation, the intervention goals are always set up with the patients as part of the patient-centered care approach. Patients are encouraged in decision making and setting goals to accomplish their rehabilitation objectives. Because adults bring a variety of experiences into the learning process, therapists can draw on these experiences to make learning relevant and functional. Teaching materials can include written patient education and audiovisual tools, as well as computer-assisted instruction that allows for self-paced learning. Group discussions can be used for interaction with others of the same age and situation, especially when related to prevention of chronic diseases/disorders such as diabetes, hypertension, and obesity.

The second phase of Erikson's developmental stages is the *middle-aged* adult. In this phase, the individual takes greater responsibility and control and attempts to produce something that makes a difference to them and society.[79] Career, work, and family are very important. Psychosocially, the middle-aged adult establishes significant relationships within the family, workplace, local church, and other communities.[79] During middle age, many individuals already have attained their desired socioeconomic status and have become highly accomplished in their careers. These adults are also ready to help younger and older persons in their family. They find satisfaction through their work or careers, as family members, or providers for the family. Also, middle-aged adults may serve as mentors for younger people or follow new undeveloped interests. Erikson considers middle age to be the time a person re-examines his or her own achievements and goals in life.[79] Additionally, individuals may be taking the responsibility to care for their older parents or for their children and grandchildren. On the other hand, when their children have grown up and left home, many middle-aged adults can slow down their regular activities and begin to attend more exciting events in the community. As a result, they pursue new social interests and leisure activities. Also, because they are close to retirement age, they may be interested to learn about financial planning or about other forms of activities they could not pursue in younger years. Many middle-aged adults may actually go back to school to learn other professions or careers that interested them as young adults.

In regard to health, middle-aged adults may feel motivated to follow health care recommendations or may deny illnesses or even abandon healthy and preventive practices altogether. When visiting health care providers, middle-aged adults want direct participation in their care to become members of the health care team. For patient education in physical and occupational therapy, the therapist must encourage the adult's decision-making, listen actively to his or her concerns, help in prioritizing, and keep the adult and his or her family informed. Middle-aged adult women can be extremely stressed because later marriages and childbearing are forcing them to take increased responsibilities later in life for their elderly parents as well as adolescent children. Seventy percent of middle-aged women between the ages of 35 and 54 are concerned about rising health care costs, and 65% about an aging parent's care or well-being.[80] Fifty-nine percent worry about not having enough time to help and support a family member.[80] Fifty-five percent have difficulty managing stress.[80] Consequently, therapists should provide referrals for counseling and other community resources to help. Additionally, during patient education, the therapist should be aware of women's misconceptions in regard to their health and well-being. These misconceptions can affect their ability to learn or be motivated during the learning process. For example, women fear that menopause represents the end of their sexual life and that forgetfulness is imminent. A majority of middle-aged adults want to know the correct information to be able to maintain their optimal health. They also need to be reassured and praised for their efforts and competencies.

Malcolm Knowles's adult learning theory (described in Chapter 11) offers a problem-centered framework that is more suitable for adult learning. This form of acquiring knowledge is totally different than the subject-centered childhood learning. Adult learning theory can be applied to all adults; however, sometimes older adults may need a different type of teaching and learning called *gerogogy*.[80] This takes into consideration the person's abilities as well as their age-related impairments and functional limitations. Knowles's theory of andragogy states that adults prefer to learn from their own experiences, which represent a rich resource for learning.[53] Adults have specific learning needs that are generated by life events. The main motivation of adult learning is to be able to apply the knowledge and skills to life or work-related situations.[53] Newer learning theories explained by Knowles and other educators recognize that learning is a lifelong process.[55]

Persons of all ages have the potential to learn, though some learn faster than others. Age may or may not affect an individual's speed of learning because people vary in the ways they like to learn.[81] It is true that a new learning situation can cause stress and confusion. Some anxiety often increases motivation to learn, but too much anxiety may cause fatigue, resentment, inability to concentrate, and other barriers to learning.[81] The teaching and learning atmosphere should foster trust and acceptance of different ideas and values.[81] The therapist as the educator must incorporate in the teaching and learning process the adult learner's experiences, observations of others, and personal ideas and feelings. The depth of long-term learning is dependent on the extent to which a learner is assisted to analyze, clarify, or articulate his or her experiences to others including the instructor, other learners, and the learner's family, friends, or social group. The depth of learning increases when new concepts and skills are useful and meet the learner's current needs or problems.[81] This allows for immediate application of the theory to a practical situation.

In regard to acquiring new behaviors, the teaching and learning program may provide only one step in an individual's progress toward changing behaviors. The adoption of new behaviors depends on the following factors:[81]

- Former knowledge and attitudes that may predispose the individual to take a particular action

- Availability of and access to resources enabling the individual to carry out new plans of action

- Environmental conditions and family characteristics helping to reinforce or hinder the behavioral changes

The best method of teaching and learning promotes the learner's active participation in the educational process. The instructor must select among several teaching methods and choose the method that best allows learning to take place.[81] Using varied methods of teaching helps the learner to maintain interest and reinforces concepts without being repetitious.

Concepts of adult learning can also be applied to children and adolescents; for example, both adults and children prefer learning experiences that are participatory.[82] They learn faster when new concepts are useful in their current as well as future lives. The role of an educator for the young and middle-aged adult is to be able to assess the audience's interest, current skills, and goals. Then, the information can guide the structuring of the learning atmosphere and selection of teaching methods that are the most satisfying and effective for the learners.

Learning is more effective when the environmental conditions support an open exchange, sharing of opinions, and problem-solving strategies. As discussed earlier, the learning environment is important for adult learning because it involves physical factors, emotional factors, and learning factors. For example, individuals react differently to such factors as room temperature, arrangement of the furniture in the room, time of day, brightness of the lighting, and sound. Adults differ in regard to whether they prefer to work alone or in groups. Physical factors in the learning setting also include the noise level, lighting, temperature, structure of learning, and time of day. Emotional factors involve social needs such as learning alone or with others, and the learner's motivation (including extrinsic and intrinsic). The learning factors have to do with the learning styles such as auditory, visual, or kinesthetic.

The most important attributes of an effective teacher for adults are to be knowledgeable, to show concern for student learning, to present material clearly, to motivate, to emphasize relevance of class material, and to be enthusiastic.[82] Additionally, the teacher's role is to actively involve the adult learner in the educational process. The teacher must obtain the adult learners' perspectives about the topics and allow them to work on projects that reflect their interest. Adult learners want to assume responsibility for their learning. The teacher's role is to create a comfortable learning atmosphere and to adapt to meet the diverse needs of his or her students. The learner has already established his or her goal that needs to be attained during the learning experience. Thus, the educator is expected to help the student attain his or her goal. This classification of goals and course objectives must be done early in the beginning of the lesson.

Respecting the young and the middle-aged adult is very important because it reflects the instructor's acknowledgement of the student's wealth of experiences that he or she brings to the classroom. Adults as learners should be treated as equals in experience and knowledge and be allowed to voice their opinions freely during the teaching process.

## Teaching and Learning for the Late Adult Stage of Development

The late adult stage is calculated to last from 55 or 65 years old to the end of life. Erikson's late adult stage includes reflection about the meaning of life and valuable contributions to society.[79] Erikson considered the major psychosocial developmental task at this stage in life as ego integrity versus despair.[62] Older individuals contemplate their accomplishments. If they see their lives as unproductive, they feel guilty about the past and become dissatisfied with life.[62] At that point, they can develop despair, depression, and hopelessness. For those who experience major depression, the most likely predictors are multiple losses over a short period of time with respect to a previous support network of home, friends, family, and job. Additionally, the unsuccessful ending for those adults perceiving failures means despair and fear of death while still struggling to find a purpose to their lives. The phase of late adulthood includes dealing with the reality of aging, the acceptance of death, the reconciliation of past failures with present and future concerns, and developing a sense of growth and purpose for those years remaining.[62] A successful late adulthood is characterized by wisdom and acceptance of death as the completion of a satisfied life.

The most common psychosocial tasks of aging involve changes in lifestyle and social status as a result of retirement, death of a spouse, illness, or relocation of children, grandchildren, and friends.[79] Any losses signify a threat to the older adult's autonomy, independence, and decision making, and may result in isolation, financial insecurity, diminished coping mechanisms, and a decreased sense of identity, personal value, and societal worth.[79] With aging, some individuals, particularly the oldest adults, begin to question their perception of a meaningful life being the potential for further enjoyment, pleasure, and satisfaction.

Typically there are three classifications of old adults: the young-old adult, between 65 and 74 years of age; the old-old adult, between 75 and 84 years of age; and the oldest-old adult, 85 years of age and older.[5] By 2010 in the United States there will be an estimated 21.5 million people in the 65- to 74-year-old age group, 17 million in the 75- to 84-year-old age group, 2.1 million in the 85- to 99-year-old age group, and a small number in the 100 years and older age group.[83] As of 2003, there were nearly 36 million people in the United States age 65 or older.[83] When discussing health and older adults, the growth in the aging population and increase in life expectancy cause concerns about disease and disability; however, disease and disability are not considered an inevitable part of the aging process. The prevalence of physical disability in older individuals decreased from 26% to 20% between 1982 and 1999.[83] The reasons for this decline include better medical interventions, positive behavioral changes, more widespread use of assistive technologies, rising patient education levels, and improvements in socioeconomic status.

Although disability rates have been reduced, many older individuals suffer from at least one chronic condition. On average, older adults are hospitalized longer than persons in other age categories and require more patient education. Education programs for older individuals can improve their health and prevent chronic diseases such as heart disease, type 2 diabetes, high blood pressure, stroke, and many respiratory problems. However, in the United States, preventative care is not regularly offered to older people. Screening for life-threatening diseases and conditions is provided commonly to younger individuals, but older individuals are routinely left out when it comes to prevention and different types of interventions such as cancer treatments.[58] Furthermore, some health care professionals believe that chemotherapy is not a choice of treatment for an older patient.[84] When providing health care to older patients, many health care providers are not trained to appropriately meet the needs of older people or they do not feel that the older individual is important enough to deserve better care.

The American media stereotype older adults, portraying them as helpless, unproductive, dependent, and demanding. In reality, the majority of older individuals are self-sufficient, independent adults ready to use their talents and skills productively for the benefit of American society. Media stereotyping takes place because many older adults unfairly receive societal discrimination called *ageism*. Ageism is a widespread practice found in every segment of American society including health care.[85] Unfortunately, ageism is reported to affect over 50% of American households with older people.[85] Ageism can be compared to the discriminatory attitudes of racism and sexism. The effects of ageism are negative labels hurtful to older people. Ageism should be eliminated through funding, training, and federal policies supporting more research in geriatrics. Training health care practitioners and students is also essential. In health care, ageism can be so harmful that it may shorten an older individual's life. As an example, some health care professionals may decide not to run certain tests or prescribe certain medications and interventions because they do not consider the older patient's health important enough to receive these procedures. Another reason may be that health care practitioners may consider certain tests and procedures to be very tedious and difficult on the older patient's tolerance. As an example in oncology, some older patients have been denied chemotherapy because the side effects are so negative.[84] Nevertheless, when asked about trying these medical interventions, older patients wanted to go through the procedures and receive the needed care to improve their health. In certain situations when living with chronic disorders and pain, some older patients who were not able to receive the treatment committed suicide.

The health care provider's attitude is a big factor in providing care to an older person. If the attitude of the health care professional is inclined against providing indispensable health care, the older person will suffer the consequences. The American health care system needs to work harder to remove its prejudice against providing adequate and equal health care to older people. All health care students need education to understand the variations occurring in aging and how to properly work with the older adult. Additionally, patient instruction to help the older adult learn to manage his or her irreversible losses can also combat the ageism bias and unfairness.

## TEACHING AND LEARNING USING GEROGOGY

In physical and occupational therapy, patient education for older patients is different than for their younger counterparts. As mentioned earlier, the teaching of older persons involves gerogogy, which is different from andragogy. For teaching to be effective, gerogogy must accommodate the normal physical, cognitive, and psychosocial changes that occur at this phase of growth and development.[86] For example, because older individuals have diminished functional and sensory abilities, nurses were able to effectively teach patients in a nursing home using visual art-based strategies in bulletin board design.[86] This method allowed older individuals to learn at their own pace and also to develop specific questions for health care professionals.[86]

When teaching older adults, health care providers must consider physiological changes that begin in middle adulthood and some even in young adulthood. These changes can progress significantly in the older adult stage of development.[87] Using gerogogy, physical and occupational therapists and assistants need to note these changes and adapt their teaching to meet the patient's learning needs. For example, when teaching patients with visual impairments, one must consider the older adult's visual impairments that affect visual acuity when reading and writing.[87] Impairments such as the inability to focus properly and blurred vision (called presbyopia), visual changes such as cataracts, macular degeneration, reduced pupil size, and decline in depth perception must all be carefully considered, especially when relating written information.[87] For example, glossy paper and small print should never be used on written material. Other considerations in teaching and learning of the older adults may be disorders such as stroke or certain prescription medications such as steroids, tranquilizers, or antidepressants that can be detrimental to the learner's vision and also to the correct understanding of the material.[87]

Other changes as a result of the aging process also should be considered when imparting verbal information to older individuals. For example, hearing alterations such as presbycusis can occur in the inner ear affecting the middle-aged or older adult's understanding of consonant sounds of another person's speech.[87] This poor auditory speech discrimination and comprehension can be very frustrating for the older learner, especially when teaching takes place in a noisy environment. Additional hearing losses could be associated with pathologies such as Paget's disease (causing osteitis deformans) or hypothyroidism.

Older patients may learn at a slower pace than younger adults. The learning may be affected by cautiousness, anxiety, and cognitive impairments such as short-term memory loss. These cognitive deficits can begin in the mid-60s and can be observed more significantly by the early 80s.[87] They contribute to the older learner's decreased information processing ability. Furthermore, short-term memory impairment can be task dependent and may appear with novel conditions and new learning. For information processing, the therapist should search for alternative methods of interaction to increase the effectiveness of message delivery. It is important to remember that older adults have the capacity to learn; however, their learning may be affected by environmental, medical, cognitive, and psychological factors (**Table 12.2**).

Another important concept when teaching the older adult population is health literacy. Health illiteracy is a nationwide issue that affects the entire American population; however, certain groups, such as the older population, are more at risk than others. A large portion of the adult population is unclear about personal health facts. Patient barriers to health knowledge are individual, technological, and social. With age-related decline, as well as

| Table 12.2 | |
|---|---|
| **General Characteristics of Older Adult Learning[84]** | |
| Older adults tend to learn new material more slowly than younger adults. | |
| Age-related changes are not the only factor involved in learning effectiveness. | |
| Individual differences in learning ability are important. | |
| Instruction and practice can improve the older adult's learning performance. | |
| Older adults learn more effectively when the information is related to information they already know. | |

potential chronic illness, older patients are left more susceptible to increased morbidity due to inadequate communication. Older individuals must receive adequate patient education to decrease potential health disparities that may arise from inadequate management of chronic illness caused by lack of understanding of health care advice.

Many health literacy problems among older adults may be caused by physiological and cognitive changes related to aging. For example, as the individual's vision decreases, they may choose not to read as much, and therefore their reading skills are compromised. In such situations, the therapist must use other approaches such as active listening, creating an environment that is nonjudgmental, and encouraging the patient to participate in the teaching and learning process as much as possible.

In general, the therapist must be acquainted with indicators to identify, address, and progress toward resolving the issues of low literacy patient populations throughout health care. Patient education topics such as communication, active listening, clarity of language, and sensitivity to possible patient impairment and functional limitation must be considered by the therapist and addressed properly. The gerogogy model of teaching emphasizes message length, demonstration, adjusting the teaching pace to the learner, tying the message or topic to the previous experiences of the patient, repetition, and concreteness of the information.

## TEACHING AND LEARNING CONSIDERING CRYSTALLIZED/FLUID INTELLIGENCE

Intelligence is not a singular phenomenon but has two pertinent aspects identified as crystallized and fluid intelligences.[88] Crystallized intelligence is learning from past experiences and previous learning.[89] For example, reading comprehension and vocabulary exams are situations when crystallized intelligence is necessary.[89] This type of intelligence is based upon facts and experiences.[89] Crystallized intelligence becomes stronger as people age accumulating new knowledge and better understanding. Elements of crystallized intelligence may include arithmetic reasoning, social interaction, and the application of skills and knowledge to solving problems.[88] Crystallized intelligence continues to grow throughout adulthood. Fluid intelligence, also called native mental ability, is the ability to think and reason abstractly and also problem-solve.[89] Learning, experience, and education are not part of fluid intelligence.[89] Fluid intelligence also is the individual's capacity to perceive relationships and perform abstract thinking.[89] Elements of fluid intelligence may include the speed with which information can be analyzed, as well as attention and memory capacity.[88] Fluid intelligence peaks in adolescence and starts to decline in the 30s and 40s.[89] Fluid and crystallized intelligence are complementary to each other. Some learning tasks can be mastered mainly by exercising either fluid or crystallized intelligence.[89] Additionally, fluid intelligence, or reasoning, has been viewed as an individual's aptitude for learning.[88] As people age, they become somewhat less adept as learners, with learning ability beginning to taper off at about age 20.[88] Fluid intelligence is more likely to decline with age than crystallized intelligence.[89] In fact as mentioned before, crystallized intelligence may continue to improve with age. Many people continue to gain expertise and skills in particular areas throughout life. Additionally, from a cognitive perspective, an individual's fluid intelligence regarding information processing may decline with age.[90] Nevertheless, familiar information and tasks that are well-practiced may not necessarily be affected by age. This means that physical and occupational therapists should connect new information and skills to activities and material the learner already knows. However, complex tasks that require taking in new information and analyzing it may become more difficult as a person ages.[90] This deficiency can also be attributed to impairments that may occur in an individual's attention, speed of information processing, and memory.

## TEACHING AND LEARNING CONSIDERING COGNITIVE ABILITIES

Attention is necessary for new information to be acquired.[90] Certain changes in the learner's attention ability have been reported with older age. This difficulty in sustaining attention may be related to the general overall slowing of information processing.[90] Mental processing and reaction time become slower with age. As the American Federation of Aging Research describes:[90]

> This slowing of information processing speed actually begins in young adulthood (the late 20s), although imperceptibly at first.
>
> By the time people are past 60 or older, they will generally take longer to perform mental tasks than younger people. For example, on tests of intelligence that require the person to perform tasks within a short time frame, older adults often do worse than younger people. This was wrongly considered (in the past) to be a measure of decreased cognitive functioning.
>
> However, on intelligence tests with liberal time limits, older adults are often able to perform just as well as younger individuals.
>
> Therefore, it is clear that older adults don't lose mental competence. It simply takes longer to process the necessary information.

Memory is a complex function that has been divided into different types.[91] Only some of these are affected by age. Difficulties that occur with memory are usually small and vary widely from person to person, making generalizations difficult. Short-term memory or working memory is commonly believed to be affected by age.[91] Short-term memory is the retention of information that must be manipulated or transformed in some way. Conscious mental processing goes on in working memory.[91] It requires taking in information from the environment and from memory stores and accomplishing a mental task. Every person has limits on how much they can keep in their short-term memory at one time. As people get older, complex mental tasks can become more difficult if they require too much information to be held in memory in order to process it.[91] Another method to classify memory is the categorization of implicit and explicit memory. Implicit memory is the retention of skills and reflexes that have been acquired, such as the procedures for driving a car.[90] Implicit memory generally remains intact throughout life. Explicit memory is the conscious memory of facts and events.[90] These memories are more vulnerable to age-related decline. Additionally, older adults may have increasing difficulty with word retrieval such as recalling the name of a familiar person or object.[90] The reason for this may be slowed processing speed.[90] The information is not forgotten altogether but they need more time for retrieval. The physiological explanation may be related to prefrontal cortex atrophy.

For example, brains of older adults showed a pattern of decline and also of preservation.[90] This means that decreased mental activity in older adults is a combination of factors. These may include deterioration of neurons, shrinkage of frontal lobe and hippocampus, or/and decline in the utilization of dopamine.[90] As a result, many older adults may experience difficulties with word finding or sometimes being absentminded.[90] However, the research is still investigating brain repair by using plasticity when the death of neurons due to damage such as from a stroke can be compensated by surrounding neurons.[90]

## TEACHING AND LEARNING CONSIDERING THE OLDER ADULT'S AUTONOMY

An important aspect of learning for the older adult is the ability to be independent. Independence or autonomy gives the older individual a sense of self-respect, pride, and self-functioning. Autonomy is an important factor of the older adult to be able to make independent choices. Older individuals need control and choices in their abilities to be independent and have self-esteem. Consequently, effective patient education for the older adult must help him or her maintain or regain their autonomy. For example, patients found education in regard to impairments of hearing, vision, depression and urinary incontinence to be useful helping them with decision-making abilities and also self-management of the impairments.[92] Social acceptability is another major goal of older adults, allowing them to receive approval and acceptance from others. Social acceptability is derived from health, a sense of vigor, and feeling and thinking young. Despite declining physical attributes, the older adult often has residual fitness and functioning potentials. Thus, patient education can help to channel these potentials. For effectual patient education, the therapist must assess a patient's life patterns including habits, physical and mental strengths, and economic situation in order to determine how to incorporate teaching to complement existing regimens and resources with new required behaviors. The ability to cope with change during the aging process is indicative of the person's readiness for patient education, especially for preventive health. Positive coping mechanisms allow for self-change as older individuals draw on life experiences and knowledge gained over the years. Negative coping mechanisms indicate a person's focus on losses and show that their thinking is immersed in the past. The therapist as the teacher must emphasize exploring alternatives, determining realistic goals, and supporting large and small accomplishments.

## TEACHING AND LEARNING CONSIDERING VISUAL IMPAIRMENTS

When teaching an older adult, the teaching environment should be brightly lit but without glare to accommodate vision changes. The American Printing House (APH) for the Blind recommends specific guidelines for people with low vision. APH's guidelines were implemented in research studies showing optimum readability for persons with low vision.[93] When teaching older individuals who may have vision problems, therapists must include large print materials with headings that are bolder and bigger than regular large print (**Table 12.3**).[93]

## TEACHING AND LEARNING CONSIDERING HEARING IMPAIRMENTS

When teaching older individuals who have hearing impairments, the therapist must create an environment where the learner has a clear and direct view of the teacher's mouth and face and speaks from a well-lighted area of the room.[87] The instructor should not stand in front of windows or light sources that may show only a silhouette and hinder the necessary visual cues. The instructor must face the light source and keep his or her hands away from the face when speaking.[87] Any background noise must be turned off and the therapist must speak clearly at a normal to slower (if necessary) pace. People who have mustaches need to have them trimmed so the lips show clearly. If the learner uses hearing aids, these must be checked for working batteries.[87] The therapist needs feedback from the patient (client) to determine whether he or she is speaking too fast, too slow, or not clearly enough. Nonverbal cues such as leaning forward or cupping hands to his or her ears means the learner has difficulty hearing or understanding the message.

During patient education, the therapist must obtain feedback at every opportunity as an indicator of the student's level of understanding. If the learner does not understand, the educator must repeat the information, rephrase it, or use a different word succession.[87] For correct reinforcement, the new information must be repeated by the instructor in different contexts.

The topics should be sequenced so that new material is related to previously learned facts. All information must be written in detail and provided to the patient (client). When writing the material: (1) use simple vocabulary, (2) use short sentences, (3) reduce concept density, (4) keep cause and effect expressions in a very simple form, (5) do not omit words (such as "that") to clarify a sentence, (6) use simple coordinating conjunctions (such as

| Table 12.3 | |
|---|---|

### *Guidelines for Large Print Material for Older Adults*[93]

The font for large print materials should be at least **18 points** in size.

The typeface should not have serifs (such as CENTURY GOTHIC).

Spacing between lines of print should be at least 1.25 spaces.

Headings and subheading should be larger and bolder than regular large print text.

Paragraphs should be block style and use 1-inch margins. The left margin must be justified and the right margin must not be. There should be no first-line indentations to delineate paragraphs.

Printed materials should not have columns or divided words.

Use black print on white, ivory, cream, or yellow paper with a dull finish to inhibit glare.

The print should not use a background design or other graphical material.

Graphic materials such as graphs and charts are not recommended; however, if they need to be used, they must be enlarged and have good contrast, clarity, and coloration.

When art is used, full-color or high-quality black line art must be used (instead of gray-scale or shaded drawings).

"but," "for," or "so"), and (7) avoid transitional words (such as "however" or "although").[87] Certain language forms should always be avoided including verbs in passive voice, negative forms of verbs and other expressions of negation, and colloquial and idiomatic expressions.

For patients with hearing impairments, visual material needs to be used as much as possible. Only one source of visual information should be presented at each teaching session, however. Before starting the teaching process, the attention of the learner must be engaged. Interpreters in sign language or sign English can be used for patients (clients) who are deaf or hard of hearing.[87] If an interpreter is used, the therapist needs to go over the specialized vocabulary prior to starting the patient education session. Videos or film presentations need to include captioning. Audiotapes, videotapes, and other auditory rehabilitation materials can be translated into print format to make them accessible for older adults with hearing impairments.

## OTHER CONSIDERATIONS REGARDING OLDER ADULTS' TEACHING AND LEARNING

In physical and occupational therapy, teaching and learning must be concerned with the older adult's physiological needs and their level of *concentration and alertness*. Certain medications or interventions could cause exhaustion and loss of concentration. As an example, a simple antihypertensive medication such as Tenormin can cause dizziness, weakness, cold extremities, and extreme tiredness. The patient would not be able to concentrate and would be too fatigued to attend a learning session. Before teaching a rehabilitation intervention to a patient, the therapist must also be acquainted with the patient's level of knowledge in regard to that specific intervention. Basic material should be understood before more complex facts.

The older patient's ability to learn may be affected by the *methods and materials* chosen for teaching. One-to-one instruction can be the best teaching method, especially in rehabilitation, because it provides a nonthreatening environment in which to meet the older adult's needs and goals.[87] For some individuals, group teaching can be more beneficial because they can work together with others with the same experiences. Additionally, the family members or caregivers can be included in the teaching sessions, if the patient is agreeable to involving them and having them as support. Teaching older adults can be directed at helping them to use the talents and skills they have acquired over their lifetime.

*Readiness* to learn and *motivation* to master new information are also critical factors in effective learning by older adults. Therefore, desire to learn is a precursor to effective learning by elderly patients, and care should be taken to demonstrate the relationship between the individual's motivation for learning and the manner in which information is presented. As a result, the *selection of content* that is meaningful and appropriate to the older adults is important.

Another important aspect of patient education in general and with older adults in particular is effective *communication*. Clear communication between the therapist and the patient prevents medical errors, strengthens the patient-therapist relationship, increases interaction, and can lead to improved health outcomes. Physical and occupational therapists must establish a relationship based on respect by addressing the patient formally. The patient can be asked about his or her preferences in being addressed. Familiar terms such as "dear" and "hon" tend to patronize and can be annoying and upsetting for older adults.[87] When interviewing the patient and gathering important information about patient history, the therapist should allow enough time for the patient to respond to questions. Patients who feel rushed through the initial interview believe they are not heard or understood.[94] Patients should not be interrupted early in the interview. On average, health care professionals have been found to interrupt patients within the first 23 seconds of the initial interview.[94] Once interrupted, patients are less likely to reveal all of their concerns.[94]

Moreover, patients may be afraid that their complaints will be dismissed as trivial or that if they complain too much about minor issues, they will not be taken seriously later on. Some older patients do not mention symptoms because they are afraid of the diagnosis or treatment. They may worry that the health care professional will recommend costly diagnostic tests or suggest to them to stop some of their daily activities such as driving.

*Clear explanations of diagnoses* are critical. Uncertainty can be disturbing. When patients do not understand their medical conditions, they tend not to follow the interventions. Some patients refuse medical interventions because they do not understand how they will improve their health. Interventions that involve lifestyle changes such as exercises can be very disturbing and unacceptable for some patients. Encouraging the patient to make his or her own goals and take an active role in planning interventions can increase the patient's satisfaction, motivation, and compliance with interventions. In patient education, goal setting can increase the patient's self-regulation and self-efficacy.

## OLDER ADULTS' LEARNING STYLES, RATE OF LEARNING, AND GOAL SETTING

Educational programs for older adults must consider their learning styles as well as the rate of learning.[95] Typically, older adults learn at a slower pace and have a longer response time compared with younger people.[95] For example, when learning motor skills, older adults required more time to process nervous system information. Also, their response times to motor and sensory stimulation were affected, particularly when performing "complex motor movements."[95(p.1)] However, older adults were able to improve their performance on motor tasks with practice.[95] This observable fact also happens in younger adults. When planning programs for older adults, the therapists must know that the quantity of information may need to be decreased, and the time may need to be extended for people to integrate information and to respond with questions.[95] Additionally, older adults appear to benefit from a variety of learning techniques, with most older adults responding best to information presented in a visual format.[95] Furthermore, teaching older adults in a group setting may improve problem-solving skills.[95] Also, it is important to incorporate active learning into a variety of teaching methods such as handouts, overhead transparencies, demonstrations, problem-solving activities, home diaries, and peer evaluation and feedback.[95]

Goal setting is an integral component of self-regulation, especially for older patients with chronic disabilities.[18,96] Goal setting can be used in patient education as well as in health education of older adults. Community-based health education programs for health promotion initiated by rehabilitation professionals are essential to decrease the incidence and severity of many chronic conditions that affect older adults. Additionally, community-based health education programs have the potential to decrease the incidence and severity of many chronic conditions that affect older adults.[96] Similar to patient education, the educational programs must fulfill the needs of older individuals as well as their families. Consequently goal setting related to medical, preventive, and health maintenance interventions are essential. In this context, the following elements must be considered in the rehabilitative plan of care: (1) collaborative definition of problems, in which patient/patient's family problems are identified; (2) goal setting and planning, in which the patient and therapist can focus on a specific problem, set realistic objectives, and develop an action plan for attaining those objectives in the context of patient preferences and readiness; and (3) patient's access to services that teach skills needed to guide health behavior changes.[96]

Goal setting is also part of the self-efficacy theory stating that individuals must make a commitment to attain a goal.[30] Goals motivate people to exert the effort necessary to meet task demands and persist over time. Goals direct individuals' attention to relevant task features, behaviors to be performed, and potential outcomes.[30] Goals can also affect how people process information. Effective goal setting requires that older individuals set a long-term goal; break it into short-term, attainable subgoals; monitor progress and assess capabilities; adjust the strategy and goal as needed; and set a new goal when the present one is attained.[30] This multi-step plan is a key to promoting healthier human functioning, higher motivation, and perceived self-efficacy.

In chronic illness, day-to-day care responsibilities fall most heavily on patients and their families. Effective collaborative relationships with health care providers using a patient-centered care approach can help patients and families better handle self-care tasks. Collaborative management is care that strengthens and supports self-care in chronic disabilities while assuring that effective medical, preventive, and health maintenance interventions take place. Self-care and medical care are both enhanced by effective collaboration among patients and their families and health care providers.[96] Collaborative management occurs when patients and health care providers have shared goals, a sustained working relationship, mutual understanding of roles and responsibilities, and requisite skills for carrying out their roles.[96]

Moreover, setting small and attainable goals and giving regular feedback about these goals can increase the likelihood of successful performances on any given task. Generally, individuals across the lifespan have reported that observing patients who are successfully performing tasks or who have been in a similar situation encourages them to succeed in rehabilitation. For the older adult patient, role modeling of patients of similar age and illness may be enough to prompt him or her into action and increase his or her participation in the rehabilitation process. For example, exposing the older adult to videotaped sessions that focus on the positive aspects of rehabilitation by showing the progression from dependence to independence is beneficial.

## TEACHING AND LEARNING CONSIDERING FAMILY/CAREGIVERS

The role of the family must be considered as an important variable in patient education. Family can influence positive outcomes, especially for chronic disabilities and multiple disorders that are common with older individuals. Family and caregivers play an important role in the lives of their loved ones. They also play an increasingly important role in how the health care system functions. Family and caregivers may be able to offer essential information about the patient. By communicating with all the individuals involved in the patient's care, the physical and occupational therapist can provide more effective interventions.

In many cases, the family or caregiver can be a facilitator, helping the patient express concerns and reinforcing the health care provider's information. The family or the caregiver can also decrease the stress of interventions, positively influencing the patient. Also, the patient's family and/or caregivers can provide emotional, physical, and social support to the patient. The entire health care team can be involved in the family/caregiver education. However, to protect the patient's privacy, the therapist must confirm with the patient that the family's/caregiver's involvement in the rehabilitation process is acceptable. Sometimes, families may want to make decisions for a loved one. Adult children especially may want to step in for a parent who has cognitive impairments. The therapist has to be sure that the family member has been named the health care agent or proxy and has the legal authority to make health care decisions. Without this authority, the patient must make his or her own choices.

The therapist needs to set clear boundaries with family members and encourage the entire health care team to respect them. Families or caregivers face profound emotional, financial, and physical challenges. They often provide help with household chores, transportation, and personal care. An older spouse may find it hard to make time for him- or herself. The therapist must encourage the spouse to take a break from the loved one (if possible). The health care provider's encouragement and praise can help to sustain a family member or caregiver.

The therapist must determine the family's/caregiver's learning style preferences, cognitive abilities, and fears and concerns. Perceptions of the problem by both the family and the health care team must be determined to identify similarities and differences so that effective teaching can be provided. Additionally, especially with patients in the hospital or a skilled nursing facility, the family/caregiver can prepare the patient for discharge, help them to become more independent (or keep their independent status), and play a large role in the patient's continuity of care. The patient's family/caregiver becomes the most significant determinant of the success or failure of the continuation of rehabilitation at home (**Table 12.4**).

Regarding the patient's and family's/caregiver's cultural diversity, the therapist must be open to suggestions about incorporating religious practices or alternative medicine in the patient's plan of care and interventions. Appreciating the richness of cultural and ethnic backgrounds among older patients can help to promote good health care. The therapist must recognize how different cultures view health care and tailor questions and plan interventions to meet the patient's needs. The use of alternative medicines, herbal treatments, and folk remedies is common in many cultures. Also, showing respect to native healers on whom the patient may rely helps to build a trusting relationship with the patient and family/caregiver.

Older immigrants or non-native English speakers may need a medical interpreter. Federal regulations require health care providers to create a plan for serving their non–English-speaking patients. Guidance for accommodating people with limited English proficiency is available through federal, state, or community resources. Medical interpreters are more reliable and accurate translators than are family members or friends, who may inadvertently misinterpret the information.[87] Although the patient may choose to have a family member translate, they should be offered access to a professional interpreter.[87] Patients

| Table 12.4 | Examples of Rehabilitative Topics for the Family/Caregiver |
| --- | --- |

Specific information about the patient's illness and care needs. The materials can be pamphlets, videos, and other educational data. The material must match the family's reading level and language, and also consider cultural diversity. The family/caregiver may also need to learn relaxation techniques to reduce anxiety and modes to cope with the patient's illness.

The patient and the family should be encouraged to take notes and ask questions. Active involvement in the teaching and learning process promotes the patient's/family's/caregiver's retention and adherence. Key points should be repeated at each instructional meeting.

Plan the intervention goals and outcomes together with the patient and family/caregiver. For chronic illness, evaluation of the patient's ability to perform activities of daily living (ADLs) is important. The family/caregiver needs to receive education to encourage the patient's independence in ADLs.

Provide information on support groups and group education programs (and also suggest those that can be found on Internet).

When discharging the patient from physical or occupational therapy, involve the family/caregiver early in the discharge plan. Provide additional help with referral for home health or alternate care if necessary. Identify equipment needed for the patient at home. Work with the family/caregiver to develop schedules of outpatient rehabilitation, environmental evaluation of the patient's home, and specific exercise or patient care routines for home use.

Involve all members of the rehabilitation team early in the discharge process. A social worker needs to participate with other members of the team in home evaluation to identify various needs such as oxygen, a hospital bed, assistive and adaptive devices, and a wheelchair.

also need appropriate translations of written materials. When working with patients from other countries who speak English, the therapist must always ask about the patient's language preference.[87] Additionally, nonverbal communication related to body language and gestures should be considered. For example, some cultures point with the entire hand, because pointing with a finger is extremely rude behavior.[87] For other cultures, direct eye contact is considered disrespectful.[87]

## TEACHING AND LEARNING CONSIDERING PATIENTS' ACTIVE PARTICIPATION

Members of the rehabilitation team should encourage each patient to take the initiative in his or her rehabilitation. Promotion of engagement and active participation will decrease the feeling of powerlessness that often accompanies aging. Additionally, increasing the patient's sense of competence by having the patient assume greater responsibility for his or her progress and engaging him or her in self-challenging, problem-solving behavior can increase motivation. Increasing elderly patients' knowledge about rehabilitation issues and injuries, as well as tapping into any prior experience they may have had in the rehabilitation process, often encourages the patients to see themselves as skilled experts in their own care. Older patients are anxious to get back to their way of life. This need will often encourage patients to do whatever is required to return to their previous lifestyles. Physical and occupational therapists and assistants have the responsibility to encourage patients' participation in rehabilitation by reducing negative experiences, increasing rapport with the patient, and establishing and maintaining a safe and trusting environment. All of these factors, in conjunction with appropriate goals, will serve to increase motivation in the older adult population and thereby increase the likelihood of success and establishment of an appropriate discharge plan. The resultant increase in motivation will also serve to improve overall functional performance and quality of life for these patients.

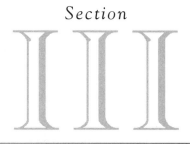
# CONCLUSIONS

## Section III Summary

This section described the importance of teaching and learning theories and principles in physical and occupational therapy patient education. Motivational strategies for teaching and learning were discussed in relation to enhancement of patient instruction. Learning theories were identified for implementation in patient education programs. The importance of Social Cognitive Theory to patient teaching and learning was emphasized in addition to other teaching and learning theories such as behaviorism, cognitivism, constructivism, andragogy, gerogogy, VAK, humanism, experiential learning, multiple intelligences, and Bloom's taxonomy. Section III concluded with application of Erikson's and Piaget's developmental stages to teaching and learning strategies in physical and occupational rehabilitation.

## Section III Case Study

### HEALTH EDUCATION PROGRAM FOR OLDER ADULTS

Per the APTA's *Guide to Physical Therapist Practice*,[1] the patient physical therapy diagnostic classification pattern is:

Impaired motor function and sensory integrity associated with progressive disorders of the central nervous system

ICD-9-CM Codes: 332 Parkinson's disease

APTA's *Guide to Physical Therapist Practice*[1] recommendations for patient-related instruction:

Instruction, education, and training of patient and caregivers regarding:

- Current condition (pathology/pathophysiology, impairments, functional limitations, or disabilities)
- Enhancement of performance
- Health, wellness, and fitness programs
- Plan of care
- Risk factors (pathology/pathophysiology, impairments, functional limitations, or disabilities)
- Transitions across settings
- Transitions to new roles

## Patient Description

The patient, Mr. S., is a 76-year-old man with a medical diagnosis of idiopathic Parkinson's disease (PD). He has a 10-year history of PD. He is taking Sinemet and bromocriptine. Mr. S. lives at home with his wife of 49 years, a healthy 70-year-old retired teacher. They have three children and six grandchildren. His wife is the main caregiver. In the past 6 months, he fell in his home twice. The first time he fell, Mr. S. was treated in physical therapy for bruises and a muscle tear in his right shoulder. This time, after his second fall, Mr. S. has no musculoskeletal complaints. Both falls happened in the morning when he tried to sit down on the kitchen chair to have breakfast. After the first fall, Mr. S. started to take his medication (as per his physician) prior to going into the shower. As suggested by the physical therapist at that time, he bought a walking stick used by trail walkers to use for support when walking. The stick allows him to maintain an upright posture. After his second fall, he visited the neurologist explaining that he also has been experiencing freezing episodes and forward falling (propulsion). Mr. S. explained that freezing occurred when starting to walk after a period of sitting, on turns, at doorways, and when approaching a target, such as a chair. The neurologist increased the dosage of Sinemet to help reduce the freezing episodes.

At this time (after his second fall), the plan of care in physical therapy was targeted at preventing falls. A home evaluation was scheduled by the physical and occupational therapist. The home evaluation resulted in removal of loose mats and cords. The occupational therapist recommended a set of handrails to be installed in the shower recess, and a shower chair and handheld shower hose were provided for showering. A rail also was installed at the back door steps (which led to the terrace). Mr. S. was encouraged to maintain regular physical activities, such as walking with a partner present. He received a falls diary and was trained in how to record the date, time, location, and perceived reason for each fall.

The physical therapy clinic that treated Mr. S. decided to hold a fall prevention health education program. Mr. and Mrs. S. and many other older adult patients and their families and caregivers were invited to participate. The educational program was organized by the rehabilitation team and was called "How to Prevent Falls: A Team Approach."

*Guiding Ideas to Prepare a Health Education Program for Fall Prevention*

The room where the education will be conducted must:

- Be a large room
- Control noise
- Eliminate distractions
- Use natural light and different levels of lighting throughout the facility (to mimic the home)
- Have a corner area with an easy chair and floor lamp to simulate home
- Include several types of flooring (if possible)
- Avoid clutter
- Set up several areas around the clinic with assistive devices (such as canes or walkers)
- Have in place small benches for family to watch and interact (but not to interfere)

Topics included in the educational program:

- Risk factors at home (e.g., throw rugs, lamp cords)
- Medication review (by the physician)
- Hearing check
- Vision check
- Alcohol intake risk
- The benefits of regular exercise
- The nutritional benefits of a calcium-rich diet

# *Section III References*

1. American Physical Therapy Association. *Guide to Physical Therapist Practice*. 2nd ed. Alexandria, VA: APTA; 2001.
2. American Occupational Therapy Association. *Occupational Therapy Practice Framework: Domain and Process*. Bethesda, MD: American Occupational Therapy Association Press; 2002.
3. Jette DU, Bacon K, Batty C, et al. Evidence-based practice: beliefs, attitudes, knowledge, and behaviors of physical therapists. *Phys Ther*. 2003;83(9):786–802.
4. Shepard KF, Jensen GM, eds. *Handbook of Teaching for Physical Therapists*. 2nd ed. Woburn, MA: Butterworth-Heinemann; 2002.

5.  Bastable SB. *Essentials of Patient Education.* Sudbury, MA: Jones and Bartlett; 2006.

6.  Falvo DR. *Effective Patient Education: A Guide to Increased Compliance.* Sudbury, MA: Jones and Bartlett; 2004.

7.  Pawar M. Five tips for generating patient satisfaction and compliance. *Fam Pract Manage.* 2005;12(6):44–46.

8.  Agency for Healthcare Research and Quality. Expanding patient-centered care to empower patients and assist providers. Available at: http://www.ahrq.gov. Accessed July 2007.

9.  O'Connor AM. Patient education in the year 2000: tailored decision-support, empowerment, and mutual aid. *Qual Saf Health Care.* 1999;8:1–5. Available at: http://www.qshc.bmj.com. Accessed July 2007.

10. Deakin T. Structured patient education: who are the x-Perts? *J Diabetes Nurs.* 2006;Nov-Dec:1–8.

11. Steiner WA, Ryser L, Huber E, et al. Use of the ICF model as a clinical problem-solving tool in physical therapy and rehabilitation medicine. *Phys Ther.* 2002;82(11):1098–1108.

12. Schenkman M, Deutsch JE, McGill-Body KM. An integrated framework for decision making in neurologic physical therapist practice. *Phys Ther.* 2006;86(12):1681–1702.

13. Randall KE, McEwen IR. Writing patient-centered functional goals. *Phys Ther.* 2000;80(12):1197–1204.

14. Habel M. Getting your message across: patient teaching. *Nurs Spectr.* 2005;2:Spring. Available at: http://www.patienteducationupdate.com/2005-05-01/article6.asp. Accessed March 2008.

15. Rankin SH, Stallings KF, London F. *Patient Education in Health and Illness.* Philadelphia: Lippincott Williams & Wilkins; 2004.

16. Pine GJ, Horne PJ. Principles of learning for adult education. *Adult Leadership.* 1969;18(4):108–110.

17. Dreeben O. *Introduction to Physical Therapy for Physical Therapist Assistants.* Sudbury, MA: Jones and Bartlett; 2007.

18. Maclean M, Pound P, Wolfe C, et al. Qualitative analysis of stroke patients' motivation for rehabilitation. *Br Med J.* 2000;321:1051–1054.

19. Catania AC. *Learning.* 2nd ed. Englewood Cliffs, NJ: Prentice-Hall; 1984.

20. Redman BK. *Advances in Patient Education.* New York: Springer Publishing Company; 2004.

21. SIL International: Partners in Language Development. *Developmental Theories of Learning.* Available at: http://www.sil.org/lingualinks/literacy/implementaliteracyprogram/Developmental TheoriesOfLearning.htm. Accessed May 2008.

22. Ferster CB, Skinner BF. *Schedules of Reinforcement.* New York: Appleton-Century-Crofts; 1957.

23. Wood D. *How Children Think and Learn.* 2nd ed. Oxford, England: Blackwell; 1998.

24. Svinicki MD. *Learning and Motivation in the Postsecondary Classroom.* Bolton, MA: Anker; 2005.

25. Martin G, Pear J. *Behavior Modification: What It is And How to Do It.* Upper Saddle River, NJ: Prentice-Hall; 2007.

26. Glanz K, Rimer BK, Lewis FM. *Health Behavior and Health Education: Theory, Research and Practice.* San Francisco: Wiley & Sons; 2002.

27. Hetherington EM, Parke RD, Locke VO. *Child Psychology: A Contemporary Viewpoint.* New York: McGraw-Hill; 2002.

28. Huitt W, Hummel J, Kaeck D. Assessment, measurement, evaluation, and research. *Educational Psychology Interactive.* Valdosta, GA: Valdosta State University; 2007. Available at: http://chiron.valdosta.edu/whuitt/col/intro/sciknow.html. Accessed March 2008.

29. Bandura A. Social cognitive theory: an agentive perspective. *Ann Rev Psychology*. 2001;52:1–26.
30. Bandura A. *Self-Efficacy: The Exercise of Control*. New York: W.H. Freeman; 1997.
31. Kaufman DM. ABC of learning and teaching in medicine. *Br Med J*. 2003;326:213–216.
32. Schunk DH, Zimmerman BJ, eds. *Self-Regulation of Learning and Performance: Issues and Educational Applications*. Hillsdale, NJ: Erlbaum; 1994.
33. Anderson ES, Winett RA, Wojcik JR. Self-regulation, self-efficacy, outcome expectations, and social support: social cognitive theory and nutrition behavior. *Ann Behav Med*. 2007;34(3): 304–312.
34. Daniels JA, Larson LM. The impact of performance feedback on counseling self-efficacy and counselor anxiety. *Couns Ed Superv*. 2001;41(2):120–130.
35. Spivey NN. *The Constructivist Metaphor: Reading, Writing, and the Making of Meaning*. San Diego, CA: Academic Press; 1997.
36. Kozulin A. *Vygotsky's Psychology: A Biography of Ideas*. Cambridge, MA: Harvard University Press; 1990.
37. Byrnes JP. *Cognitive Development and Learning in Instructional Context*. Boston, MA: Allyn & Bacon; 1996.
38. Hilgard ER, Bower GH. *Theories of Learning*. 4th ed. Englewood Cliffs, NJ: Prentice-Hall; 1975.
39. Brunner J. *Acts of Meaning*. Cambridge, MA: Harvard University Press; 1990.
40. Downing K. Information technology, education, and health care: constructivism in the 21st century. *Educational Studies*. 2001;27(3):229–235.
41. Herman WE. Humanistic influences on a constructivist approach to teaching and learning. Paper presented at: Annual Meeting of the American Educational Research Association; April 18–22, 1995; San Francisco, CA. Available at: http://www.eric.ed.gov. Accessed February 2008.
42. Smith MK. Humanistic orientations to learning. *Encyclopedia of Informal Education*; 1999. Available at: http://www.infed.org/biblio/learning-humanistic.htm. Accessed February 2008.
43. Rogers C, Freiberg HJ. *Freedom to Learn*. 3rd ed. New York: Merrill; 1993.
44. Hjelle LA, Ziegler DJ. *Personality Theories: Basic Assumptions, Research and Applications*. New York: McGraw-Hill; 1981.
45. Kolb DA. *The Learning Style Inventory: Technical Manual*. Boston, MA: McBer and Company; 1976.
46. Kolb DA, Osland J, Rubin I. *The Organizational Behavior Reader*. 6th ed. Englewood Cliffs, NJ: Prentice-Hall; 1995.
47. Schön D. *The Reflective Practitioner*. New York: Basic Books; 1983.
48. Gardner H. *Frames of Mind*. New York: Basic Books; 1983.
49. Campbell L, Campbell B, Dickinson D. *Teaching and Learning Through Multiple Intelligences*. 3rd ed. Boston, MA: Allyn & Bacon; 2003.
50. Dunn RS, Dunn KJ. *Educator's Self-Teaching Guide to Individualized Instructional Programs*. West-Nyack, NY: Parker Publishing; 1975.
51. Bloom BS. *Taxonomy of Educational Objectives, Handbook I: The Cognitive Domain*. New York: David McKay; 1956.
52. Clark D. Learning Domains of Bloom's Taxonomy: Performance, Learning, Leadership, & Knowledge. Available at: http://www.nwlink.com/~donclark/hrd/bloom.html. Accessed June 2008.
53. Knowles MS. *The Adult Learner: A Neglected Species*. Houston, TX: Gulf; 1984.
54. Green J. Andragogy: teaching adults; In: Hoffman B, ed. *Encyclopedia of Educational Technology*. San Diego, CA: San Diego State University; 1994. Available at: http://coe.sdsu.edu/eet/Articles/andragogy/index.htm. Accessed June 2008.

55. Knowles MS, Holton EF, Swanson RA. *The Adult Learner: The Definitive Classic in Adult Education and Human Resource Development (Managing Cultural Differences)*. Woburn, MA: Gulf Publishing Company; 1998.

56. Brookfield SD. *Understanding and Facilitating Adult Learning: A Comprehensive Analysis of Principles and Effective Practices*. San Francisco: Jossey-Bass; 1986.

57. Zemke R, Zemke S. Adult learning: what do we know for sure? *Training Magazine*. 1995;25(3): 31–40.

58. Carlson ML. A learning needs assessment of patients with COPD. *MedSurg Nurs*. 2006;15(4): 1–14.

59. Lowman J. *Mastering the Techniques of Teaching*. San Francisco: Jossey-Bass; 1990.

60. Davis EC, Nur H, Ruru SA. Helping teachers and students understand learning styles. *English Teaching Forum Online*. 1994;32(3):1–16. Available at: http://exchanges.state.gov/english teaching/forum-journal.html. Accessed March 2008.

61. Felder RM, Silverman LK. Learning and teaching styles in engineering education. *Engr Education*. 1988;78(7):674–681.

62. Erikson EH. *Identity: Youth and Crisis*. New York: W.W. Norton & Company; 1994.

63. Erikson EH. *Childhood and Society*. New York: W. W. Norton & Company; 1985.

64. Ratliffe KT. *Clinical Pediatric Physical Therapy*. St. Louis, MO: Mosby; 1998.

65. Feldman, W. *Learning and Attention Disorders: A Guide for Parents and Teachers*. Toronto, Canada: Key Porter Books; 2000.

66. Kennedy RW. *The Encouraging Parent: How to Stop Yelling at Your Kids and Start Teaching Them Confidence, Self-Discipline, and Joy*. New York: Three Rivers Press; 2001.

67. Schor EL, Abrams M, Shea K. Medicaid: health promotion and disease prevention for school readiness. *Health Aff*. 2007;26(2):420–429.

68. Substance Abuse and Mental Health Services Administration, Office of Applied Studies. *The OAS Report: A Day in the Life of American Adolescents: Substance Use Facts*. Rockville, MD: SAMHSA; 2007:1–10. Available at: http://oas.samhsa.gov. Accessed March 2008.

69. Nigg JT, Wong MM, Martel MM, et al. Poor response inhibition as a predictor of problem drinking and illicit drug use in adolescents at risk for alcoholism and other substance use disorders. *J Amer Acad Child Adol Psych*. 2006;45(4):468–475.

70. Spear LP. The adolescent brain and age-related behavioral manifestations. *Neurosci Behav Rev*. 2000;24:417–463.

71. National Center on Addiction and Substance Abuse at Columbia University. National survey of American Attitudes on substance abuse X: teens and parents; 2005:1–73. Available at: http://www.casacolumbia.org. Accessed March 2008.

72. Martino SC, Elliott MN, Corona R, et al. Beyond the "big talk": the roles of breadth and repetition in parent-adolescent communication about sexual topics. *Pediatr*. 2008;121(3):612–618.

73. Lefkowitz ES, Stoppa TM. Positive sexual communication and socialization in the parent-adolescent context. *New Dir Child Adoles Develop*. 2006;112:39–55.

74. Santelli JS, Lindberg LD, Finer LB, et al. Explaining recent declines in adolescent pregnancy in the United States: the contributions of abstinence and improved contraceptive use. *American J Public Health*. 2007;97(1):150–156.

75. Sawyer SM, Drew S, Yea MS, et al. Adolescents with a chronic condition: challenges living, challenges treating. *Lancet*. 2007;369:1481–1489.

76. Collins SR, Schoen C, Kriss JL, et al. *Issue Brief: Rite of Passage? Why Young Adults Become Uninsured and How New Policies Can Help*. Washington, DC: Commonwealth Fund; 2007:1–16. Available at: http://www.cmwf.org. Accessed March 2008.

77. National Adolescent Health Information Center. A health profile of adolescent and young adult males: 2005 brief. Available at: http://nahic.ucsf.edu. Accessed March 2008.

78. Vanden Zanden JW, Crandell TL, Crandell CH. *Human Development*. Boston, MA: McGraw-Hill; 2007.

79. Hoare CH. *Erikson on Development in Adulthood: New Insights from the Unpublished Papers*. New York: Oxford University Press; 2002.

80. National Association of Social Workers. Challenge of aging population nearing: much of social work workplace also aging, retiring. *NASW News*. 2005;50(10):1–54. Available at: http://www.socialworkers.org. Accessed March 2008.

81. Hammond C. Impacts of lifelong learning upon emotional resilience, psychological and mental health: fieldwork evidence. *Oxford Rev Ed*. 2004;30(4):551–568.

82. Donaldson JF, Flannery DD, Ross-Gordon JM. A triangulated study comparing adult college students' perceptions of effective teaching with those of traditional students. *Continuing Higher Ed Rev*. 1993;57(3):147–165.

83. National Institutes of Health, National Institute on Aging. U.S. population aging 65 years and older: 1990 to 2050 (in millions). Available at: http://www.nia.nih.gov. Accessed March 2008.

84. Poon LW, Gueldner SH, Sprouse BM. eds. *Successful Aging and Adaptation with Chronic Diseases*. New York: Springer; 2003.

85. McMann P. Ageism in America: discrimination against older people in health care. *Ezine Articles*. 2007. Available at: http://EzineArticles.com/?expert=Patti_McMann. Accessed June 2008.

86. Thomas CM. Bulletin boards: a teaching strategy for older audience. *J Gerontol Nurs*. 2007;33(3):45–52.

87. Dreeben O. *Physical Therapy Clinical Handbook for PTAs*. Sudbury, MA: Jones and Bartlett; 2008.

88. Beier ME, Ackerman PL. Working memory and intelligence: different constructs. *Psychological Bull*. 2005;131(1):72–75.

89. Colman AM. *Oxford Dictionary of Psychology*. New York: Oxford University Press; 2006.

90. The American Federation of Aging Research. Health and Age: Exploring the Secrets of Aging. Neurobiology of Aging Information Center. Available at: http://www.healthandage.com/html/min/afar/index.htm. Accessed March 2008.

91. Christensen H, Mackinnon A, Jorm AF, et al. Age differences and interindividual variation in cognition in community-dwelling elderly. *Psychology Aging*. 1994;9(3):381–390.

92. Van Eijken M, Wensing M, De Konink M, et al. Health education on self-management and seeking health care in older adults: a randomized trial. *Patient Ed Counsel*. 2004;55(1):48–54.

93. Kitchel JE. Large print: guidelines for optimal readability and APHont™ a font for low vision. American Printing for the Blind; Louisville, KY: 2004. Available at: http://www.aph.org/edresearch/lpguide.htm. Accessed March 2008.

94. Marvel MK, Epstein RM, Flowers K, et al. Soliciting the patient's agenda: have we improved? *JAMA*. 1999;281:283–287.

95. Peel C. "Tone your bones": a model for health education for older adults. *J Phys Ther Ed*. 2001;2:1–10.

96. Von Korff M, Gruman J, Schaefer J, et al. Collaborative management of chronic illness. *Ann Intern Med*. 1997;127(12):1097–1102.

# ETHICAL, LEGAL, AND CULTURAL VARIABLES IN PATIENT EDUCATION

Section IV of this book, "Ethical, Legal, and Cultural Variables in Patient Education," identifies major ethical systems and events contributing to the contemporary expansion of bioethics in the United States. Rational morality, conflict resolution, solving clinical dilemmas, and the importance of professional values in physical and occupational therapy are emphasized. The last two chapters of Section IV examine ethical, legal, and cultural aspects of patient teaching and learning. Section IV is divided into the following four chapters:

# THE ROLE AND SIGNIFICANCE OF ETHICAL SYSTEMS FOR HEALTH CARE

## Objectives

After completing Chapter 13, the reader will be able to:

- Identify major ethical systems.

- Compare and contrast teleological and deontological ethics.

- Appreciate virtue ethics in relation to moral decisions.

- Explain the role of care ethics in health care.

- Discuss the historical perspectives of bioethics in the United States.

- Identify the events contributing to the contemporary expansion of bioethics in the United States.

## The Significance of the Major Ethical Systems

Ethical systems represent comprehensive philosophical ideas on which guiding ethical and legal principles are based. These systems attempt to be coherent and systematic, trying to answer the fundamental practical ethical question that frequently emerges in every health care setting: "What am I supposed to do in this situation?" Contemporary ethical principles stem from systems that go back to earliest recorded history. All of these ethical systems represent altruistic and noble attitudes toward people. These attitudes exemplify health care providers' distinctive qualities. In clinical settings, the ability to recognize an ethical situation requires physical and occupational therapists to have knowledge of bioethical theories and issues that can apply to clinical situations. The multifaceted health care environment can produce issues that inevitably involve fundamental bioethical systems as described in this chapter.

Ethical principles represent moral values or standards governing a person's conduct.[1] The word *ethics* is derived from the Greek word meaning moral character; *morality* is derived from the Latin word for custom or manner. From a philosophical perspective, ethics is the theory of the right action whereas morality is its practice.[1] Both ethics and morals have to do with the customs or the manners in which people do things. Also, because ethics is part of philosophy, it can be defined as the study of moral philosophy or moral conduct.[1] Ethics is divided into three broad areas: (1) descriptive ethics, (2) normative ethics, and (3) metaethics.

Descriptive ethics, also known as comparative ethics, explains the moral systems of a group or culture.[1] It is specifically the study of people's beliefs about morality. The philosophical question for descriptive ethics would be: What are a group of people's beliefs about right or wrong or justice and injustice?[1] Normative (or prescriptive) ethics studies ethical theories, establishing moral systems for people to be able to make moral decisions. The philosophical question for prescriptive ethics would be: How should an individual act in a specific situation?[1] Metaethics or analytical ethics is the study of ethical terms and theories.[1] The philosophical question for metaethics would be to ask an individual: What is the meaning of right or wrong?[1]

In addition to these three broad areas of ethics, there is another type of ethics called applied ethics.[2] This form of ethics attempts to apply ethical theory to actual life situations.[2] The philosophical question for applied ethics would be: How does one take moral knowledge and apply it to practice?[2]

## THE PHILOSOPHIES OF THE MAJOR ETHICAL SYSTEMS

In ethics, five major ethical systems are predominant: ethical relativism, divine command theory, teleological ethics, deontological ethics, and virtue ethics.[3] The sixth system of ethics, entitled ethics of care or care ethics, is a normative ethical theory about what makes actions right or wrong.[2,4,5] It has been adopted by many health care professions including physical and occupational therapy.[2,4,5]

The first major ethical system, called *ethical relativism*, promotes the idea that all moral principles are equally valid relative to cultural preferences (**Table 13.1**).[3,6] The rules of society serve as a standard. In relativism, the individual determines what is "true" and "relative" in regard to their philosophical ideas. Relativism theorizes that truth is different for different people, not simply that different people believe different things to be true.[6]

Ethical relativism states that no moral principles are true for all people at all times and in all places.[6] The position of relativism is that there are no moral absolutes and no moral right or wrong.[6] It means that people's morals evolve and change with social norms over a period of time. This philosophy allows people to transform ethically as the culture,

| Table 13.1 | *The Main Philosophical Ideas of Ethical Relativism*[3,6] |
|---|---|
| There are no moral absolutes. | |
| What is right for one individual's culture may not necessarily be right for another individual's culture. | |

knowledge, and technology change in society.[6] Additionally, this view places the individual's will subordinate to the will of the cultural majority. From a positive point of view, some ethicists believe that relativism encourages tolerance and acceptance of other cultures.[3] From a negative perspective, most ethicists reject this theory because they believe that although the moral practices of societies may differ, the fundamental moral principles underlying these practices do not.[3] As a theoretical example of relativism, let's say one society's common practice is to kill one's parents after they reach a certain age. This could stem from that society's belief that people are better off in the afterlife if they entered in it while still physically healthy. Such a practice would be condemned in the United States, where the underlying moral principle is the duty to care for parents. Also, if certain practices depend on cultural beliefs, others such as torture or political repression may be governed by universal moral standards and be wrong regardless of the differences that exist among the cultures.

The *divine command theory* of ethics states that ethical standards depend solely on God.[6] It means that any act that conforms to the law of God is right whereas acts that break God's law are wrong (**Table 13.2**).[6]

A modified version of the divine command theory postulates that an ethical act is wrong if and only if it is contrary to God's commands.[6] For example, persecuting someone just for amusement would be wrong because it is contrary to the commands of a loving God.[6] Although the divine command theory is very controversial, some ethicists believe that its standards offer reasons for people to behave morally and also give equal importance to all individuals.[6] From a negative perspective, other ethicists state that the standards are arbitrary and depend on subjective interpretations.[6] Also, because there are no other moral principles apart from the ones promulgated by God, some consider the divine command to be a form of ethical relativism.[6] Rather than grounding the objectivity of ethics, this

| Table 13.2 | *The Main Philosophical Idea of Divine Command Theory*[6] |
|---|---|
| A moral act is obligatory if—and only if—it is commanded by God. | |

ethical theory completely undermines it by insisting that God's command (the same as those of societies) does not require justification in terms of external principles.[6] If there is no standard of being morally right apart from God's commands, then God could literally command us to do anything and it would be right for us to do it by definition.[6] As a theoretical example, if God commanded one person to torture another, the divine command theory considers the torture to be moral because doing the right thing is logically equivalent to doing what God commanded.

*Teleological ethics*, also called consequentialism or utilitarianism, states that the moral worth of an action is solely determined by its contribution to its overall utility in maximizing happiness among all persons (**Table 13.3**).[6]

Consequentialism believes that the moral worth of an action is determined by its outcomes.[6] This type of ethics judges the rightness of an action in regard to an external goal or purpose. Simply stated, the ends of an action justify its means. Positively, many consequentialist ethicists prefer to explain the theory by defining utilitarianism as good, pleasure, satisfaction, or preferences.[6] Actions are judged right or wrong based exclusively on their consequences. Right actions produce the greatest balance of happiness over unhappiness.[6] Also, each person's happiness is equally important. In the end, happiness or unhappiness is the same for everyone. Critically, this theory depends on the individual's own concept of happiness.[6]

Consequentialists advocate that when taking action, an individual is always required to consider the consequences of the act.[6] Furthermore, from an affirmative perspective, consequentialists promote human well-being and attempt to lessen human suffering.[6] Consequences can determine the moral value of the act. Negatively, the main question of some consequentialists remains the measurement of the moral worth of consequences.[6] One individual's moral action or happiness can become another individual's immoral act or unhappiness. Additionally, from a critical perspective, it is difficult to accurately predict all the consequences of an action.[6] As the ethical situation involves more people and alternatives, it becomes more difficult to determine which action would produce the best consequences. Also, many actions that normally would be considered wrong may cause good consequences. This theory can also undermine trust in others and intimate relationships because one can never be sure that the consequences might not justify a betrayal of trust, and in many cases, each individual is treated the same regardless of one's relationship.[6]

| Table 13.3 | ***The Main Philosophical Ideas of Teleological Ethics*[6]** |
|---|---|
| An action is right if—and only if—it promotes the best consequences. |
| The best consequences are those in which happiness is maximized. |

*Deontological ethics* focuses on the rightness or wrongness of the action itself as opposed to the rightness or wrongness of the consequences of that action. It is a form of ethics based on the duty or obligation of the action (**Table 13.4**).[3]

In deontological ethics, the emphasis is on moral rules, duty, autonomy, justice, and kind acts.[3,6] An individual must adhere to independent moral rules or duties. In order to make the correct moral choices, individuals must understand their moral duties and the rules regulating these duties.[3] An individual behaves morally only when he or she follow his or her duty.[3] When an individual does not follow his or her duty, he or she behaves immorally. Critically, this theory depends on the individual's own concept of rationality or of understanding of God's will.[3]

Deontological ethics also states that the moral value of an action is wholly independent from the consequences of an action.[3] This duty-based ethics treats people as ends and never as means.[3,6] From a positive perspective, deontological ethics provides a special moral status for people. The morals are universal. Deontological ethics also emphasizes the reasons why certain actions are performed.[3] From a negative point of view, some ethicists criticize deontological ethics for being too legalistic and not providing an accurate account of human motivation.[6] In some situations the correct motivation and duty can cause immoral consequences. Deontologists who are also moral absolutists believe that some actions are wrong no matter what consequences follow from them.[3] These ethicists argue that it is always wrong to lie, even if a murderer is asking for the location of a potential victim.[3] The consequences of an action such as lying may sometimes make that action the right thing to do. For example, during the Nazi's anti-Semitic aggression, a person would probably be acting immorally if they lied to Nazis about where Jewish families were hiding. Another criticism of deontology says that in many situations the rules of duty can be so abstract and conjectural that they may not be able to relate to the living entities.[3]

The fifth major ethical system is *virtue ethics*. Virtue ethics theories focus on helping people develop good character traits,[6] such as kindness and generosity. These character traits will, in turn, allow a person to make correct decisions later in life (**Table 13.5**).[6]

Virtue ethicists emphasize the need for people to learn how to stop destructive personality behaviors such as anger or greed. Virtue ethics considers morals to be within the

| Table 13.4 |
| --- |
| ***The Main Philosophical Ideas of Deontological Ethics[3,5]*** |
| An action is right if—and only if—it is in accord with a moral rule or principle. |
| A moral rule is a rule placed on people by God and by reason, and it would be chosen by all rational beings. |

| Table 13.5 | |
|---|---|
| ***The Main Philosophical Ideas of Virtue Ethics[6]*** | |
| An action is right if—and only if—it is what a virtuous agent would do in the circumstances. | |
| A virtuous individual is one who exercises the virtues. | |
| A virtue is a character trait a human being needs in order to flourish and do well. | |

individual.[6] The ethical principles seek to produce good people who act well because of their innate goodness. It emphasizes living well and achieving excellence. Critically, virtue ethics depends on an individual's own concept of being able to flourish and do well.[6]

From a positive point of view, because virtue ethics emphasizes the role of motives in moral decisions, it can make an important contribution to understanding morality and moral behaviors.[6] Virtue ethics teaches that certain virtues are required for certain moral decisions and that correct moral decisions need correct motives. For many people, especially children and young adults, encouraging them to choose morally and make the right decision becomes an important component of moral learning. Correct decision-making can increase the young person's motivation.

Ethicists consider virtue ethics important because they can teach moral conduct for people to become moral individuals, methods to make moral decisions, and the process by which moral attitudes develop. On the other hand, the critiques of virtue ethics consider that it offers no guidance for resolving ethical dilemmas.[6] Although many common moral decisions may come more easily to certain individuals, many moral dilemmas require a great deal of careful reasoning and thinking to make the right decision.[6] Also, the idea that having the "right" character helps to make the correct moral decision is not acceptable to many people. Ethicists question the "right" type of character a person must have to be able to make the right decisions.[6] Virtue theorists have treated the answer to this question as self-evident, but others do not think the same because the question had no response.[6]

The sixth type of ethics, the *ethics of care* (also called care ethics), addresses the physiological and psychological needs brought about by illness (**Table 13.6**).[4,5] Critically, in practical situations, ethicists consider that in care ethics a person must ask what each of the virtues listed in Table 13.6 requires one to do, rather than asking what would be the right moral act. Care ethics emphasizes the importance of relationships.[4,5] In health care, the main or primary relationship that needs to be maintained and fostered is that between the health care provider and the health care recipient.[5] This primary relationship is situated in a network of the patient's other relationships that must also be sustained for the primary relationship to continue.[5]

| Table 13.6 | **The Main Philosophical Idea of Care Ethics[4,5]** |
|---|---|
| | There are four virtues of caring: attentiveness to people's needs, responsibility, competence, and receptiveness. |

Ethics of care contrasts with deontological and teleological ethics, which stress the importance of universal standards and impartiality.[4] Ethics of care is a philosophical concept of ethics that emerged in the 20th century, challenging the idea that morality was just a domain of rules, laws, and duties.[4] Care ethics draws from the traditional female experiences of caregiving and being partial to persons who have needs and vulnerability.[4] The fundamental moral commitments of ethics of care expand the aims of medical practice to include caring and trying to cure patients, as well as the willingness, as a health care provider, to maintain a continual relationship with these patients.[4]

For many health care providers, the ethics of care increases the concept of clinical practice to a broader moral requirement of maintaining a relationship with the patient.[5] Because caring relations are not limited to the clinical setting, ethics of care raises questions regarding who will care for the patient at home.[5] It tries to ensure that the responsibility of care does not disproportionately fall on only one individual or only one group of individuals.[5] This could harm the individual caregiver and strain the network of caring relations. Thus, the moral obligation of the health care provider includes the commitment to arrange for a network of individuals (including family or social assistance) to care for the patient's well-being after discharge from an acute episode of care.[5] This concept demonstrates in a practical way care ethics' contribution to the field of medicine supporting patients' continuity of care after the discharge.

Philosophically, the ethics of care also promotes a dynamic caring relationship between the health care practitioner and the patient.[4,5] It involves receptivity or openness by receiving the individual who is cared for and understanding their reality.[5] The clinician is also able to show emotional reciprocity by having a caring and compassionate relationship with the patient.[5] From a realistic perspective, ethics of care increases medical practitioners' efforts to support chronically ill patients.[4] Modern medicine and technology has difficulty treating chronic patients because there are no miraculous interventions to offer.[4] As a result, many health care practitioners feel powerless and distance themselves from chronic patients.[4] The ethics of care morality allows these practitioners to address the needs of chronically ill patients by listening to their fears and concerns, providing support and encouragement, and tending to their physical and emotional comfort.[4]

The critics of ethics of care feel that it advocates partiality by stating that a person's obligations to care are stronger towards those to whom the individual feels closer.[4] This partiality is difficult to apply, especially in institutional settings, where institutional obligations to care may conflict with one's felt obligations to care. Also, ethics of care tends to assume that the caregiver knows what is in the best interests of the patient.[4] This principle can undermine the patient's autonomy.[4]

 # The Historical Role of Medical Ethics/Bioethics

Medical ethics had its origins in the Hippocratic Oath and in rabbinic and Christian knowledge.[3] One of the earliest medical ethics pledges is from an ancient East Indian manuscript.[3] It called upon the scholar studying medicine to follow a path of personal sacrifice and commitment to duty to his patient.[3] In western medicine, the Hippocratic oath remains the most important text of medical ethics. The Hippocratic ethic, also called the traditional medical ethic by physicians, has guided medical practitioners for hundreds of years.[7,8] It began in 500 B.C. in Greece and continued throughout the Roman Empire, Moslem medicine, and medieval Europe.[8] Medical ethics, as a philosophical Hippocratic theory, promotes deontological principles of duty representing a covenant between a competent physician and a sick patient.[8] It addresses the moral issues arising in the personal relationships between a treating physician and a suffering patient.[8] Hebrew medical manuscripts reveal Hippocratic influences against administering poisons to patients, giving potions to abort fetuses, committing adultery, and betraying practitioner confidences.[8]

## THE PERCIVALIAN CODE OF ETHICS

Medical ethics came into the American health care system from England between the late 18th and early 19th centuries.[8] Toward the late 18th century, Thomas Percival (1740–1804), who was the leader of the Manchester Philosophical Society, was called upon to regulate the relationships among three different groups of practitioners (physicians, surgeons, and apothecaries) at the new Manchester Royal Infirmary.[9] For the first time, these three different groups of professionals had to work together in one place giving care to patients. Percival, a physician himself, had to address the ethical conflicts among the three groups, in part because he was well known and had published on various topics in ethics already.[9] As a result of his involvement, in 1803 Percival drafted the first modern code of medical ethics called the "Code of Institutes and Precepts Adapted to the Professional Conduct of Physicians and Surgeons."[9] This code, following in the tradition of the Hippocratic oath, was to later influence the development of the American codes of medical ethics.[9]

The Percivalian code asserted the moral authority and independence of physicians in service to others, affirmed the profession's responsibility to care for the sick, and emphasized individual honor.[9] In 1847, the American Medical Association (AMA) adopted Percival's code, embracing patient autonomy concepts as well as medical jurisprudence ideas.[7]

The AMA Code of Ethics was founded in 1847 at the Academy of Natural Sciences in Philadelphia.[7] This was the first code in American health care to be adopted by a national professional organization.[7] The AMA code of medical ethics transformed American physicians' relationships with their patients and other professionals.[7] Through its early years, the AMA code went through dramatic changes and growth to improve the medical profession. The code gave medical doctors the obligation to respect patients and fellow professionals and offered a means of assessing the conduct of other physicians and surgeons as well as their superiors, employers, and other medical practitioners.[7]

## AMERICAN MEDICAL ETHICS

Today, the AMA code stresses the responsibility of the doctor to the patient and support for universal access to medical care.[7,8] The code also shows commitment to medical education and responsibility for better public health. Other features of the AMA code are: dedication, competence, compassion, and respect; honesty and duty to report fraud or deception; respect for the law and the rights of patients and colleagues; duty toward privacy and patient confidentiality; commitment to continued education, study, and consultation with other professionals; freedom of association and environment in the practice of the art of medicine; and the responsibility to make efforts to improve community health.[7]

After the implementation of the AMA code, up to the end of the 20th century, other codes of ethics strongly influenced American medical ethics. These included the Nuremberg Code (published in 1947), the Declaration of Geneva (1948), the World Medical Association International Code of Medical Ethics (1949), the Declaration of Helsinki (1967), the Patient's Bill of Rights (1973), and the Vatican's Instruction on Respect for Human Life (1987).[9] The Nuremberg Code issued 10 principles of ethics in medical research and medical subjects' rights. It originated as an international condemnation of the Nazi's World War II (WWII) crimes against humanity that were committed in the name of research.[9] The Declaration of Geneva was also established by the World Medical Association in response to the Nazis' atrocities in the concentration camps.[9] It also updated the Hippocratic oath to be more applicable to the modern era. The World Medical Association International Code of Medical Ethics of 1949 attempted to develop international standards of medical ethics. The Declaration of Helsinki was created as another response to unethical medical experiments of the Nazis in WWII.[9] The 2000 revision of the declaration includes principles of medical research such as use of placebos, ongoing trials, and conflicts of interest.[9] Many of these principles are already incorporated in American regulatory research ethics.

## THE PATIENT'S BILL OF RIGHTS

The Patient's Bill of Rights of 1973 was very important for introducing medical ethics in American hospitals and health institutions to meet the needs of their specific patient populations and make patient rights and responsibilities understandable to patients and their families. The Patient's Bill of Rights was first adopted by the American Hospital Association with the expectation that hospitals and health care institutions would support these rights in the interest of delivering effective patient care.[9] It was also written partly as a response to the growing consumer health movement.

The last major influence on American medical ethics of the 20th century was the Vatican's Instruction from 1987.[9] It related to medical interventions in the initial phase of life and the process of procreation and the need to conform to principles of Catholic morality.[9]

## THE BELMONT REPORT

Following WWII, many ethical issues found their way into American health care and health research, such as health care delivery to the elderly and to impoverished patients.[9] For American health research, crimes against humanity in human subject research constituted the primary condition for the emergence of bioethics. The ethical issues of informed consent and human experimentation represented intense ethical problems encountered in research studies. Abuses during the Nazis' atrocities of WWII, the U.S. Tuskegee syphilis experiments,[10] and Willowbrook hepatitis studies[10] indicated the need to prevent further abuses and adopt guidelines and rules in these complicated areas of morality and justice. The Doctors' Trial in Nuremberg in 1946 after the fall of the Third Reich showed the world the atrocities perpetrated by Nazi medicine and the crimes against humanity Nazi physicians committed. Additionally, the Tuskegee experiments involved denying treatment for syphilis to 399 African American men in order to investigate the disease.[10] The Willowbrook hepatitis study experimented on institutionalized children with mental retardation by intentionally infecting them with hepatitis so that the investigators could determine the effects of a hepatitis vaccine.[10] As consequences of these horrific research abuses and additional abuses of poor people and the elderly, the initial discussions to form the field of bioethics emerged. On July 12, 1974, the U.S. Congress created the National Research Act and the National Commission for the Protection of Human Subjects of Biomedical and Behavioral Research.[11]

The National Commission's responsibilities were to identify the basic ethical principles that should underlie the conduct of biomedical and behavioral research involving human subjects and to develop guidelines to assure that such research was conducted in accordance with those principles.[11] In order to accomplish these responsibilities, the commission considered the following: (1) boundaries between biomedical and behavioral research and the accepted practice of medicine, (2) appropriate guidelines for the selection of human subjects for participation in research, (3) the role of assessment of risk-benefit criteria determining the appropriateness of research that involves human subjects, and (4) the nature and definition of informed consent in various research settings.[11] After almost 4 years of discussions and intense consideration, the commission developed a minimal set of ethical principles and guidelines to prevent future research abuses. These principles that summarized the basic ethical standards identified by the commission in the course of its deliberations are known as the Belmont Report.[11]

The Belmont Report was important in the development of American medical ethics because it included three ethical standards of human research: respect for autonomy of the person, beneficence, and justice.[11] Respect for the autonomy of the person required moral assurance that participants in research experimentation would be treated as autonomous individuals, and those with diminished autonomy would receive protection. Beneficence promoted well-being of the research participants while minimizing the risks. Justice expected fair distribution of all benefits and burdens of the experiment.[11] Later the principle of nonmaleficence was added, directing that no harm should come to the participants. In addition, the Belmont Report incorporated specific elements of biomedical research with human subjects such as informed consent, reasonable and lawful selection of subjects for research, and open explanation of research risks and benefits.[10]

## THE EVOLUTION OF AMERICAN BIOETHICS

In 1979, the first edition of *Principles of Biomedical Ethics* by Thomas Beauchamp (philosopher) and James Childress (theologian) was published.[12] The field of bioethics developed considerably during the 1980s, bringing many ethical controversies to science, medicine, politics, law, philosophy, and theology. In the early development of American bioethics, the following historical factors influenced the field's expansion to its contemporary magnitude: the major and rapid technological changes creating the need to re-examine moral issues, rising health care costs questioning resource allocation, the pluralistic context in which health care is delivered, and the increase of publicly recognized rights of self-determination.[13] Nevertheless, for bioethics to expand at today's level of cloning and biotechnology, this means that other social and political phenomena influenced its growth. These may include, among others, the availability of new medical technologies and research in ecology, genetic engineering, and environmental health (**Table 13.7**).[13]

## THE ROLE OF CONTEMPORARY BIOETHICS

Bioethics, as a philosophical study of ethics in health care, is defined as a form of civil consensual ethics regulating the health care delivery system.[3] Prominent ethicists consider bioethics to be a deontological, virtue-based ethic and a liberal utilitarian morality that emphasizes individual autonomy.[8,12–15] The principles of autonomy, beneficence,

| Table 13.7 | **Events Contributing to the Expansion of American Bioethics**[13] |
|---|---|
| | The availability of new biomedical technologies that allowed new diagnostic and therapeutic possibilities and caused moral dilemmas. |
| | The new scientific and social domains such as ecology, environmental health, genetic engineering and biotechnologies, demographic growth, technological manipulation of behavior, and reproductive medicine. |
| | The outbreak of new social movements raising questions of biomedical significance. |
| | The objection to dominant medical paradigms and to the meaning of termination (of services) when providing health care. |
| | The need for an ethics for the era of techno-science. |

nonmaleficence, and justice are the cornerstone standards of bioethics. They are considered common morality standards that all moral persons accept as authoritative. However, when these principles need to be applied, they can become ethically confusing because they do not offer straightforward solutions.

Contemporary bioethical principles may be understood and employed from different perspectives. Bioethics includes disciplines from psychology to social, economic, legal, and religious areas, just to mention a few.[14] Bioethics of the 21st century is portrayed by prominent ethicists to be a continuous string of critical issues starting with genetics and molecular biology, going through the bedside professional ethics in medicine, and continuing with social policy and the ethics of health care reform.[8,15] Trying to find solutions to these numerous ethical dilemmas, many of the philosophical questions remained unanswered, ignored, or trivialized.

For the current position of bioethics, the central philosophical issue remains the same—the philosophy of right and good conduct.[13] In the 21st century, the scope of bioethics is particularly debated.[13] Some ethical theorists want bioethics to concentrate only on the morality of medical interventions or technological innovations;[15] others aim to include in bioethics all actions that relate to medicine and biology.[13,14] The issues raised by bioethics as a distinct area of academics are largely answered by the needs of various institutions in different disciplines.[13] Bioethicists are important in today's American society because they can apply the enormous body of research and history of discussions about bioethics in a fair, intelligent, and honest manner using tools from the different disciplines that supply the field.[13]

Bioethics can be found everywhere in contemporary discourses in science, politics, medicine, research, philosophy, social science, and theology.[16] For example, in regulatory research, it is impossible to create a major medical research effort without ethicists to assist.[16] Bioethics is becoming increasingly an interdisciplinary field. Bioethical analyses are also extremely vast and divisive in their substance. The future of bioethics is becoming more controversial, including an increased number of debatable political, medical, philosophical, and theological matters and questions.[13] Although medical ethics and bioethics are separated, many bioethicists and medical ethicists have different beliefs about its future.[3,8,13–15] Some think bioethics should be integrated and form a mature, philosophically based ethics called metaethics.[14] Others think that bioethics must be totally abandoned when practicing medicine in favor of traditional Hippocratic ethics.[8,15] Alternatively, in the 21st century, bioethicists are involved in new areas of bioethics, including various ethical issues emerging from different branches of biomedical sciences. One of these (called neuroethics) encompasses ethical issues arising from clinical and basic neuroscience such as neurology, psychiatry, psychopharmacology, cognitive neuroscience, and affective neuroscience.[17] These modern ethical problems are brought about by advances in brain implants and psychopharmacology as well as increased research activity in the neurological explanations of behavior, consciousness, and even spiritual transcendence, which combines religion, science, and technology.[17] The role of bioethics is expanding to include the application of neuroimaging technology to study the injured brain while trying to understand concepts of consciousness and vegetative states of individuals with brain injury.[18] At the same time, these novel discoveries could increase health care providers' understanding of mechanisms of injury and also of recovery. Consequently, contemporary progress using science and technology and its potential clinical application may increase the possibility of future bioethical debates and conflicts in health care, including the rehabilitation sciences.

# MORALITY AND VALUES IN PATIENT EDUCATION

## Objectives

After completing Chapter 14, the reader will be able to:

- Discuss bioethical trends and principles in physical and occupational therapy.
- Classify the necessary components of rational morality.
- Outline the three general considerations when resolving a moral dilemma.
- Describe five steps for solving a clinical dilemma.
- Define moral sensitivity, moral judgment, moral motivation, and moral character.
- Apply problem-solving of an ethical dilemma to a clinical situation.
- Discuss conflict resolution skills used in patient education.
- Distinguish the roles of assertive behaviors.
- Appreciate the importance of assertive listening in physical and occupational therapy.
- List the therapist's assertive verbal and nonverbal communication skills.
- Recognize the American Physical Therapy Association's main professional values.
- Identify the American Occupational Therapy Association's main professional values.

# Bioethical Trends in Physical and Occupational Therapy

For allied health professionals, bioethics is an applied form of ethics incorporated into their professional ethics. The ethics of allied health professionals is concerned with the moral issues arising from their professional knowledge and how to use that knowledge ethically when providing services to the public. Physical and occupational therapists and assistants are part of the allied health field involved with the delivery of health-related services pertaining to physical and occupational rehabilitation. Bioethical principles are included in their codes of practice and standards of conduct, setting the members of the physical and occupational therapy professions apart from others by establishing a set of ethical principles by which to work.

Physical and occupational therapists and assistants have long subscribed to a body of ethical statements developed primarily for the benefit of the patient. When evaluating ethical knowledge in physical therapy, it is clear that in the 1970s physical therapists were focusing on several ethical issues of their practice, research, and education.[19] These major moral topics, which were discussed in peer-reviewed articles in the 1970s, are concerned with the following issues: the role of the physical therapist in decision making, the function of informed consent and research, the historical context of physical therapy ethics, and teaching ethics in the professional schools.[19] A decade later, in the 1980s, physical therapy's ethical focus appeared to be on searching for moral principles of justice in resource allocation, informed consent, and ethical standards of autonomous practice. The 1990s brought to physical therapists moral dilemmas of managed care and scarce resources, prejudice and discrimination, and the evolving relationship between physical therapists and their patients.[19] Toward the end of the 20th century, truth-telling became a significant moral matter of physical and occupational therapy clinical ethics. Additional moral concerns were directed to the application of morality and justice in clinical practices.[19] This trend over 30 years demonstrates that physical therapists, the same as other health care professionals, have been concerned with the ethical development of American health care policies and health care reform. Today, in the 21st century, physical and occupational therapy is still searching for societal identity in its partnership with the community and health care institutions, in regard to normative rights, obligations, sanctions, and also ethical decisions specific to the professions.

The American Physical Therapy Association (APTA) includes ethical guidelines to oversee the moral actions of its members: physical therapists, physical therapist assistants, and physical therapist and physical therapist assistant students (**Table 14.1**).[20]

The House of Delegates, which is the highest policy-making body of the APTA, has adopted the *Code of Ethics* containing ethical principles for physical therapists (PTs) and the *Standards of Ethical Conduct* for physical therapist assistants (PTAs). The APTA's *Guide for Professional Conduct* interprets the PTs' *Code of Ethics* and guides professional development of physical therapy students, and its *Guide for Conduct* interprets the PTAs' *Standards of Ethical Conduct* and guides professional development of physical therapist assistant students.

| Table 14.1 | |
|---|---|
| ***General Principles of Ethics in Physical Therapy***[20] | |
| Physical therapists, physical therapist assistants, and physical therapist assistant students are guided by their professional organizations' ethical principles and standards in their relationships with patients, other professionals, the community, and all individuals in general. | |
| They also recognize responsibility to patients first and foremost as well as to society, to other health care professionals and providers, and to themselves. | |

The American Occupational Therapy Association (AOTA) includes its *Occupational Therapy Code of Ethics* as a public statement of promoting and maintaining high standards of conduct within the occupational therapy profession (**Table 14.2**).[21]

The AOTA's *Code of Ethics* addresses occupational therapists' and assistants' professional mission related to use of everyday life activities and occupations to help individuals participate in their functions in home, school, workplace, community, and other settings. The codes of ethics and standards of conduct in physical and occupational therapy promote discussions of ethical issues and improve ways to deal with ethical questions, dilemmas, and gray areas encountered in physical and occupational therapy work. These ethical standards and principles increase the level of confidence and trust among the members of the physical and occupational therapy professions and the public they serve.

| Table 14.2 | |
|---|---|
| ***General Principles of Ethics in Occupational Therapy***[21] | |
| Occupational therapy professionals and providers are guided by a common set of values and principles used to promote and maintain high standards of behavior in occupational therapy. | |
| Occupational therapy personnel—including all staff and personnel who work and assist in providing occupational therapy services, such as aides, orderlies, secretaries, and technicians—have a responsibility to provide services to recipients in any stage of health and illness who are individuals, research participants, institutions and businesses, other professionals and colleagues, and students as well as the general public. | |

## The Significance of Ethics of Care

In physical and occupational therapy, the ethics of care is a critical concept for patient teaching and learning because it allows the professional and provider to construct a relationship with patients and also promote patient-centered care. The ethics of care is described as an appropriate moral grounding of the physical therapy profession.[5] The physical therapist and the patient get involved in a partnership based on a caring relationship. This assists in the determination of the patient's goals for interventions. Care ethics places great emphasis on the importance of listening and respecting the patient. The therapist has to become engrossed or absorbed in the patient,[5] trying to really hear what the patient is saying. The therapist as the health care provider does not come into the conversation with a fully formed set of categories or rules for judgment. The ethics of care promotes empathy by making a connection with the patient and preserving that bond throughout and after the therapy.[5] Consequently, the ethics of care encourages continuity of care with physical and occupational therapy interventions.

The ethics of care helps therapists to make ethical decisions based on maintaining a relationship with the patient and not using detached judgments built only on principles and rules (such as in deontology; see Chapter 13).[5] The ethics of care advances wellness and behavioral modification for disease prevention. It requires therapists to have excellent communication skills to be able to receive the feelings of the patient and understand the patient's concerns, wants, needs, and fears.[5] It also demands increased time and energy from the therapist and the patient, and, if the therapist does too much for the patient, can minimize the patient's role in the intervention process.

When applying the ethics of care, institutional structures and greater administrative demands may cause ethical dilemmas. For example, conflicting demands may occur when an insurance company decides to discontinue interventions contrary to the recommendations of the therapist. Advocating the ethics of care to legislators and insurance providers can help continue to make quality services available and to protect the rights of patients/clients. Therapists need to be able to confront the conflicts generated among the dominant political, economic, and social forces and contemporary medical care. Therapists need to be in the forefront to incorporate ethics of care principles into all physical and occupational therapy practices.

## Moral Dilemmas and Strategies in Clinical Settings

Morality has a number of sources in a morally pluralistic democracy such as the United States. These may include laws, religions, schooling, family values and traditions, history, professional education and training, and personal experience.[22,23] The sources of morality can be in conflict regarding matters of human character and human and institutional behavior. Ethicists recommend that ethical conflicts be settled through rational discourse free of personal opinion.[22,23] The arguments and analyses must be clear, logical, and consistent.[22,23]

## ELEMENTS OF RATIONAL MORALITY

Health care professionals must always be prepared to solve ethical conflicts and difficult dilemmas in order to justify their medical decisions and actions. These decisions must be defended not only from a scientific, evidence-based perspective, but also from an ethical one. Ethical principles and standards, especially for health care professionals, represent a major part of such a clinical rationalization. This rationalization is also called a moral discourse and is described by philosophers and bioethicists as rational morality.[22,24] An individual's rational morality must include fairness or justice, well-founded and defensible reasoning, and the ability to reflect on his or her actions (**Table 14.3**).[22]

## STRATEGIES TO SOLVE AN ETHICAL DILEMMA

When considering deontological or teleological ethical systems, moral or ethical dilemmas can be resolved by taking into consideration the following elements: (1) the full range of options or alternative courses of action; (2) the positive and negative consequences

| Table 14.3 | *Necessary Components of Rational Morality*[22] | |
|---|---|
| Fair-mindedness | Fairness toward people and appreciation of the perspectives of various moral viewpoints. |
| Valid reasoning | A logically sound argument when making an analysis and considering key terms elucidating the concept. It can also identify similarities between moral concepts. Reasoning should be applied that considers principles and theories. The logical decision must have consistency and compare with other moral cases. |
| Reflective equilibrium | Movements between specific moral intuition and general ethical theories and principles. It also involves having a dialogue with other individuals. |

associated with different paths of action; and (3) the analyses of each path of action in relation to moral principles, social and economic environments, the importance of each ethical principle, and other variables involved.[22] After the ethical dilemma is solved, the individual must act on their option and assume full responsibility for their decision. The person must also be able to justify their choice of action. The last step of resolving a moral dilemma is to identify the circumstances that led to the problem and remove the conditions for a potential future dilemma.

When trying to resolve an ethical dilemma in physical and occupational therapy settings, the clinician has many variables to consider, such as the patient's preferences and choices, the family's choices, psychosocial issues, other members of the health care team's concerns and opinions, the work environment, personal values, and each person's emotional considerations. A person's feelings and emotions are of high importance in particular moral situations.[22,24,25] These feelings can contribute to the clinician's intuition. They are also based on personal and professional values. An individual's intuition can be influenced by family, education, society, and many other emotional elements and values. When there is a mismatch between the ethical theory and the individual's own intuition, feelings, or values, the moral dilemma becomes extremely challenging.

The health care professional may require consideration of several identifiable moral values for appropriate ethical decision making. These ethical standards may include protection of one's pride, doing one's civic duty to society, acceptance of gender roles, treating others in a caring and benevolent fashion, protection of patients' rights and lives, assurance of quality care, smooth collaboration with other members of the health care team, observation of legal standards, and respect for the community and societal needs.[24] One recommendation for solving ethical dilemmas in the clinical setting is to follow five steps: (1) clarifying the facts, (2) analyzing the issue, (3) addressing psychosocial questions, (4) trying to reach an agreement, and (5) looking for assistance (**Table 14.4**).[26]

Although each health profession's code of ethics includes a specific statement of responsibilities for members of that profession, ethical principles or standards do not give precise answers for how to handle particular situations. Their role is to provide a useful framework for understanding conflicts. When moral values are in conflict, the result may be an ethical dilemma or crisis. Discussions, analysis, problem solving, and decision making are critical to moral resolutions. Ethical conflicts could involve an individual's multiple personal values, the basic moral principles and the need to achieve the desired outcome, or disagreement between the patient's and the provider's conflicting values. Sometimes no good solution to a moral dilemma exists and, occasionally, the values of the medical community may conflict with the values of the patient, family, or larger nonmedical community. As examples in emergency medicine or during surgery, the principles of autonomy and beneficence can conflict when patients refuse a life-saving blood transfusion.[27] As a result, health care professionals and providers must understand that professional and personal ethical principles do not determine absolute law. They just *make guidelines available* by which health care professionals and providers can make decisions in particular situations considering all applicable issues.

| Table 14.4 | *The Five Steps Approach for Solving Ethical Dilemmas*[26] |
|---|---|

1. Clarifying the facts of the case. Questions to ask are: What is the clinical situation involved? Who is the primary decision maker? What are the patient's concerns, values, and preferences?

2. Analyzing the ethical issues. Questions to ask are: What are the pertinent ethical issues? How should the ethical guidelines be applied to these issues?

3. Addressing psychosocial issues. Meeting with the patient and the patient's family. Meeting with the members of the clinical team. Questions to ask are: What are the psychosocial variables involved? How are these variables affecting the dilemma? What are the practical issues that complicate this dilemma?

4. Negotiating to reach an agreement.

5. Seeking the necessary assistance to reach an agreement.

Physical and occupational therapists and assistants face moral issues and dilemmas on a daily basis.[25] Ethical decisions are part of their clinical judgments. Similar to other rehabilitation interventions, patient education can also involve difficult moral conflicts and concerns. These require the health care provider to choose the best or right course of action. It may not always be easy to make the right choice because one moral obligation may be in disagreement with another different but equally righteous moral duty in a given situation.[25] Nevertheless, ethical problems can be managed if the physical or occupational therapist and assistant have high moral personal values as well as higher order decision-making and problem-solving skills. These skills may include empathy, active listening, questioning techniques, verbal and nonverbal communication, and reasoning.[25]

Cognitive psychology proposes that solving moral dilemmas requires an integrated model of moral behavior overlapping the four components of moral action: moral sensitivity, moral judgment, moral motivation, and moral character.[2,28] For each moral dilemma, the therapist's ability to make an ethical decision is dependent on these four components. Moral sensitivity allows the therapist to identify and interpret an ethical situation; moral judgment analyzes and makes good moral decisions.[28] Moral motivation is the value the therapist can give to the ethical factors and the related factors.[28] Moral character represents the therapist's strength and courage to act on the moral decision.[28]

This model of solving an ethical dilemma and arriving at an ethical action is not a linear problem-solving pattern.[28] For example, an individual's moral character may limit his or her moral motivation, or moral sensitivity may affect moral motivation. The components of the model are interactive and dependent on each other.[28] In this four-component paradigm (**Table 14.5**), the moral or ethical action is dependent on a person's cognition, affect, and behavior.[2,28] Affective and cognitive processes influence identification of a situation that is ethical or unethical.[28] Moral or ethical action is complex. It requires people to be assertive, help others, show leadership skills, manage their fears, stand up under pressure, be steadfast in their moral convictions, overcome obstacles, use resources judiciously, and take charge of their actions.

In physical therapy, when two or more ethical principles conflict with each other, the problem-solving method can incorporate the four ethical systems of deontology, teleology, virtue theory, and ethics of care (**Table 14.6**).[2] The deontological morality would stress the importance of the therapist's duty toward the patient, understanding his or her obligations as a health care provider and the rules that regulate his or her work.[2] The therapist's judgment would follow the ethical principles and standards of the profession as well as those of the institution and society. Teleological ethics would consider the consequences of the therapist's action, whereas virtue theory would place emphasis on helping the patient by showing kindness and generosity.[2] The teleological focus would be on understanding

Table
14.5

## *The Moral Action Approach*[2,28]

***Moral or ethical sensitivity*** is defined as evidence of concern for others and awareness of the consequences of one's actions. The individual must have the ability to identify and interpret a moral situation and understand how his or her actions will affect others. As a result, moral sensitivity involves imaginatively constructing possible scenarios, knowing cause and consequence chain of events, and having empathy and role-taking skills. Moral sensitivity is necessary to become aware that a moral issue is involved in a situation. Moral or ethical sensitivity includes the following abilities: to interpret a situation correctly; to have moral awareness of one's actions; to have empathy; to be aware of a moral issue; to understand patients' emotions; to express correctly one's own emotions; to find prejudice and to stop it; to communicate effectively in different settings with different people; to become culturally sensitive and competent; to care for other people; and to be unbiased and flexible.

*(continues)*

Table 14.5

## *The Moral Action Approach*[2,28] *(continued)*

*Moral or ethical judgment* is defined as evidence of a person's character in deliberating about ethical choices. The individual must be able to analyze the situation and make the correct moral decision. Once a person is aware that various lines of action are possible, that person must ask him- or herself which line of action is more justified morally. Moral or ethical judgment includes the following abilities: to be able to think critically; to problem solve; to reflect on choices and decisions; to know the ethics of right and wrong, justice and injustice; to make the correct choices; to understand the consequences of certain actions or decisions; to cope with disappointment and anger; and to be resilient.

*Moral or ethical motivation* and commitment is defined as being able to prioritize moral principles over personal ones. When reaching a decision, the individual must also be able to consider all the moral values involved in the ethical dilemma. These values need to be prioritized before making a decision. Ethical values need to take priority over personal values or interests. Moral motivation includes the ability to want to care and do the beneficent action over the self-interest action.

*Moral or ethical character* and competence is defined as having the strength of personal convictions, courage, persistence, overcoming distractions and obstacles, showing ego-strength, and possessing implementation skills. It includes the ability to have set goals and self-discipline, be able to control impulses, and also maintain strength and skill to act in accordance to one's own moral goals. In many situations, a person may be sensitive to moral issues, have good judgment, and prioritize moral values, but if he or she is lacking moral character and competence, the individual may weaken under pressure and not follow through, or he or she may be distracted and discouraged, causing moral behavior to fail.

the result of the therapist's choice of action.[2] Acting ethically brings correct consequences. Virtue morality would not permit the therapist to problem solve using their anger or greed.[2] Additionally, ethics of care would prompt the therapist to show respect for the patient's uniqueness and to establish a close interdependent relationship with the patient.[5] Finally, the therapist's moral decision would have to consider the essentials of care ethics such as compassion, collaboration, accountability, and trust.[5]

| Table 14.6 | *A Problem-Solving Approach Specific to Physical/Occupational Therapy*[2] |
|---|---|

1. Gather all the factual information in regard to the situation. The therapist must be able to ask him- or herself whether the situation is ethical.

2. Find the main area of the situation. This area can be related to the three domains, the individual, the organization, or the society.

3. Decide which component (or components) of moral action will be the most appropriate to apply. There are four components: sensitivity, judgment, motivation, or character (see Table 14.5).

4. Decide what type of ethical situation is involved. The ethical types (situations) can be: issue, problem, temptation, distress, or dilemma.

5. If the ethical situation is within the organization or society, the resolution may focus on identifying the needed policy and systems changes. Suggestions are necessary in regard to the involved values and the organization's policies and procedures contributing to the ethical problem. Organizational or societal situations may need a blending of all components of moral action. Situations at the organizational or societal level may require moral actions at a large scale such as organizing people, demonstrating, or writing letters to congressmen and senators.

6. If the situation is an ethical dilemma at the individual level, the resolution may focus on:

   • Applying the involved ethical principles such as beneficence, nonmaleficence, justice, autonomy, confidentiality, veracity, or fidelity.

   • Applying professional duties (from the American Physical Therapy Association's *Code of Ethics* or *Standards of Conduct* or from the American Occupational Therapy Association's *Code of Ethics*).

   • Deciding which outcome is the most beneficial.

   • Questioning the consequences and relating them to the patient, colleagues, other professionals and providers, and self.

   • Finding practical solutions and evaluating the consequences of the moral resolution.

   • Considering everything involved in the resolution, such as the law, disputed facts, resources, efficiency, cultural values, risks, psychosocial elements, code of ethics, standards of conduct, and other variables.

# Emotions, Reasoning, and Assertiveness During Ethical Dilemmas

Moral resolutions involve professional and personal obligations and duties. Finding moral solutions can cause tension and anxiety. Additionally, when solving ethical dilemmas, the individual's personal values, expressed as positive or negative emotions, can influence moral sensitivity, judgment, motivation, and character.[25]

## EMOTIONS AND REASONING

In regard to emotions, neuroethics (a new form of bioethics) reveals a strong relationship between emotions and reasoning.[25,29] The relationship between emotion and logic can result in empathetic decision making and problem solving. Neuroscientifically and philosophically, an individual's emotions are caused by normal brain functioning and are able to mediate cognitive tasks during interactions.[25,29] This means that emotions and thinking reflexively work together. Feelings, as expressions of emotions, arise from neural patterns forming mental images that represent emotional responses of a person's brain functioning.[29]

"Emotions and reasoning are constantly interacting"[25(p.15)] and influencing therapists' moral behavior. In stressful situations, negative moral emotions (such as guilt, contempt, disgust, or anger) can help the therapist find corrective actions, whereas in less stressful states, positive moral emotions (such as respect, awe and elevation, or gratitude) can expand a person's moral creativity and judgment.[30]

When discussing emotions and reasoning, guilt is a negative moral emotion that can motivate an individual to help someone they have victimized or to repair a misbehavior.[31] Freud considered guilt as the traditionally central moral emotion that was said "to be caused by the violation of moral rules and imperatives."[31(p.863)] Guilt reactions seem to appear mostly in individuals involved in personal relationships' dilemmas.[31] Contempt involves looking down on someone and feeling morally superior. Contempt can be elicited by the perception that another person does not measure up to the position that he or she occupies.[31] Psychologists think that contempt motivates neither attack nor withdrawal; however, contempt can cause social-cognitive changes such that the object of contempt will be treated with less respect, warmth, and consideration.[31] In health care, contempt can undermine an important moral emotion, such as compassion. Disgust is a negative response to physical objects and social violations.[31] It influences a person's motivation to avoid or break off contact with the offending party. Disgust involves different issues in different cultures and may be expressed in situations when people morally disgrace themselves.[31] Anger is described as the most underappreciated moral emotion.[31] Anger can be a response to unjustified insults and also can be triggered on behalf of one's family or friends.[31] Anger also could help an individual to bring justice back to a certain moral situation. Generally, anger involves a motivation to attack, humiliate, or get back at the person who is perceived as acting immorally or unfairly.[31] In many cultures, anger entails "a motivation for revenge."[31(p.859)] Unjust actions such as oppression, racism, or exploitation can direct people (even the ones with no relation to the victimized group) to be angry and demand corrective measures.[31]

As a positive moral emotion, respect involves holding a person in high regard and is related to the patient's autonomy. Respect can motivate the therapist to work for the best interest of the patient. Awe and elevation also are positive emotions that may be caused by seeing manifestations of humanity's higher nature.[31] Awe is elicited by experiences such as natural beauty or exceptional human actions or abilities. Awe seems to make people stop, admire, and open their hearts and minds.[31] Elevation is an emotional state that may cause an individual the desire to become a better person.[31] Elevation seems to also open "one's heart not only to the person who triggered the feeling, but to other people as well."[31(p.868)] Additionally, elevation promotes caring, altruism, and empathy. Gratitude is described as being warm and friendly toward a benefactor prompting one to repay a favor.[31] Gratitude encourages altruism and acting in a more shared, societal manner.[31]

Emotions and feelings are important in ethical decision making because they naturally occur in clinical practices. They should always be considered when solving ethical dilemmas. Additionally, in patient education, positive emotions induce caring values, beliefs, and practices that support communication and promote adaptation by reducing stress and helping to meet the psychosocial needs of patients. The ability to care for a patient during teaching and learning can help foster the therapist's sensitivity to self and to the patient.[2] As a result, the patient experiences comfort, concern, empathy, nurturance, support, and involvement.[2] The emotion of caring is an interpersonal process and behavior that allows the therapist to listen, help, and show respect for the patient.[2] Physical and occupational therapists and assistants must attend to positive feelings and emotions. Acknowledging the emotions is normal. In stressful situations that are fraught with negative emotions, the therapist must find constructive ways to express feelings in a socially acceptable mode. Being responsible for one's own feelings and behavior can help to deal with conflicting conditions.[32] Self-control using integrity and logic is an appropriate approach to an ethical dilemma. Additionally, the therapist's self-control can be enhanced by rationally understanding other individuals' emotions and working with them to clarify the problem and find an acceptable solution.[32] Constructive efforts on the part of the therapist can dissipate negative emotions and provide the opportunity to ask questions, listen to the answers, and try to understand the other person's point of view.[32] Furthermore, using humor whenever possible can diffuse a very tense situation.[32]

## ASSERTIVENESS

Ethical dilemmas may cause emotional behaviors that translate into conflicts involving patients, clients, and their families or colleagues and associates. Physical and occupational therapists and assistants need to be able to stand up and advocate for themselves and for their patients or clients. Assertive attitudes and behaviors are at the focal point of effective advocacy and moral resolution. Ethical dilemmas require decision-making skills and assertiveness. Assertiveness is a way of thinking and behaving that allows a person to stand up for his or her rights while respecting the rights of others.[2]

Assertiveness is characterized by getting the point across without offending others and using direct and appropriate expression of opinions, beliefs, feelings, and thoughts in an inoffensive manner.[2,33] The key elements of assertiveness are self-expression, honesty, respect for others, verbal and nonverbal appropriateness, and being direct, firm, and socially responsible.[2] Assertive individuals tend to face problems promptly and focus on solutions rather than problems.

Sometimes assertiveness can be wrongly confused with aggressiveness because both types of behavior involve standing up for one's rights and expressing one's needs. The key difference between the two styles is that individuals behaving assertively will express themselves in ways that *value* the other person.[34] Assertive attitudes and behaviors are important for effective advocacy that recognizes an individual's legal and moral rights.[34] Assertive individuals respect themselves and other people, and they are willing and ready to negotiate with others.[34] Assertive individuals are able to understand others points of view, although they may not necessarily agree with them. In contrast, aggressive individuals want their feelings to take precedence over other people's feelings and ideas. They may blame others for their problems and have the tendency to behave in a manipulative and inappropriate manner.[34]

In physical and occupational therapy, assertiveness is an ethical and professional responsibility that can increase the therapist's self-control, confidence, and respect.[33] Assertiveness skills can help the therapist learn to be confident, to respect other people's rights, and also to preserve those rights. Assertiveness skills can reduce the level of conflict and enable the therapist to maintain a mutually supportive relationship with other people.[33] Nonassertive individuals can be either passive or aggressive. People in the aggressive group may demonstrate condescending attitudes, lack of respect for others, public humiliation of colleagues, temper tantrums with patients, or an open display of embarrassing remarks.[33] As previously described, aggressive individuals insist that their opinions are the only correct ones.[34] They are not capable of finding logical solutions. On the other hand, passive individuals are not committed to their own rights and are not willing to stand up for themselves or others. Passive people also may be depressed and wish to be liked and accepted by everyone. Both aggressiveness and passivity are not acceptable skills to be used in communicating with patients, clients and colleagues.[2] Also, they are totally inappropriate in clinical reasoning situations. Furthermore, aggressiveness and passivity should never be used in patient education. Health care providers must learn to communicate with patients using assertive attitudes and behaviors. When assertiveness is applied to physical and occupational therapy, the therapists must follow these successive steps: (1) informing the patient that the therapist wants to understand his or her point of view; (2) having the readiness and the ability to accurately (without bias) understand the patient's point of view; and (3) informing the patient that his or her point of view was clearly understood.[34] Situations can occur when the therapist may be tempted to apply aggressiveness or passivity in his or her relationship with patients. However, being able to recognize his or her aggressiveness or passivity can help the therapist to change and practice assertive behaviors (**Table 14.7**).[2]

| Table 14.7 | *Examples of Assertive Behaviors in Patient Education[2]* |
| --- | --- |

*Recognizing situations in which it can be tempting to communicate with others either passively or aggressively.* This requires the therapist to develop skills recognizing these communication patterns and being aware of situations in which the behavior can become passive or aggressive. As a hypothetical example, a timid and introverted physical therapist has been teaching a patient for 20 minutes to ambulate with crutches using a four-point gait. The patient's husband, who is her caregiver, is aggravated by the situation. He feels that his wife does not need therapy and that the therapist does not know how to properly teach her how to walk. He thinks that he can actually teach his wife how to walk. He states that a year ago he also had therapy somewhere else and learned how to walk using a walker. He is angry and disagrees with the therapist's walking instructions. After the patient makes 10 to 15 tries to practice the gait pattern, the therapist is exhausted and stops the therapy. Patient's husband is ready to go home. He angrily states that he will never bring his wife there for therapy. The therapist keeps quiet and does not attempt to openly discuss the situation with the patient's husband. In this example, the therapist has assumed a passive behavior. The therapist gave up managing the conflict in favor of the husband's aggressive behavior.

*Recognizing situations in which it can be tempting to attribute setbacks to uncontrollable forces such as the medical system or the institution or a powerful individual's unpleasant personality.* This requires the therapist to think of strategies to replace feelings of negativity or hopelessness. Continuing the above example, the therapist should find a strategy and replace her feelings of hopelessness when teaching the patient how to ambulate. She should not attribute her teaching failure to the power and control of the patient's husband who aggressively interrupts and disagrees with her teaching.

*Replacing negative thought patterns with positive and powerful thoughts.* This requires the therapist: (1) to confront the nature of the situation that aroused the emotion (either on her own or asking a friend or colleague for help), (2) to change the passive or aggressive behavior of that situation, (3) to find the belief behind the wrong behavior, and (4) to replace the old (wrong) belief with a confident and positive thought. Continuing the above example, the therapist must change her passivity into assertiveness and find a positive strategy for reasoning. In order to do that she may need to understand the cause for the patient's husband's aggressiveness. She may need to listen to the patient and patient's husband and recognize their perspectives of disagreement.

*(continues)*

| Table 14.7 | *Examples of Assertive Behaviors in Patient Education*[2] *(continued)* |
|---|---|

*Practicing new opinions and new reasoning and positively modifying emotions and thoughts.* This requires the therapist to acquire new thoughts and feel positive and helpful. Continuing the above example, the therapist needs to take control of the situation and explain to the patient and her husband the gait pattern and the reasoning behind it. Her explanation should be assertive but also show respect and caring behaviors. As an appropriate ending to this hypothetical example, after listening to the patient's husband's point of view, the therapist found out that he learned a different form of gait pattern from his prior physical therapy interventions. He believed that the gait pattern he already knew must be applied to every patient, including his wife. The therapist now understood the patient's and her husband's viewpoints and was able to change her negative passivity into a positive assertive behavior.

*Practicing the new behavior that goes with the ownership of the right.* Practicing the new acquired behavior helped the therapist to become assertive.

Moral reasoning and verbal communication require *assertive listening skills.* These skills can strengthen the relationships between the individuals involved in the conflict, reduce stress, and provide the necessary patient support.[2] Considering another person's point of view does not necessarily mean agreeing with that person; however, it represents the first step in resolving the moral conflict, allowing for deliberation of all variables that involve the agreement/disagreement process. The focus of the therapist is to inform the patient that he or she is interested in hearing and understanding the patient's opinions (**Table 14.8**).[2]

All individuals involved in the moral conflict must be able to listen in a relaxed manner to ensure the accuracy of information, and assertive verbal communication is crucial (**Table 14.9**). The listener should be relaxed and genuinely attentive to the other person's message.[34] Tension should not be included in the listening process because it can obstruct a clear understanding of the situation.[34] Having the therapist summarize the patient's point of view allows for verification of the correctness of the information. Correctly understanding the patient's reasoning can be a start for finding solutions. The therapist must be able to work out a solution with the patient, although some problems may remain unresolved.

Nonverbal assertiveness can be communicated through eyes, facial expression, posture, personal appearance, and gestures.[34] Nonverbal behaviors provide clues to an individual's credibility, sincerity, and emotional state. For example, a slouching posture, avoiding eye

| Table 14.8 | Examples of How a Therapist Reasons When Communicating with a Patient[2] |
|---|---|
| "I would like to hear your views on..." | |
| "Could you tell me about them?" | |
| "Would you tell me more about how you see the situation?" | |
| "I think we are approaching this situation from two different perspectives." | |
| "I am confused about your stand on..." | |
| "What does the situation look like from your perspective?" | |

contact, or using nervous gestures mean passivity and nonassertiveness.[34] In contrast, a tense and rigid posture communicates a heightened emotional state, anger, and aggressiveness.[34] Nonverbal behaviors are significant advocacy tools during the patient communication process, especially in moral conflicts. Direct eye contact with the patient or client is an assertive behavior in American culture; however, the therapist must consider cultural diversity when applying assertiveness skills.[35] In some cultures, establishing eye contact with the patient may be inappropriate. In the United States, looking down when speaking to another suggests timidity, a weak point of view, and passivity. Additionally, looking to the side and not directly at the other person may indicate avoidance of truth and insincerity.[35] An erect and relaxed sitting or standing position may demonstrate confidence, self-control, energy, and a positive outlook.[35] The therapist's leaning slightly forward when sitting shows interest in the patient and also a sense of purpose.[35] Leaning back means just the opposite—disagreement and disinterest. Furthermore, crossing arms and legs

| Table 14.9 | Assertive Verbal Communication: DESC[2] |
|---|---|
| **D**escribe the situation. | |
| **E**xpress the feelings about the situation. | |
| **S**pecify the change in regard to the situation. | |
| **C**onsequences: evaluate the consequences by reflecting on the results that may occur from communication. | |

suggests a closed attitude whereas uncrossed arms and legs show a relaxed and open attitude.[35] An individual's facial expressions also can indicate assertive, aggressive, or passive behaviors. As an example of assertiveness, the face may reveal emotions such as alertness, interest, and agreement (**Table 14.10**).[34,35]

# Personal and Professional Values in Patient Education

In patient education, physical and occupational therapists and assistants must remain open to their patients' values, which may be different than their own. Values are important determinants of human behavior (**Table 14.11**).

Values constantly influence a person's choices and actions. An individual's values are based on enduring personal beliefs about what is important and what type of action a desired outcome can bring.[2,30,33] For example, an individual's values may change based on required actions for a desired outcome. Values related to personal decisions are termed nonmoral values whereas values associated with human interaction are called moral values.[2] Moral values are included in a person's identity and can fulfill individual goals and needs.[2] People's behaviors in their interactions depend on their values and true beliefs.[2] These

| Table 14.10 | **Assertive Verbal and Nonverbal Communication Skills[34,35]** | |
|---|---|---|
| **Verbal** | **Nonverbal** | |
| Focus the patient's attention. | Maintain an erect and relaxed sitting or standing posture at the same eye level as the patient. | |
| Use simple, clear, and easy to understand vocabulary. | Lean forward slightly with uncrossed arms and legs. | |
| Use a moderate tone of voice. | Maintain eye contact (being sensitive to the patient's cultural background). | |
| Be verbally sensitive to the patient's cultural background. | Maintain facial alertness, interest, or agreement; smile or nod as necessary. | |

| Table 14.11 | **Definitions of Values**[2,30] |
|---|---|
| Standards and patterns of choice that guide persons and groups toward satisfaction, meaning, and realization. | |
| Ideas that orient choice and form action. | |
| Concepts that require moral thought and conduct that may lead to the "fulfillment of human potential"[2(p.35)] or finding new meaning in life. | |
| Philosophical concepts that are not necessarily feelings or emotions but involve desires and fears and always are mediated through particular acts. | |

philosophical concepts of individuals' values are important to consider in patient education. In the teaching and learning experiences, the patient's values are intertwined with the therapist's professional values, helping to foster an effective and efficient relationship between the therapist and the patient. Physical therapists' professional values are considered to be altruistic when related to the benevolence aspect of care and trying to enhance and preserve the patient's welfare.[2] Furthermore, respect for the individual's right to dignity, privacy, and independence while maintaining personal, societal, and social relations represent priorities of physical therapy professionals and providers.[30]

## THE THERAPISTS' PERSONAL VALUES IN CONTEXT OF AFFECTIVE DOMAIN OF CARE

In addition to adhering to professional values, moral values are necessary to develop therapists' affective domain of care. The affective domain can increase the rehabilitation provider's appreciation of the patient's life situations and promote a clear understanding of the patient's beliefs, perspectives, and priorities.[36] Effective patient education requires a teaching plan based on the values and needs of the patient.[36] Additionally, the therapist's professional values can enhance his or her understanding of the psychosocial factors involved in physical and occupational therapy practice. The affective domain encourages development of the interpersonal and communication skills necessary for effective teaching and learning in patient management. Physical and occupational therapists and assistants can adjust their verbal and nonverbal communication and teaching skills when applying the affective skills of patient observation and questioning. Therapists' ability to self-assess and improve their affective skills represents the main solution to successful patient education and patient management.[36,37] Therapists' affective skills contribute to their clinical and educational abilities in the clinical settings. For example, affective skills can increase the clinician's observation proficiency, questioning style, and verbal and nonverbal communication patterns.[37] Furthermore, the therapists' affective abilities also can prompt them to recognize whether patients are understanding the new information or/and patients' needs for therapists to modify their verbal and nonverbal communication patterns accordingly.[37]

In physical and occupational therapy formal education, the affective domain skills (such as interests, attitudes, appreciation, and values) are difficult to teach and evaluate because they contain an inherent subjectivity.[37] In physical therapy practice, a clinician can increase his or her affective skills through professional socialization, self-assessment, and by using the participant-centered problem-solving approach.[37] Professional socialization requires a moral inventory of one's own nonmoral values and acceptance of new moral values consistent with the values of the physical or occupational therapy profession.[37] Improving the clinician's affective proficiency by demonstrating appreciation and respect for the patient or client can increase the patient education aspect of care and also provide greater patient satisfaction and adherence.[37]

Educators and health care providers have been searching for ways to improve the affective domain of care for students and patients. The importance of a clinician's affective skills has been observed in the development of personal and professional relationships and value systems.[36,37] In the educational field, the affective domain of learning is associated with success in the patient's cognitive domain of receiving and retaining knowledge.[38] Newer teaching and learning theories (in the sciences) suggest that increasing the affective component—such as the learner's attitude, involvement, and values—can in fact help the cognitive part of the learning process.[38] For example, the affective-cognitive consistency learning theory examines the relationship between the learner's attitudes and beliefs and hypothesizes that learners are in an unstable state when their attitudes towards an object, event, or person and their knowledge about that object, event, or person are inconsistent.[38] This theory suggests that if the affective component of the attitude system is increased through persuasive messages, the cognitive component becomes highly enhanced.[38] It is established that once the individual goes through an attitude change, his or her cognition will be stimulated to process the new information.[38] Processing the message requires that the individual appreciates the meaning and the value of the message in order to accept it and retain it in the long-term-memory.[38]

Clinically, the best method to involve patients in the affective domain of learning is the patient-centered approach. Through patient-centered care, the patient can increase his or her cognitive part of learning by working with the therapists to integrate new values and commitments to a broader learning situation.

## THE PHYSICAL/OCCUPATIONAL THERAPIST'S PROFESSIONAL VALUES

The APTA identifies seven main professional values for the physical therapy profession: accountability, altruism, compassion/caring, excellence, integrity, professional duty, and social responsibility.[20] These values are conceptually similar to the occupational therapy ideals, which include such concepts as equality, freedom, prudence, truth, dignity, justice, and altruism.[39] The AOTA describes equality as a principle requiring all individuals to be perceived as having the same fundamental human rights and opportunities.[21] In occupational therapy, equality means for therapists to always be fair and impartial in their daily inter-actions with patients.[21] Freedom allows patients or clients to exercise choice and demon-strate initiative, autonomy, and self-direction.[21] Prudence is the ability of the rehabilitation provider to govern and discipline him- or herself using reflection and reasoning. Prudence requires the therapist to be judicious, discrete, and vigilant and use moderation, care, and circumspection when making judgments.[21] Truth means faithfulness to facts and reality. To abide by truthfulness or veracity means to be honest, forthright, accountable, and accu-rate in one's attitudes and actions. Truthfulness can contribute to the therapist's commit-ment to learning, self-understanding, and development of professional competence.[20,21] The value of dignity emphasizes the inherent worth and uniqueness of each individual. This professional value can be demonstrated in physical and occupational therapy through empathy and respect of self and others such as patients, clients, caregivers, and family. Professional values in occupational therapy also stress the importance of dignity by helping patients/clients combine their biologic and sociocultural attributes with life experiences and by respecting the interaction among the individual's mind, body, and physical and social environments.[21] The professional value of justice upholds moral and legal principles such as fairness, equity, truthfulness, and objectivity. This means that rehabilitation serv-ices should be provided to all individuals who are in need of these services. Occupational therapy practitioners must also be knowledgeable and respect patients' legal rights, and abide by the local, state, and federal laws governing the profession. Altruism is defined by the AOTA as unselfish concern for the welfare of others.[21] This moral professional concept is reflected in actions and attitudes of commitment, caring, dedication, responsiveness, and understanding of occupational therapists and assistants (**Table 14.12**).

In physical therapy, the professional value of accountability is described by the APTA as an active acceptance of responsibility for diverse roles, obligations, and actions includ-ing self-regulation and other positive behaviors contributing to the needs of patients, the profession, and society.[20] In patient education, accountability can relate to managing the patient's teaching and learning and assuming responsibility for the patient's learning. Accountability may also incorporate the responsibility to maintain professionalism and to be able to work with change.[20] The value of altruism, similar to occupational therapy, means devotion to the patients' interests including the fiduciary responsibility of placing the needs of the patient ahead of the therapist's self-interests.[20] In physical therapy practice, altru-ism also involves using evidence-based research to enhance the patient's health care needs.[20] Seeking to complete patient and professional responsibility tasks prior to personal wants represents another example of altruism. The value of compassion is the desire to iden-tify with another individual's own experience. Caring includes the professional's concern, empathy, and consideration for the values and needs of others (**Table 14.13**).[40]

In physical therapy, excellence means to practice using current knowledge and theory, integrating judgment and patient perspective, challenging mediocrity, embracing advance-ment, and always working toward new knowledge.[20] Using evidence-based research and valuing what other more experienced therapists can offer in clinical practices demon-strates excellence. Integrity as a professional value means to possess and adhere to high

| Table 14.12 | *Summary of Professional Values in Physical and Occupational Rehabilitation[20,21]* |
|---|---|
| Accountability. |
| Altruism. |
| Compassion and caring. |
| Excellence. |
| Integrity, truth, and justice. |
| Duty and responsibility. |

moral principles or professional standards.[20] Integrity may also include abiding by rules, regulations, and laws governing the physical therapy profession, being trustworthy, recognizing the limits of one's expertise, and choosing ethical employment situations. Professional duty is the commitment to provide efficient services to patients/clients, effectively serve the profession, and positively influence the health of society.[40] Social responsibility promotes mutual trust between the profession and the public and responds to the societal needs for health and wellness.

| Table 14.13 | *Characteristics of Compassion and Caring[40]* |
|---|---|
| Understanding the sociocultural and psychological needs of diverse populations. |
| Abstaining from acting on one's own social, gender, cultural, and sexual biases. |
| Demonstrating respect for the uniqueness of others. |

# ETHICAL AND LEGAL ASPECTS OF PATIENT EDUCATION

## Objectives

After completing Chapter 15, the reader will be able to:

- Describe the relationship between ethics and law.

- Differentiate between beneficence and nonmaleficence.

- Apply beneficence to physical and occupational therapy services.

- Examine the concept of negligence in clinical practice.

- Relate the principle of confidentiality to privacy and protection of information.

- Compare and contrast justice and veracity.

- Identify the relationship between veracity and patient autonomy.

- Describe informed consent and patients' requirements for informed consent.

- List the main communication concepts of informed consent in clinical practice.

- Relate the principle of autonomy to the patient-centered care model.

# The Relationship Between Ethics and Law

In the 21st century, ethical and legal principles are critical components of health care. This is largely due to the increased complexity of caring for patients and the difficult decisions that the new contemporary technologies and life events demand. Highly visible bioethical issues of the 21st century include biotechnology matters such as genetics, cloning, and patenting human tissue products; end-of-life problems such as euthanasia and physician-assisted suicide; and public health policy topics such as bioterrorism, pandemics, and access to health care. Physical and occupational therapists and assistants are confronted daily with less visible but more common ethical topics such as research ethics, managed care, or ethical clinical issues.

When making ethical decisions, all health care providers must consider the relationship between ethics and the law. The most important connection between these two disciplines, especially when related to physical and occupational therapy, is providers' concern for patients' access to medical care including informed consent, confidentiality, and provision of high standards of care. The strong association between bioethics and law can be expressed as a linear correlation in which the two are dependent on each other.[41]

Bioethics or ethics is the identification of values that "ought" to be, whereas law is the manifestation of these values as public rules.[41] Ethical standards are derived through law, institutional policies and practices, professional standards, and fiduciary obligations. Laws are a result of the federal and state constitutions, statutes, regulations, and individual cases or lawsuits.[41] Although they are interrelated, bioethics and law have different views in regard to their philosophy, function, and power. An ethical principle is a significant professional and moral guide, but is generally unenforceable by law. Conversely, a court ruling is a binding decision that determines the outcome of a particular argument or controversy. Typically, a statute or administrative code sets a general standard of conduct, which must be adhered to; civil (or criminal) consequences may follow a breach of the standard.

Frequently, lawmakers such as courts and legislatures turn to the ethical policy statements of professional organizations when creating laws affecting that profession. As a result, health care providers may greatly influence legal standards by their work in creating professional ethical standards. Furthermore, law and bioethics are dynamic and in a constant state of change due to challenges created by new technologies, laws, or other stimuli.[41]

Physical and occupational therapists may encounter situations during patient education that relate not only to ethical, but also legal issues. Typically, ethical and legal concerns cannot be separated due to their close relationship with each other. The therapist's ethical and moral beliefs can have a significant effect on a patient's legal rights. Physical and occupational therapy providers must be clear and demonstrate awareness of their personal ethical and legal beliefs in relation to patient teaching and learning. In health care, many providers believe it is normal for them to influence patients based on their own values, which they consider to be correct and best for their patients. Nevertheless, by doing so, they can inadvertently infringe on patients' autonomy and freedom. Ethical issues such as informed consent, confidentiality, justice, or autonomy can easily become legal problems, especially when violating a patient's rights or the federal laws of self-determination and confidentiality. Assuring that each rehabilitation intervention, including patient education, has a patient's informed consent is an important ethical and legal obligation. For the patient to be able to make an informed consent on a physical or occupational therapy intervention, the therapist needs to provide enough information. Additionally, understanding health care policies and the legislative processes are important parts of delivering high-quality physical and occupational therapy in contemporary health care.

The more demanding and costly the medical care becomes, especially in rehabilitation, the more patient instruction may be needed to assist patients to assume increased responsibilities for their own health. Teaching patients in rehabilitation is a process of training them in skills and tasks as part of the usual interventional process. Additionally, patient instruction provides patients with the necessary abilities to improve their health, wellness, and fitness, and effect changes in their lifestyles and societal roles. Typically, matters related to behaviors, prevention, and lifestyle modifications that impact others can result in moral and legal dilemmas. An example of a setback could be the discontinuation of physical therapy interventions when the therapist perceives the patient to be nonadherent to his or her teaching about lifestyle modifications. The attainment of the patient's goal to change his or her behavior and achieve the maximum degree of health can become an ethical dilemma when considering the conflicting views of the patient and therapist. Eventually, this can become a legal issue.

As an example of a moral issue that could become a legal issue, teaching a 48-year-old patient smoking cessation after a myocardial infarction can be different than instructing an 83-year-old individual. The therapist may be more successful with the 48-year-old patient, whose values are different than those of the 83-year-old individual. Educating the younger patient regarding smoking cessation may be successful using positive reinforcement instruction and taking into account the patient's personal rewards, social support, and self-esteem enhancement. On the contrary, the same patient instruction may not be successful with the older individual who lives alone, has no friends, and is depressed. Additionally, more problems can arise when the therapist's ideals and values are totally different from those of the patient or client. The therapist's personal principles may be in conflict with the elderly patient's values. Consequently, a moral concept could change into a legal one if the therapist tries to force his or her principles to alter the patient's values.

The world is changing rapidly. Modern society is more unpredictable and complex than ever before. This causes more pressure when trying to find right answers and actions. Resolving ethical dilemmas requires critical thinking and continuous ethics checks to decide what is right and at the same time what is legal.[41] Questions in regard to violating either civil laws or the institution's policy may occur. Contemporary ethical dilemmas require all health care professionals and providers to be equipped with increased individual responsibility and special critical-thinking and problem-solving skills. Twenty-first century ethical and legal abilities may include empathetic listening by paying attention to the patient's complete message and responding appropriately to their needs, and being able to evaluate risks by recognizing and managing ethical and legal issues in the clinical practices. Physical and occupational therapists and assistants are required to be accountable to uphold and consistently act in concert with their professional values and principles.[20,21] They need to advocate for organizational decisions that are driven by the needs of their patients and patients' families. They must act with integrity by communicating openly and honestly, keeping promises, honoring commitments, and promoting loyalty in all their relationships. They must collaborate with all essential stakeholders in interprofessional relationships to promote common interests and shared values and to address opportunities and challenges. When providing interventions in rehabilitation, including patient instruction, physical and occupational therapists and assistants must always take into consideration their moral decisions and actions and relate them to ethical and legal principles of health care.

# Interrelated Legal and Ethical Principles in the Context of Patient Education

Ethical principles are important for all health care providers when making health care decisions. By disregarding ethical principles, health care providers also could break legal rules and regulations found in the local, state, or federal codes of law. Many would argue that, in patient education, there are no challenges involving ethical and related legal concerns. However, others would say just the opposite, indicating that patient education poorly done can create harm to the patient such as "loss of confidence and incapacitated confusion."[42] In addition, inaccurate patient education, paternalistic attitudes of the health provider, or declining (for unfounded reasons) patient's opportunity to receive instruction also could breach ethical as well as legal principles and tenets.[42] Interrelated legal and ethical principles presented in this subchapter are beneficence, nonmaleficence and negligence, confidentiality, justice, veracity and autonomy, informed consent, truthfulness, and patient autonomy.

## BENEFICENCE

Traditionally, beneficence is the first principle of morality to "do good and avoid evil" (**Table 15.1**). Beneficence is a moral obligation to promote good and prevent or remove harm and to promote the welfare, health, and safety of society and individuals in accordance with their values, preferences, life goals, and beliefs.[16]

Ethicists argue that beneficence is partially dependent for its content on how an individual defines the concepts of good and goodness.[16] Beneficence is not consider a specific moral rule and cannot by itself instruct an individual as to what concrete actions constitute doing good and avoiding evil.

For health care professionals and providers, beneficence is the moral principle of having the duty to act for the benefit of the patient or client (**Table 15.2**).[16,35] Under the principle of beneficence, the physical and occupational therapy professionals and providers' primary obligation is service to the patient and the public at large. In rehabilitation, the most important part of beneficence is the provider's obligation to deliver rehabilitation services in a competent and timely manner demonstrating patient care and support. The

| Table 15.1 | **Concepts of Beneficence in Clinical Practice[16,35]** |
|---|---|
| Promotes what is best for the patient. |
| Emphasizes the moral importance of doing good to the patient. |
| Highlights the provider's respect for the patient. |
| Stresses the patient's autonomy. |
| Ethical dilemma of beneficence: when a competent patient chooses a course of action that is not in their best interest. |

therapist's beneficent intent has to be without an ulterior motive or benefit that would not be experienced by the patient but by other individuals.

In addition, in regard to patient education, physical and occupational therapists and assistants must provide and promote appropriate instruction to patients, clients, families of patients and clients, caregivers, and the community at large. The instruction must be accurate, reflect the most current information (from the evidence-based research), and produce good outcomes for the recipient(s).

| Table 15.2 | **Applications of Beneficence in Physical and Occupational Therapy[16,35]** |
|---|---|
| Provide high-quality services in an appropriate, equitable, and just manner. |
| Strive to ensure that fees are fair and reasonable; commensurate with services provided; and in accordance with local, state, and federal requirements. Also consider the patient's individual ability to pay. |
| Advocate for patients to obtain needed interventions and services through their available resources. |
| Recognize and appreciate each patient's cultural components related to race, economics, ethnicity, geography, religion, politics, sexual orientation, gender, age, and marital status. |
| Promote the public health, safety, and well-being of all individuals, communities, and the public at large. |

Sometimes, the rehabilitation professional's/provider's understanding of benefit for a patient can differ sharply from that of the patient, client, family, or caregiver. Consequently, beneficence should be applied with caution, not to legally breach patients' rights. Care has to be taken not to use certain interventions that the patient or client does not want and that may take over the patient's or client's autonomy. Particularly with patient education, it can be very easy for the therapist to become paternalistic by coercing the patient into the necessary activity. The therapist may sincerely believe that the information is in the best interest of the patient; however, the patient's point of view regarding the recommendations should also be considered. As an example, a physical therapist gives patient education about smoking cessation to a patient who is 83 years old and is in the hospital after a recent second myocardial infarction. The patient tells the therapist that he has been smoking for more than 67 years and does not want to stop smoking at this point. The patient insists that at this time he wants to go outside and smoke. He keeps stressing that he is alone and does not care if he lives or dies. Trying to force this patient to comply with what the therapist thinks is "best" for him would significantly infringe on the patient's autonomy and personal values. The principle of autonomy requires the therapist's respect for the patient's decision-making capacity as a competent adult. In this example, the patient is an 83-year-old competent adult. This patient has the right to refuse physical therapy education in regard to smoking cessation.

Other legal aspects of beneficence in addition to respecting the patient's autonomy involve the therapist's adherence to the tasks and duties of his or her job description, his or her professional organization's ethical codes/standards of conduct, and the rehabilitation facility's policies, procedures, and protocols.

## NONMALEFICENCE AND NEGLIGENCE

Traditionally, the second bioethical principle is *nonmaleficence*. It means "first, do not harm." Beneficence and nonmaleficence are not directly related. Beneficence requires taking action to benefit others whereas nonmaleficence involves refraining from action that might harm others.[35] Nonmaleficence can be interpreted to imply that if a health care provider cannot do "good" without also causing harm, then he or she should not act at all in that particular circumstance (**Table 15.3**).[16,35]

| Table 15.3 | *Concepts of Nonmaleficence in Clinical Practice*[16,35] |
|---|---|
| Do not harm the patient. |
| Weigh any probability of potential harm to the patient/client and apply the *prima facie* ("by first instance") duty not to cause injury. |

Physicians interpret nonmaleficence to exclude the practice of euthanasia, when the physician directly and intentionally administers a substance to cause death. Perhaps the most extreme example is the violation of the nonmaleficence dictum by Dr. Jack Kevorkian, who was convicted of second-degree homicide in Michigan in 1998 after demonstrating active euthanasia on the television news show *60 Minutes*.[43] American medical ethicists have been engaged in a large debate over the issue of physicians subscribing to the physician-assisted suicide instead of euthanasia. The reason is that, with physician-assisted suicide, the physician may not consider him- or herself responsible for administering the lethal medication. Physician-assisted suicide occurs when a physician provides a medical means for death. Usually it involves the physician giving to the patient a prescription of a lethal amount of medication that the patient takes on his or her own.[44] The patient, not the physician, administers the lethal medication. Euthanasia means that the physician would act directly, for instance by giving a lethal injection, to end the patient's life.[44]

Physician-assisted suicide continues to be a national debatable ethical issue in regard to its legalization in the United States. Many medical doctors feel that laws concerning or moral objections to physician-assisted suicide and even euthanasia should not prevent physicians from honoring a patient's (or authorized patient surrogate's) decision to refuse life-sustaining treatment. It means that doctors in medical clinical practices can in appropriate situations withhold or withdraw medical interventions by allowing competent patients the opportunity to guide future health care decisions. Competent patients can convey their decision about end-of-life care ahead of time by using "advance directives." These are legal documents providing a way for patients to communicate their wishes to health care professionals, family, and friends in order to prevent misunderstandings later when they may not be able to do so.[44]

From a legal aspect, nonmaleficence can cause negligence and malpractice. *Negligence* is a term used when a health care provider's conduct falls below the standard established by the law for the protection of others.[35] Negligence describes a form of conduct that often results in injury to a patient. Negligence is the provider's failure to conduct himself or herself in the same manner as would another provider in the same or similar circumstances (**Table 15.4**).[35]

Negligence is considered an actionable behavior when it falls below the standard of care or is in direct violation of a statute, rule, or ordinance that prescribes the acceptable behavior. In health care, the most common example of negligent care may be the deficiency of well-trained, properly supervised nursing staff in long-term facilities such as nursing homes.[45] The Congressional Government Accountability Office (GAO) has revealed many negligence violations in nursing homes ranging from severe bedsores to overuse of prescription medications and even malnutrition resulting in patient death.[45]

Negligence in health care typically ends up in court as a malpractice suit. The medical malpractice plaintiff must establish the "appropriate" standard of care to be able to prove that the standard of care was breached. The most common legal definition of *standard of care* is how a similarly qualified practitioner would have managed the patient's care under similar circumstances.[35,46] In most medical malpractice cases, both the standard of care and its breach are established through the testimony of expert witnesses.

| Table 15.4 | *Concepts of Negligence in Clinical Practice*[35] |
|---|---|

Negligence is a type of tort (meaning civil wrong); however, negligence can also be used in criminal law.

Negligence is culpable conduct because the health care provider falls short of what other providers would do to protect the patient from a predictable risk of harm.

Through civil litigation, if an injured patient proves that the health care provider acted negligently to cause their injury, he or she can recover damages to compensate for the harm.

Sometimes there may be a situation when negligence occurred and the plaintiff has to establish the standard of care and breach without an expert witness. Although rare, the law calls this response *res ipsa loquitur* meaning the thing speaks for itself.[16,46] In medical negligence cases, *res ipsa loquitur* can occur when: (1) the patient suffered an injury that is not an expected complication of medical care, (2) the injury does not normally occur unless someone has been negligent, and (3) the defendant was responsible for the patient's well-being at the time of the injury.[16,46] As a hypothetical example, a patient who had a total hip replacement was found to have a shoulder fracture immediately after performing gait training with the physical therapist. This is not an expected complication of a hip replacement, and the physical therapist as the defendant was responsible for the patient's well-being at the time the injury occurred. Because there are no other explanations for the patient's injury other than that the therapist mishandled the patient during transfer and gait training, the plaintiff does not need expert testimony to establish the standard of care and its breach.

Negligence in a malpractice case is based on the defendant's violation of a law. The plaintiff must show that the law was violated, that the law was intended to prevent the type of injury that occurred, and that the plaintiff was the class of persons intended to be protected by the law.[46] The plaintiff may claim negligence "per se" even if the defendant has not been convicted or administratively sanctioned under the law in question. Negligence per se claims are a threat to health care providers who disregard laws intended to protect patients.[46]

In physical and occupational therapy, negligence and malpractice acts are typically rare, especially when compared to physicians' litigations. However, in modern health care, malpractice acts in physical therapy can occur in the latest area of practice of occupational health. Essentially, occupational health services relate to preventive services and establishing/maintaining safe and healthy working environments. Occupational therapists have long been involved in occupational health; however, physical therapists also have recently been participating in identifying and assessing risks in the workplace, advising and organizing ergonomically correct working practices, and providing training and education on health and safety and proper use of protective equipment.[47] In occupational health, patient education is an important aspect of rehabilitation. After an individual experiences an injury, he or she needs rehabilitation and a transition period to recover and be able to perform the same tasks as before or learn new tasks. Occupational and physical therapists are able to provide client instruction for safety in job coaching, functional training, work hardening and conditioning, and injury prevention. The therapists can evaluate the client while on the job to determine the client's capability to complete the tasks safely by applying ergonomic and functional guidelines. During this type of instruction, which involves risk management strategies and also prevention and wellness programs, physical and occupational therapists are prone to increase their liability for negligence and malpractice litigations.

Specific legal and risk management guidelines should be followed by the physical therapists involved in occupational medicine.[46] The legal issues that can lead to malpractice if not properly followed may include ethical issues, adverse administrative actions, financial risk exposure, and operational safety concerns.[46] For example, when performing a functional capacity evaluation, the therapist is responsible and liable for ensuring he or she is practicing within his or her scope of practice by performing testing in a nondiscriminatory and safe manner and informing the clients of the risks associated with the tests. When performing prevention services, the therapist needs to ensure that the activities taught to clients fall within the state practice acts for physical and occupational therapy.[46] The prevention activities included in the client's teaching must be objectively documented including specific interventions that were taught and practiced, and the time spent in each activity. The records of such services must be maintained for the time period required by state and federal laws. Potential immunity from negligent or malpractice acts must also consider worker's compensation statutes dependent on the state and federal requirements.[46] For example, depending on the specific state laws, physical therapists may not be able to legally perform all environmental evaluations that are essentials for an individual's job performance. These evaluations may not be under the jurisdiction of physical therapy practice in the state where the evaluations are performed. As a result, the therapists may need to consider the opinions of other professionals when making recommendations related to assessments of temperature, lighting conditions, or noisy environments.

In physical and occupational therapy, proper standards of conduct can be violated (resulting in negligence and malpractice) when the therapist fails to do what another competent provider would have done under similar circumstances.[16,35] The negligence is proven when harm occurred to the patient or client.[16,35] To avoid negligence and malpractice, therapists should maintain a therapeutic relationship with the patient and not exploit the patient in any manner, either physically, emotionally, financially, or socially. Negligence that can cause intentional harm to the patient can also be caused by nonmaleficence. It is difficult to think about nonmaleficence acts in patient education intentionally causing harm to the patient; however, nonmaleficence can occur in certain situations when the patient instruction encourages harmful behavior or when information to prevent injury is purposefully withheld. Additionally, during patient instruction, the same as in a classroom setting, the patient as the student can be harmed by having the teacher gossip about the student's poor performance.

If, during patient education, a therapist discloses the patient's perceived weakness in learning a skill to a third party, it can cause harm to the patient. As a hypothetical example, the physical therapist is working with a 67-year-old client, T.L. The client had a right rotator cuff tear more than a year ago and received excellent results with physical therapy. A few months after completion of physical therapy treatments, T.L. participated in a golf fitness program in the same clinic, which helped him to increase the speed and distance of his golf game. Currently, T.L., an avid golfer, wants to improve his golf game again. After several sessions, T.L. is making small gains and the therapist seems puzzled about the situation. A friend (and neighbor) of T.L. has been receiving physical therapy interventions at the same clinic. During one therapy session, the therapist discloses T.L.'s perceived learning weaknesses to his friend (and neighbor), trying to find a better teaching solution for T.L. By disclosing T.L.'s learning weaknesses to his friend, the therapist violated the principle of nonmaleficence. The therapist cannot guarantee what the third party (T.L.'s friend and neighbor) may do with the information and how much harm he may cause to T.L. And in this case, harm was caused to the patient. The patient's friend disclosed the information to three other individuals who usually played golf with T.L. As a result, the patient physically confronted his friend and neighbor and in the scuffle he suffered severe injuries to his right shoulder. At this time, T.L. needs surgery for his right shoulder. Consequently, T.L. could try to sue the therapist for negligence. The negligence in this case was caused by the therapist breaching the ethical concept of nonmaleficence.

## CONFIDENTIALITY

In the prior example, in addition to nonmaleficence, the therapist also violated the legal principle of patient *confidentiality* by sharing private information with a third party without the patient's consent.[16,35] The therapist divulged confidential information about the patient's learning weaknesses to the patient's friend. By doing so, the therapist breached the confidentiality standards. Perhaps the therapist did not consider patient education as a form of physical therapy intervention and consequently overlooked the privacy issue.

Confidentiality relates to the concept of privacy and protection of privileged information. Bioethics and the law require that information in the patient's medical record be kept confidential, and not shared or divulged to a third party except with the patient's written permission (**Table 15.5**).[16,35] Confidentiality is a fundamental ethical principle in health care, including in physical and occupational therapy. Confidential information is individually identifiable data regarding a patient's medical history, cognition, physical condition, and interventions as well as other material related to test results, patient education, discussions with the patient and/or family, and financial and billing information.[35] These confidential records may be disclosed when patients and/or their legal representatives agree to disclosure, when mandated by law, or when there exists overriding and compelling grounds for disclosure, such as the prevention of substantial harm to the patient or identifiable other persons. Health care providers may be mandated to disclose confidential information for

| Table 15.5 | **Concepts of Confidentiality in Clinical Practice[16,35]** |
| --- | --- |
| | Confidentiality is the right of the patient to have personal, identifiable medical information kept private. |
| | The patient's private medical information should be available only to the health care professionals and providers and insurance personnel as necessary. |
| | The patient's private medical information should not be disclosed to others unless the patient (or his or her legally authorized representative) has given specific permission for such release. |
| | The patient or his or her legally authorized representative must provide written informed consent for any and all releases of private medical information. |
| | If the patient's private medical information is disseminated without the patient's permission (or the legally authorized representative's permission), the health care professional or provider is liable for legal action. |

specific problems such as cases involving minors, drug testing, employee health, perpetrators and victims of violent crimes, the media, and communicable and sexually transmitted diseases. Such cases can require an extraordinary degree of sensitivity, discretion, and judgment on the part of the health care provider. The federal law called the Health Insurance Portability and Accountability Act (HIPAA) and other individual state laws govern the release of identifiable patient information by hospitals and other health care providers.[35] All of these laws establish protections to preserve the confidentiality of medical and personal information. As a result, all medical records must be maintained in a secure, locked location. The computerized database should be accessible only to health care providers and must not be shared with anyone without the written permission of the patient.[35]

In physical and occupational therapy, confidentiality is, in addition to an ethical obligation, a matter of respecting the privacy of patients as well as encouraging them to seek rehabilitation and discuss their problems openly. Confidentiality is not absolute.[48] It can be overridden to protect individuals or the public or to disclose or report information when the law requires.[48] When breaching confidentiality is legally necessary, it should be done in such a way as to minimize harm to the patient and also comply with federal and state laws.[48]

Patient education information goes into the medical record the same as other interventions material. Ethically and legally, the patient has the right to examine his or her medical records. The actual chart is the property of the therapist (or the institution where the therapist is employed), but the information in the chart is the property of the patient.[35] Whenever the patient requires a copy of that information, the therapist is obligated to release it to the patient or to a third party at the request of the patient.[35] To protect the confidentiality of the information, the therapist must release the copy only with the written permission of the patient (or the patient's legally authorized representative).[35]

Additionally, confidentiality represents significant ethical and legal concepts because it supports and also encourages patient autonomy. To provide for patient's confidentiality and also be able to respect patient's autonomy, the therapist may need to: (1) protect all patient's information; (2) collaborate with patients using a patient-centered care approach; (3) disclose fully the risks, benefits, and potential outcomes of interventions; (4) obtain informed consent from patients, assuring that they understood potential risks and outcomes; and (5) respect the patient's rights to refuse interventions.[35]

## JUSTICE

Justice or integrity is a bioethical principle meaning that a health care provider distributes equal and fair interventions. In physical therapy, justice as a general concept can be exemplified by the therapist's integrity and dependability of doing the right thing at all times. Three types of justice may be considered in health care: legal, rights-based, and distributive. Legal justice requires health care professionals and providers to follow ethically acceptable laws. Therapists must abide by applicable rules, regulations, and laws; adhere to high professional standards; articulate ideals (such as universal health care); and always take responsibility for their actions. Ethically acceptable laws represent legal guidelines that need to be observed by all licensed physical and occupational therapists and assistants. In health care in general, when the legal guidelines or laws are not morally acceptable to the licensed professionals or providers, these professionals/providers are not obliged to observe them. For example, a physician who morally disagrees with abortion is not required to perform the procedure; however, he or she is required to arrange for the patient to see another professional who will be able to perform the abortion.

In addition to legal justice, there also are rights-based and distributive justice. Rights-based justice requires professionals and providers to abide by patients' rights.[16] In the United States, patients' rights are guaranteed by state and federal laws. Individual healthcare facilities also often have their own patient bill of rights. Distributive justice applies to the distribution of limited resources.[16] From the ethical aspect of care, distributive justice is concerned with the distribution of scarce health resources and how decisions are made when the interest of one person or a group of people competes with the interest of another person or another group of individuals.[16,35] When decisions are made, distributive justice requires that all individuals be treated fairly and not in an unpredictable manner.[35] An individual's right to health care resources should not be affected by his or her age, race, gender, quality of life, and socioeconomic status. People who are rich or poor should be treated equally and receive the same amount of care and attention from their health care providers (**Table 15.6**).

| Table 15.6 | **Concepts of Justice in Clinical Practice**[16,35] |
|---|---|
| | Justice requires that patients in similar clinical situations have access to the same health care. |
| | Health care professionals and providers should distribute the limited health care resources fairly. |

An example of distributive justice in occupational and physical therapy is therapists' commitment to serve patients with disabilities. Their contributions can be demonstrated by their dedication to teach children and adults with developmental and physical disabilities by using fair and equal modes of interventions for all and providing the necessary amount of time regardless of compensation. The therapists are instrumental to create home adjustments that help individuals with disabilities to remain in their own homes in the community instead of being forced into institutionalized care.[49] The therapists are strong advocates for legislative assistance to advance technological developments. Scientific progress could enhance the skills of patients with disabilities to independently continue to function at home, at school, or in the community. Additionally, the therapists apply explicit empowerment and justice requirements to develop state and federal policies to create flexible working conditions to accommodate people with disabilities. Furthermore, occupational and physical therapists and assistants always provide quality patient education in addition to other physical therapy interventions to produce distributive justice in rehabilitation.

Failure to make available occupational or physical therapy or supplying less than quality care (including insufficient patient instruction) based on patient diagnosis or discriminating on the basis of an individual's culture, sexual orientation, or national origin can result in being liable for violating the ethics of justice. Therapists continuously advocate to insurance companies, regulatory agencies, and the legislatures regarding the need to provide access to health care services to all individuals.

## VERACITY/TRUTHFULNESS AND AUTONOMY

Veracity (or truthfulness) is an ethical principle that promotes honesty and telling the truth. Veracity binds both the health care provider and the patient in an association of truth.[35] The patient must tell the truth to receive the appropriate health care. The health care provider must disclose factual information so the patient can exercise his or her personal autonomy (**Table 15.7**).[35]

Physical and occupational therapists and assistants must always represent truthfully their credentials, qualification, experience, education, and competence. Also, any personal or financial affiliations that may cause conflict of interest when working with patients or

| Table 15.7 | **The Relationship Between Veracity and Autonomy[35]** |
| --- | --- |
| | Veracity is linked to the patient's autonomy. |
| | Not telling the truth undermines the principle of respect for the patient's autonomy. |

clients must be fully disclosed. Veracity or truthfulness is also based on the principle of respect for the patient. The adherence to veracity fosters trust between the therapist and the patient. Lying and inadequate disclosure violates respect for the patient and obstructs a trusting relationship. Nevertheless, veracity or truthfulness is not an absolute ethical concept.[35] Truthfulness deals with information, the meaning of information, and its scope. As a result, it can be difficult to determine its validity. For example, a conflict of interest can arise in a physical therapy practice when the physical therapist has a financial stake in the profit of a referring orthopedic surgeon's company. In the physical therapist's patient education, he or she may try to persuade the patient to have orthopedic surgery. This act can cause a conflict of interest for the therapist.

Being truthful in the daily interactions with patients or clients is an important responsibility for all health care providers. A patient's perceptions of caring and empathy account for more that 50% of a health care provider's trustworthiness and credibility.[38] Also, a patient's awareness of competence and expertise helps to determine the clinician's level of trust and credibility. The provider's communication skills are vital when conveying truthfulness, objectivity, and sincerity. Nonverbal cues, such as eye contact and facial expressions, often make more of an impression on the patient or client than do verbal messages.[38]

In patient education and physical therapy, truthfulness is closely connected to teaching patients about the correct performance of interventions and also being truthful about the risks and benefits involved in various rehabilitation procedures.[35] Truth and integrity are patients' rights. Regardless of the patient's age, sexual orientation, gender, physical disability, or race, the patient has the right to receive truthful interventions including patient education. All therapists must clearly describe to the patient: the proposed intervention, the reasonable alternatives, and the risks, benefits, and uncertainties related to interventions. The patient's understanding of interventions must also be assessed.[35] Legally, all these elements of veracity also are representatives of informed consent.

As a theoretical example of truthfulness, Mrs. N., who is a kindergarten teacher, was referred to physical therapy with low back pain. She came to the clinic because her friend had the same type of pain and got better in just 2 weeks by having ultrasound treatments, deep massage, and stretching of her tight muscles. At her evaluation she requested the same type of interventions. The physical therapist explained to Mrs. N. that ultrasound could not be used for her back pain because she was 4 months pregnant. She also emphasized that ultrasound is contraindicated in pregnancy. She offered other interventions to help relieve her back pain. However, Mrs. N. did not accept the alternative interventions recommended by the therapist and refused the therapy. Later that day, Mrs. N. called the owner of the clinic and complained about the therapist not treating her properly. The owner, who was not trained as a physical therapist, told the therapist that in the future she should never refuse patients the treatments they desire. Additionally, he felt that it was not necessary to discuss with the patient "possible risks" because these may not really happen. Shortly after the incident, the therapist quit working at the clinic. The therapist had the right to tell the patient the truth and not perform a contraindicated type of procedure that could have caused harm to the patient and her unborn fetus.

The key to successful truth-telling is effective communication between the patient and therapist in which the individual patient's needs and concerns are identified and addressed. Although in the above example the therapist told the patient the truth, it is not known whether the information exchange between patient and therapist was a continuing flow of two-way information. Perhaps the therapist was not clear enough in her explanation about the ultrasound, preventing the patient from understanding the material or interpreting the idea correctly. It also is possible that some inconsequential detail may have confused more than enhanced the patient's ability to make a decision.

In patient education, therapists may be tempted to make their own choices about which information is necessary for the patient. They can be reluctant to afford the patient autonomy, instead imposing their own values on the patient and deciding in a paternalistic way what is best for the patient to know. Ethical dilemmas also may arise between the primary health care provider's lack of candor explaining to the patient a grave condition and prognosis and the therapist's truth-telling about the same condition, which is tempered with compassion. Cultural differences must be considered with patients who are not willing to know about the factual diagnosis and prognosis. For example, some eastern European cultures are reluctant to know the truth about their diagnosis and prognosis. One all-purpose method of respecting the patient's right to information is to ask the patient what he or she would like to know as the intervention progresses.

## Informed Consent

The concept of informed consent requires the health care professional and provider to describe all relevant treatment options to the patient, noting the benefits and risks (**Table 15.8**). The Patient's Bill of Rights gives patients the right: (1) to receive considerate and respectful care; (2) to know the name of their health care provider; and (3) to obtain from their provider complete information in understandable terms about their diagnosis, prognosis, and interventions.[16,35] Giving informed consent is an ethical value and a legal doctrine. Ethically it is based on the health care provider's truthfulness and respect for the patient and patient's right to determine their own goals and how to achieve these goals. A patient's autonomy is considered the ethical basis for informed consent—that the patient can come to their own decision.[16,35] The role of the health care professional and provider is to make available enough information for the patient to be able to make the decision.

| Table 15.8 | *Patients' Requirements for Informed Consent*[16,35] |
|---|---|
| Competence | Patient's capacity to make a reasonable decision. |
| Comprehension | Patient's ability to understand or to be able to intellectually grasp the meaning of the information. |
| Deliberation | Patient's ability to reflect on the information and only after that make a decision. |

The amount and type of information enables the patient to make an informed decision and give their informed consent to interventions.

In informed consent, the health care provider must disclose truthfully all information to the patient so he or she can make a rational decision and also must not use coercion or force (from themselves or from others) to determine the patient's choice.[35] In health care, even if all these elements are satisfied, some patients may still reject the interventions due to high costs or certain personal, religious, or cultural beliefs.

The 21st-century doctrine of informed consent can become very complicated, focusing not only on the patient's/family's consent but also on the content of information and the process of consent. The health care professional must provide enough information that is understandable, logical, and includes recommendations.[35] The patient's or family's concurrence must be free and uncoerced. Many patients and their families have to make critical medical decisions based on neutrally presented statistics that are as free as possible from the influences of health care professionals' judgments. Because health care professionals such as physicians ethically must withhold their recommendations and give patients/families the choice of interventions, many feel that patients and families may not be able to make the correct decision.[16,35] Furthermore, many times, the principles and practice of informed consent rely on patients to ask questions, to think carefully about their choices, and to be forthright with their health care providers about their values, concerns, and reservations about specific recommendations. In ambiguous situations, the hospital ethics committees or the legal authorities must intervene to try to solve ethical dilemmas and also comply with state or federal legal doctrines.

Informed consent requires three elements to promote patient's autonomy and rational decision making: information, voluntariness, and competency.[50] The health care provider should give the patient all necessary information to make a reasonable informed decision. Voluntariness means that for an informed consent to be legal, the patient must give the consent freely and without any coercion, fraud, or duress. The third element of consent, patient's competency, can be assessed by a health care provider by determining patient's cognitive capacity.[50] In situations, when the patient is incapacitated cognitively, the clinician must obtain substitute consent to treat the patient.

In general, the doctrine of informed consent can become slightly relaxed in four situations: incompetence of the patient, emergency situations, therapeutic privilege, and waiver.[16] If a patient lacks the capacity to consent to treatment, the local jurisdiction's laws regarding substitute decision makers come into play. In emergencies, a physician can administer a treatment without patient consent.[16] Therapeutic privilege can be used by a physician when he or she feels that disclosure of information would actually harm the patient and will negate the benefits of an autonomous and informed decision. The concept of therapeutic privilege allows the physician to slightly modify the degree of disclosure; however, the treatment still needs to be explained in detail to the patient.[16] Physicians and especially psychiatrists may use the therapeutic privilege in emergency situations to treat patients who lack capacity to make decisions or when a patient's disorder influences the patient's ability to tolerate detailed explanations. For example, in emergency situations in psychiatry, a patient with schizophrenia may be physically unable to make an informed decision in regard to risks and benefits to take the medication.[50] However, the patient's condition could worsen without the medication. Therapeutic privilege allows the physician to circumvent the legal requirement and immediately initiate treatment.[50] However, legally, therapeutic privilege "cannot be used as a means of circumventing"[50(p.365)] the requirement to obtain patient's informed consent before starting the treatment. Another exception to informed consent is the waiver. This happens when the patient has voluntarily, competently, and knowingly waived his or her right to be informed.[50] An example would be when a patient taking chemotherapy would not want to be informed of chemotherapy drug risks. By not knowing the drug risks (and side effects), it may help the patient in his or her psychological recovery.

As previously described, the informed consent right can be effectively exercised only if the patient possesses enough information to enable an intelligent choice. Only then can the patient make a determination about interventions. During patient teaching, physical and occupational therapists must communicate to the patient the findings of their initial examination and evaluation by using a thorough professional judgment in informing the patient of any substantial risks of the proposed interventions. Therapists should include in their information a description of the intervention, a clear explanation of the risks and benefits, anticipated time frames, anticipated costs, and reasonable alternatives to the recommended therapy.

When obtaining informed consent, the therapist's attitudes and feelings can influence the way the information is presented to the patient and also the patient's receptivity to the material. The legal doctrine of informed consent is dependable on good clinical care. Informed consent allows the patient to become a partner in making treatment decisions dependent on their needs and values. Additionally, the therapist' verbal and nonverbal communication are important. For example, nonverbal cues that indicate disapproval or hesitance when explaining an intervention can alter the patient's view of the verbal information. Also, giving the material and rushing the patient into making a decision can create pressure and conflict for the patient. When obtaining informed consent, the therapists should not rush the patient and should offer an atmosphere as free of distraction as possible, allowing enough time for the patient's questions and concerns. The involvement of the patient's family in decision making is also important. From the beginning of rehabilitation, the family can provide additional support and encouragement and enhance communication between the therapist and the patient. Family members can help to clarify information that the patient may be hesitant to ask or that may be difficult to understand. Nevertheless, prior to involving the patient's family in the process of informed consent, the therapist needs to discuss all applicable issues with the patient in advance. Some individuals may be reluctant to have the spouse or family involved with their health care decisions and treatment.

In the process of informed consent, the patient must know the therapist who will apply the intervention. If assistants and/or students are to implement parts of the plan of care, this should be included in the information given to the patient as part of the consent. Patients may feel offended and become distressed if they are treated by students without being informed. Failure of the health care provider to acquire informed consent before initiating treatment legally constitutes battery, leaving the provider open to civil litigation and/or professional disciplinary proceedings. Treatment given to a patient on the basis of an invalid informed consent because it was not voluntary or was obtained by misrepresentation also constitutes battery. Additionally, even in the absence of negligence or malpractice, the therapist as the health care provider can be held liable for not properly informing the patient about the treatment.

Because the informed consent laws differ regarding the information required to be provided to the patient, therapists must be aware of their specific state laws.[35] Due to statutes established through litigations, some states call for particular types of information to be supplied in order for the patient to be sufficiently informed.

Therapists are also liable for disciplinary action by their licensing board if they fail to provide the patient with the information they need to make an informed decision in relation to the treatment. For example, in physical therapy, the most common injuries occur due to falls associated with interventions.[35] As a result, physical therapists and assistants should teach patients (especially older adults) about the risk of falling and accurately document their patient education. Patients need to be able to understand the information and consent to the proposed intervention. Obtaining the patient's signature on a copy of the presented material is very helpful, but not always infallible in a court of law. If the patient is diagnosed with dementia or is under the legal age for giving consent, therapists must consult their state laws about advance directives and turning to the family or patient's surrogate for medical decision making.

In regard to informed consent in physical therapy, it also is recommended that physical therapists and assistants know and comply with state law and practice act requirements. Physical therapists as health care providers must consider the World Confederation of Physical Therapy's *Declaration of Principle* on informed consent, which asserts the therapist's obligation to provide the patient (who is a competent adult) with adequate, intelligible information about the proposed therapy (**Table 15.9**).[51]

## PATIENT AUTONOMY

Patient autonomy refers to the capability and right of patients to control the course of their own medical treatment and participate in the treatment decision-making process.[44]

| Table 15.9 | **Concepts of Informed Consent in Clinical Practice[51]** |
|---|---|
| | A clear description of the intervention(s) that will be provided. |
| | A clear explanation of the risks associated with the proposed intervention(s). |
| | The expected benefits of the proposed intervention(s). |
| | Anticipated time frames and costs of the proposed intervention(s). |
| | Reasonable alternatives to the proposed intervention(s). |

Autonomy gives the patient the right to refuse or choose their treatment.[44] Autonomy recognizes individuals' right to self-determination and their ability to make informed decisions about personal matters.[44] Autonomy can be classified as the autonomy of thought (thinking for oneself), autonomy of will (doing something based on one's own deliberation), and autonomy of action (an individual acting as they wish).[44] Historically, patient autonomy emerged as a reaction to a paternalistic tradition within health care. The concept of informed consent or the freedom to act on one's own behalf is based on the principle of autonomy.

Philosophically, respect for a patient's autonomy is a complicated process (**Table 15.10**). The idea of autonomy is an individual personal ruling to understand that being autonomous requires total freedom from other people's controlling influences. Autonomy is the same as self-determination. Autonomous patients have the capability and right to control the course of their medical treatment and participate in their treatment decision-making process. To be autonomous, a patient or client must have the ability to exercise control over their own actions and circumstances.[35] Autonomous patients must be able to make decisions without coercion and any undue influences, also demonstrating competence and understanding of the information.[44] This prioritizes the patient's wishes over their best interests. The patient has control over his or her life. This is a libertarian point of view regarding autonomy, and subscribes totally to the patient's desires; however, this view does not prevent the patient from making decisions that may be more harmful than beneficial.

Respect for autonomy is the basis for informed consent and advance directives.[35] Legally, a patient's autonomy rights are easiest to defend and implement in the context of a well-informed adult of sound mind. The most familiar tool for extending autonomy is the advance directive. Advance directive is a living will that allows a person who is of sound mind to exercise autonomy over the care they will receive should they become unable to communicate their wishes.

The concept of autonomy is extended in health care to empower others to speak on behalf of the patient. This can be done formally, through a durable power of attorney, or

| Table 15.10 | *Concepts Included in the Principle of Respect for Autonomy*[35] |
|---|---|
| Privacy. | |
| Self-mastery. | |
| Doing something voluntarily. | |
| Free choice. | |
| Choosing one's own moral position. | |
| Accepting responsibility for one's choice. | |

informally, when the family and others serve as the patient's surrogates. The extension of autonomy at the end of life causes many ethical and legal conflicts in American health care. Many of the ethics cases that have inspired national debates, such as Schiavo, Quinlan, or Cruzan, have involved surrogate decision makers and extended autonomy. Those cases, similar to some European nations' substituted judgments for incompetent patients, are considered totally paternalistic, ignoring the main ethical concept of health care, "to do good" for the patient. However, in some situations, aggressive care for a terminally ill patient may not necessarily lead to recovery but a prolonged dying. For example, hypothetically, a patient with terminal cancer prefers to live the rest of her life without receiving any cancer treatments, especially medications that make her constantly ill. The physician may convince the patient and her family to take chemotherapy treatments because the medications will prolong her life. In this situation, the physician used his authority to manipulate the patient to choose the treatment that will benefit the patient best medically. One drawback of the autonomy principle, as seen in this example, is that the paternalistic individual may not always have the same ideals as the dependent person and will deny the patient's autonomy and ability to choose her treatment. As a result, this decreases the amount of beneficence. The patient with terminal cancer feels that her quality of life, even a shorter life, may be better without the ill effects of medications.

In physical and occupational therapy, the patient-centered care model encourages patients to actively make decisions, promoting an intense collaboration between patient and therapist. The patient can autonomously make choices that are informed by both the evidence-based facts explained by the therapist and the therapist's clinical experience. Additionally, the patient-centered model can lessen the patient's uncertainty and fear and may enhance healing and patient satisfaction. Autonomy requires the patient to have liberty of action, freedom of choice, and effective deliberation. The patient or the patient's legally authorized representative should be able to formulate appropriate goals, establish priorities, determine the best means for the goals, make appropriate changes in goals, and have access to all pertinent information. For physical and occupational therapy providers, the concepts of beneficence and autonomy must always outweigh self-interest.[2] As health care providers, the therapists must remember that they are ethically obligated to make moral judgments and decisions. They also must consider their important roles in providing the best services and support to their patients.

# CULTURAL FACTORS IN PATIENT EDUCATION

## Objectives

After completing Chapter 16, the reader will be able to:

- Define and contrast culture from the perspectives of the nursing, medicine, and allied health professions.
- Analyze all characteristics of culture.
- Evaluate cultural dimensions in patient education.
- Identify verbal and nonverbal cultural communication variables.
- Discuss five constructs to achieve cultural competence.
- Illustrate stereotyping in teaching and learning.
- List the four levels of cultural awareness.
- Determine the importance of cultural knowledge and cultural skills in teaching and learning.
- Apply the modified ESFT model.
- Recognize the LEARN model to achieve effective communication.
- Explain specific cultural strategies for teaching Hispanic American, African American, Asian American, and Native American patients.

# Concepts of Culture in Patient Education

Patient education is highly influenced by patients' needs and expectations. In the multicultural United States, health care providers must always consider culture when delivering interventions, including patient education. The patient's culture has a major influence on health behaviors and the patient's interest in learning more about his or her health. Patients' principles of health and illness vary considerably among cultural groups. As a result, in the past, many health care providers experienced difficulty caring for patients whose cultural beliefs differed from their own.[52] Lack of cultural sensitivity resulted in wasted time and interventions and even tragic and dangerous consequences caused by misdiagnosis of health problems.[52] Sadly, even today, in the 21st century, some providers remain unaware of the complex factors influencing their patients' responses to health care. Ethnocentrism, or the belief that one's culture is the best, is still much more common than cultural openness. The more health care providers know about different cultures, the more they realize that one culture is neither superior nor inferior to another but they are simply different. Understanding different cultures and the impact they have on health care beliefs and behaviors is vital for all health care professions.

The United States stands as a model of multiculturalism, encouraging people of multiple ethnic cultures to blend into one society while simultaneously maintaining their original culture. As a result, health care providers have the great privilege of working with people from many diverse cultures. With this opportunity also arises the obligation to learn about the cultural values and mores of each group with whom they work, adapting their clinical skills to accommodate the differences in health principles and values. This is complicated, ongoing, and challenging work.

In physical and occupational therapy, cultural competence is a critical component of professional practice.[35] Each patient's culture impacts that patient's health, interventions, recovery, and continuity of care. Physical and occupational therapists and assistants have been making a strong effort to achieve cultural competence and provide culturally competent care to their patients and clients. Acquiring cultural competence requires each person to go through an intrinsic developmental process to attain the knowledge, attitudes, and behaviors specific to culture, language, and communication. The effectiveness of patient education in physical and occupational rehabilitation is enhanced when the therapist includes the patient's cultural perspectives. Physical and occupational rehabilitation, similar to other health care professions, necessitates cultural training for the therapist so he or she can understand the diversity of patients' needs.

Patients and therapists teach and learn cultural knowledge from each other. This knowledge is important for both the patient and the therapist to understand information and beliefs about disease or disorder, treatment expectations and personal preferences, tolerances, or other influences. Overall, therapists' cultural awareness and sensitivity can influence patients' ability to receive and apply information regarding their health care. Also, the ways in which the information is communicated can affect patients' learning and their ability to adhere to recommended interventions.

## CHARACTERISTICS OF CULTURE

Defining culture is a difficult task because there is no single accepted definition (**Table 16.1**). Different definitions of culture can be found in varied areas of health care such as medicine, nursing, or allied health. In nursing, the term *culture* can be generally described as shared beliefs, values, and behaviors of members of a specific group that can influence the presentation of symptoms by patients, the assessments made by health care providers, and the patient's receptivity to recommendations for treatments.[53] Another nursing description involves the idea that culture is a dynamic point of view of an individual in relation to his or her interpretation of the world, such as in the treatment decision-making.[54] In certain

| Table 16.1 | *Characteristics of Culture*[59,60] |
|---|---|

Culture is socially constructed, allowing people to connect with each other. Through culture people can share knowledge, attitudes, and values with each other. This characteristic permits unity and continuity of a group of people.

Culture can be demonstrated in subjective and objective ways. Examples of subjective ways are peoples' attitudes, beliefs, and values; their learning styles; their behavioral norms; or their hierarchy of roles. Examples of objective ways include physical artifacts people create such as clothing, food, or furniture.

Culture can be either internalized in unconscious ways or articulated in conscious ways. For example, a patient unconsciously does not like exercises. The patient's perception remains internalized until he or she needs physical therapy and consciously expresses his or her dislike of exercises.

Culture is dynamic because it continuously changes depending on environmental circumstances or group associations. Individuals go through an ongoing learning and relearning of their culture due to constant changes in their lives. As an example, an individual who had an amputation because of an accident finds comfort in learning the cultural cues of people with disabilities.

Culture can belong to various social groups or subgroups. Culture cannot be considered uniform in terms of whole societies. Culture can be viewed as a series of interactive social levels. At each level there are a number of subgroups influenced by the larger culture. In most cultures, the family and community levels have the greatest and most direct influences.

cultures when becoming ill, an individual will typically have another member of the family making treatment decisions. In medicine in general, culture is represented as learned and shared rules, knowledge, and attitudes, that individuals use to interpret experiences and to generate behaviors.[55] As a result, culture in medical primary care can be a compelling factor behind the behaviors, actions, and their related consequences associated with individuals.[55] As an example, in certain Eastern European countries, adolescent males' smoking is considered a socially acceptable behavior and a sign of adulthood. Therefore, within that society, patient education for smoking cessation will not be an acceptable or appreciated form of intervention.

In regard to occupational and physical therapy, the therapists' role is to respect and value culture, understand patient's cultural beliefs, and develop effective and culturally appropriate interventions.[56] Similar to other health care professions, physical and occupational therapy recognize culture to be dynamic and interactive.[57] Thus, the therapists acknowledge patients' uniqueness and their sociocultural values and beliefs.[56] Patients' cultures are an intrinsic part of the physical and occupational therapy rehabilitative system including examination, evaluation, diagnosis, prognosis (including the plan of care), and interventions.[56] As a whole, the dynamics of culture are integrated in physical and occupational therapy practice, education and research.[57] Additionally, physical and occupational therapists and assistants have been continuously incorporating the unique needs of individuals, children, and families into their culturally-driven interventions.[57]

Culture matters because it can shape people's identity. Many processes, conditions, enabling and constraining factors, and subjective experiences contribute to culture. During patient instruction in occupational and physical therapy, culture can have a profound influence on a patient's values, beliefs, and behaviors.[56] Culture can affect a patient's perception of illness and health, view of therapy, and the meaning ascribed to what one does and how that fits into the context of one's life.[56] The impact of culture on a patient's response to therapy cannot be underestimated. In physical and occupational therapy, culture profoundly can affect patients' diagnosis, interventions, and responsiveness to interventions.[58] Another important point in understanding culture is for the therapist to be able to identify his or her own culturally based predispositions.[58] This can be a long process that takes commitment and self-reflection. Therapists should seek to understand their "own culturally mediated values and biases"[58(p.4)] in order to identify ways to gradually change them.

The influences of culture in the teaching and learning process are based on specific characteristics such as: (1) culture is socially constructed; (2) culture is subjective and objective; (3) culture is conscious and unconscious; and (4) culture is continuously shifting and adapting.[59,60] Culture can also be patterned and provide sources of identity for individuals, groups, and subgroups.[59,60] Understanding these influences and characteristics can help physical and occupational therapists and assistants identify their assumptions and values upon which their own behaviors and worldview rest. This knowledge can increase their appreciation and acceptance of differences and enhance their cultural sensitivity and awareness.

For physical and occupational therapists and assistants, being able to teach a patient from a different culture means shifting perspectives and gaining knowledge of how the culture dictates the teaching and learning process.[59] This process is very difficult and cannot be learned immediately. Cultural sensitivity and awareness is a continuing lifelong progression.[59] The most important aspect of using a cultural perspective in health care is the health care provider's willingness to acknowledge their own culturally biased tendencies. This requires the provider's ongoing critical contemplation and readiness toward change.[58] Therapists must recognize their own cultural values, biases, and misconceptions before being able to model cultural sensitivity to patients or clients. In teaching and learning, exploring and clarifying the teacher's cultural biases can influence the degree of consideration, openness to, and acceptance of the learner's culture.

# Cultural Dimensions in Patient Education

Physical and occupational therapists and assistants need to be aware that cultures tend to vary across a number of cultural dimensions. Cultural dimensions can be described as psychological dimensions or value constructs, which can be used to portray or explain a specific culture.[59] To be able to reflect on their own cultural values and conceptions, therapists have to understand the unique significance of their patients' cultural dimensions. These dimensions play an essential role in the patients' daily interactions. For example, the main dimensions of diversity when people meet and interact are generally gender, physical makeup (appearance), ethnicity, physical and mental limitations, age, sexual preference, income level, geographical location or region, occupation, religion, and education.[61]

When acquiring cultural sensitivity, the therapist may not realize that knowledge of various diversity dimensions can expand his or her cultural perspectives. The process of examination of thoughts, behaviors, experiences, and reactions, called *cultural deliberation*,[60] can increase the therapist's ability to create and support positive relationships with his or her patients and clients. In addition to the main dimensions, there are other dimensions of diversity that play an important role in patient interventions by challenging the relationship between the therapist and the patient. These cultural dimensions that clearly relate to patient education may include individualism and collectivism, egalitarianism and hierarchy, monochronic and polychronic time, proxemics, the roles of men and women across cultures, and verbal and nonverbal communication practices (**Table 16.2**).[61]

## INDIVIDUALISM VERSUS COLLECTIVISM

Individualism and collectivism are two opposite cultural dimensions.[62] Individualistic cultures, such as the European and North American cultures, value self-reliance, equality, and autonomy of the individual.[62] Patients from individualistic cultures make their own decisions about interventions, sometimes with input from members of the immediate family. Opposite to individualism, collectivism values group effort and harmony in the group.[62] For choices and actions, the collectivist group members reach beyond the nuclear family to the extended family in order to support the group.[62] For example, patients or clients from collectivist cultures such as the Latin American, Asian, or African cultures make their decisions based directly on the members of their group.

| Table 16.2 | Cultural Dimensions Applied to Patient Education[61] |
|---|---|
| Individualism and collectivism. |
| Egalitarianism and hierarchy. |
| Monochronic and polychronic time. |
| Proxemics. |
| The roles of men and women across cultures. |
| Communication practices: verbal (e.g., semantics, phonology, syntax, high context, low context) and nonverbal (e.g., eye contact, gestures, space, silence, touch). |

In regard to patient teaching and learning, individualist learners work alone, are comfortable with an equal status relationship, value personal accomplishments and recognition, and place little importance on gender and age. Collectivist learners prefer to work in groups or teams and feel more comfortable with authority and titles.[62] In teaching and learning, individualistic cultures appreciate the learner's initiatives and expression whereas collectivist cultures tend to value those collectivist efforts that reinforce social connections and norms. Patients from a collectivist culture also may appreciate a vertical relationship in which the person who has a higher position (such as the health care provider) has higher importance.[62] This means that the person who is in a lower position will have a harder time winning in any discussion and the teaching aspect can become paternalistic. For example, an Asian American learner with a Chinese background may consider his or her role in rehabilitation to be highly dependent upon the therapist. The patient's cultural belief assumes a lower status in relation to the therapist as the health care provider/teacher in charge. In such a situation, questioning the teacher can be viewed by the patient as questioning the teacher's competence. Also from a collectivist perspective, when teaching and learning takes place with a patient from a Hispanic culture, the therapist needs to understand concepts such as *familismo*, indicating that the patient's family relationship is the most important. Learners from Hispanic cultures learn better with informal learning approaches linked to their family and community life.[35] For them, terms such as *respeto* or *personalismo* also are significant, demonstrating respect for authority figures (such as parents, elders, or priests) as well as the need to show personal interest in a relationship, especially when learning.[35] Personalized teaching by providing instruction tailored to the Hispanic American learner's interests and learning styles can be the best approach in patient education.

# EQUALITY VERSUS HIERARCHY

In regard to equality versus hierarchy, in collectivist cultures, equality may not be there. Relationships are typically long term and good relationships continue in the future. Use of the first name is very slow to develop and titles are important. Gift giving is also part of collectivism and can solidify relationships. Contrarily, in individualistic cultures, equality and fairness are critical, hierarchy being always connected with rigidity.[61] Collectivist cultures value hierarchy as a means of acknowledging innate differences and inequalities.[61] Hierarchy in collectivism can facilitate communication through the recognition of various social levels, titles, and roles.[61] Individuals of higher class or status may expect privileges. As examples, Asian American patients, who value professional achievements and who are comfortable with status distances and hierarchies, are likely to prefer health care professionals to use their titles and display their degrees. However, a patient who is Native American may not be impressed by professional degrees and may be more interested in the therapist's personal qualities and relationships to his or her own family.

# MONOCHRONIC VERSUS POLYCHRONIC TIME

When relating to monochronic and polychronic time, monochronicity occurs when a person engages in just one activity at a time whereas with polychronicity a person engages in two or more activities during the same block of time. In the monochronic perspective, time is a scarce resource,[61] which must be rationed and controlled. In the polychronic perspective, time is flexible, and used for the maintenance of harmonious relationships. These concepts have become increasingly relevant in cultural differences in health care when discussing people's "time personalities."

Typically, patients with monochronic time adhere to their goals, emphasize promptness, and take time commitments (such as schedules) seriously. They feel their time is tangible and can be saved or spent carefully. The patient with a polychronic view, however, believes personal interaction is more important than being "on schedule." Patients with polychronic time prefer to do many tasks at once, are highly distractible, are committed to people and relationships, and base their promptness on the relationship. For them, the involvement of people and the completion of transactions are the most important aspects.[61]

Cultures can often be distinguished by how strictly their members adhere to a schedule of being monochronic or polychronic. Monochronic cultures, such as the American culture, organize their days around clocks and daily planners, and emphasize punctuality. Other cultures, including Native American and Hispanic American, are more polychronic. Rather than adhering strongly to schedules, they emphasize completion of one event (regardless of how long it takes) before beginning another. In patient education, issues can arise when patients from event-oriented (polychronic) cultures do not adhere to appointment schedules[35] or respond vaguely when asked questions about temporal events.

# PROXEMICS AND GENDER ROLES

Other equally important cultural dimensions may include the use of personal space or proxemics. Patients vary in how comfortable they feel when talking with health care providers in clinical settings. In the United States, the zones of spatial distance or interpersonal distance are typically 0 to 18 inches for intimate interactions, 18 inches to 4 feet for general personal interactions, 4 to 12 feet for social interaction, and 12 to 15 feet for public interaction (**Table 16.3**).[61] For example, patients from Asia prefer a greater conversational distance than Americans, who, in turn, may feel uncomfortable with the closeness of stance of individuals from other cultures such as Middle Eastern or African American.

Additionally, the roles of men and women vary substantially across cultures, influencing access to education, ownership, and choice of profession. In many cultures, it is the man who makes decisions for the woman. For individuals from certain Middle Eastern countries, gender roles may even affect whether a woman can receive interventions without a male family member being present.[35] Interventions may have to be established with the patient's spouse or an older member of patient's family. Including patient's family and community members in health care decisions may also be a usual practice. Gender roles can also affect the degree to which a woman's body can be exposed during a clinical examination.

Furthermore, health care providers must understand that there is a difference when interacting with men and women from other cultures. Psychological research showed that in medical interactions, in most cultures, female patients show warmth, agreeableness, openness to feelings, and sometimes a high level of neuroticism (as negative emotions) whereas male patients are open to ideas and communicate assertiveness.[63] Women also do not like to complain and are fearful about unfamiliar things.[63] Fear and concern could be the reasons why so many women from other cultures are afraid to discuss with health care providers sensitive issues such as sexual assault or intimate partner violence. Therefore, during the physical and occupational therapy examination, it is important for the therapist to learn about the patient's culture and to try to screen the patient for other health problems that may not necessarily be directly related to rehabilitation. These may include depression, hypertension, substance abuse, sexual diseases, or diabetes. When working with patients from another culture, the therapists should not make wrong assumptions, but work with the patient and patient's family. Learning about other cultures can also help the therapist to

| Table 16.3 |
|---|
| **_North American Proxemics_**[61] |
| Distance of intimate interactions: 0 to 18 inches. |
| Distance of general personal interactions: 18 inches to 4 feet. |
| Distance of social interaction: 4 to 12 feet. |
| Distance of public interaction: 12 to 15 feet. |

choose the rehabilitation interventions (including patient education) that are most appropriate for the patient's culture and socioeconomic status.

# *Culture and Verbal Communication*

Communication is an important variable in understanding and observing cultural differences during the patient education process. Communication is an essential requirement underpinning any successful encounter including patient education.[59] Communication is the product of a verbal code and nonverbal acts. Depending on the situation and the words used, verbal communication can transfer information during the teaching and learning process and also convey empathy to establish a therapeutic relationship with the patient. Communication during patient education must be framed or presented in very different ways in order to be effective and convincing to patients from different cultures.[59] Consequently, individual and cultural differences in health beliefs, perception, attitude, and level of education are among the most important factors to consider when verbally communicating with a patient. Additionally, it is important to consider not only the information provided to the patient, but also the manner in which the information is conveyed. As a result, health care providers must be aware of how the semantics, phonology, syntax, and pragmatics aspects of language influence interpersonal communication.

During patient teaching and learning, semantics must be considered when using different words to get an idea across.[16] Semantics involves the variety of different ways the meaning of a word can change. A word can become wider in meaning or narrower, or can have a positive or negative meaning. For example, semantics can have a narrow and negative meaning, such as when asking an 80-year old patient who has difficulty walking, "Have you played sports?" To change the meaning, the question should be, "When was the last time you were able to do some physical activity involving any type of game playing?" Phonology, which involves listening and pronunciation, is also important to understand the meaning of words. Syntax typically concerns the rules that dictate how sentences are formed. Pragmatics is the ability to communicate to another person more information than what can be plainly and simply stated. For example, plainly (without using pragmatics) a patient can be asked, "Raise your arm." However, this short sentence does not tell the patient how to raise his or her arm, especially if the therapist wants the patient to raise his or her arm up above his or her shoulder at approximately 90 degrees with the palm facing forward. In physical and occupational therapy, pragmatics are difficult to use with patients, especially in the beginning of therapy. The therapists must always state the information in simple and plain terms. After learning the material for a period of time, some patients may be able to understand the intended meaning of the topic well. This is called "pragmatic competence." In rehabilitation, pragmatic or procedural knowledge is difficult to acquire and needs practice and experience.

Another fundamental concept of communication is the degree to which context becomes essential in deriving meaning. Communication differs among cultures in the amount of information implied by setting or context. Cultures differ on a continuum ranging from high to low context.[61] The terms *high context* and *low context* are used to describe broad-brush cultural differences between groups of people or societies. High context refers to groups where people have close connections over a long period of time.[61] Many aspects of cultural behavior are not made explicit because most members know what to do and what to think from years of interaction with each other. A family or a small religious congregation is an example of a high context environment. In a high context setting the contribution of the context, in addition to the words themselves, is very important to communicating meaning.[61] High context is characterized by less verbally explicit communication, less written/formal information, and more internalized understandings of what is communicated. Members of the group have long-term relationships and strong boundaries.[61] Knowledge is situational and relational. Decisions and activities are based around personal face-to-face relationships, often around a central person who has authority.

Low context refers to groups where people tend to have many connections but of shorter duration or for some specific reason.[61] In these societies, cultural behavior and beliefs may need to be clearly explained so that those coming into the cultural environment know how to act. Examples of low context places are airports, libraries, and supermarkets. Low context is rule oriented and task centered. Decisions and activities focus around what needs to be done and division of responsibilities.[61] The knowledge is more often transferable. It is also codified, public, external, and accessible. The connections between people are many, interpersonal, and of shorter duration. In low context cultures the words themselves are fundamental. Computer language, in which every statement must be precise, is an extreme example of a low context language.

People function in both low and high contexts, but some cultures are more prone to one or another. Generally, low context environments are easier to access as an outsider because the environment contains much of the information that a person needs to participate.[61] Also, an individual can form relationships fairly quickly in a low context environment. Low context allows task completion and not necessarily entering into a relationship. However, high context environments or cultures are difficult to enter for an individual who does not belong to the group.[61] Outside individuals do not carry the context information internally and cannot create close relationships instantly.[61]

Health care providers must always try to provide in every clinical setting, including home health, a low context environment that emphasizes explicit verbal information. Many times, patients who are ill prefer to be in a high context environment. As a result, miscommunication can occur. Low context environments supply clear, simple, and explicit information so that no miscommunication occurs. However, in physical and occupational therapy, patients' high context environments are important for the therapists to understand cues and prompts related to patient's impairments and disabilities and to try to correct them. The therapists should make every effort to include in the examination and evaluation process the patient's high-context cultural environment, especially in situations when the patient cannot speak English. Using certified and experienced translators may be helpful as well as trying to acquire the support of members of the patient's family. These individuals could provide clear and unambiguous information about the patient's problem to establish a correct diagnosis. From the cultural perspective, the therapist should always ask himself or herself if cultural differences may be causing difficulties understanding the patient.[2] The following three questions can be asked to avoid generalizations and stereotypes:[2(p.156)]

1. How is this patient like all human beings?

2. How is this patient like some human beings?

3. How is this patient like no other human being?

# *Culture and Nonverbal Communication*

It is more difficult to interact with patients or clients who are settled in their high context cultures and reject outsiders. In such situations, nonverbal dimensions of communication are very important. These nonverbal communication strategies that therapists can use include eye contact, gestures, space, silence, and touch.[35] Eye contact in general conveys a positive message in American culture. Eye contact is therapeutic because it promotes a favorable treatment outcome, increases the patient's confidence, and shows the therapist's interest in the patient's condition.[64] Looking directly in a patient's eyes without staring can also convey honesty and integrity. However, intent eye contact such as staring may impart disagreement and anger.[35] Continuous eye contact, though considered professionally therapeutic, can also be wrongly interpreted as sexual in nature. The therapist must consider whether to maintain direct eye contact, with whom he or she should have eye contact, and for how long eye contact should be maintained. For this decision, gender differences and cultures are essential. For example, patients from Middle Eastern, Asian, Native American, and Appalachian backgrounds regard eye contact as impolite or aggressive. Hispanic Americans believe that using downcast eyes is proper to show respect toward others based on age, gender, social position, or economic status.

*Physical touch* as an intrinsic part of occupational and physical therapy interventions can become a problematic cultural issue. Touching in physical therapy is subdivided into instrumental touch, such as performing a manual therapy intervention; demonstrational touch, such as using demonstrations to cue patients into effective performance of tasks; and affective touch to make connections with the patient or indicate support (**Table 16.4**).[64]

Physical touch communicates a diversity of meanings and may show comfort, healing, respect, or disrespect. Touch must be used cautiously considering the patient's cultural beliefs.[35] For example, patients from Southeast Asia may not allow a therapist to touch their child's head because it forecasts poor health. Patients from a Mexican culture also may regard touching by a stranger to make them ill. In Hispanic and Islamic societies, touching when using interventions is acceptable only between patients and therapists of the same gender. Even within middle class European American society, some patients are uncomfortable with touching or being touched by another. As a result, it is always necessary to discuss patients' expectations of touch to prevent misunderstanding and miscommunication.

In regard to the *use of silence*, there are many variations among cultures. Typically, in a conversation between two European Americans, when one stops speaking, the other starts talking. Among Hispanic Americans, there is typically overlap so that before one person

| Table 16.4 | Forms of Touching in Physical and Occupational Therapy[64] |
|---|---|
| Affective touch to make connections, show empathy, increase a therapeutic relationship, and indicate support. | |
| Instrumental touch for performing physical/occupational therapy direct interventions. | |
| Explanatory or demonstrational touch for cuing, reminders, promptness, and effectiveness of tasks. | |

is finished, the other person begins.[61] Among Asian Americans, when one stops speaking, the other waits in silence a few minutes to clarify the meaning before beginning to speak again. For many European Americans silence, after someone stops speaking, is considered rude and shows disinterest. Among Arabic and English cultures, silence conveys respect for privacy. For the French culture, silence is a sign of agreement.

# Cultural Competence and Strategies in Patient Education

Cultural competence is as an "awareness of, sensitivity to, and knowledge of the meaning of culture."[35(p.121)] It includes one's openness and willingness to learn about cultural issues and the ability to understand one's own biases, values, attitudes, beliefs, and behaviors. Cultural competence is also represented as a set of congruent attitudes,[65] behaviors, and policies that come together among health care professionals and providers to enable them to perform effective work in cross-cultural situations. Cultural competence is a developmental process to achieve the ability and availability to effectively work within the cultural context of the patient, the patient's family, or the community.

## FACTORS CONTRIBUTING TO THE DEVELOPMENT OF CULTURAL COMPETENCE

Cultural competence is a critical process in patient education and needs to be cultivated within the individual through acquisition of knowledge, behaviors, and attitudes specific to culture, language, and communication.[53] Factors contributing to the development of cultural competence include the ability to value diversity, having self-awareness of cultural dynamics, being able to culturally self-assess, integrating cultural knowledge in daily activities, and developing specific adaptations that reflect cultural understanding (**Table 16.5**).[57,65]

| Table 16.5 | ***Essential Factors for the Development of Cultural Competence***[57,65] |
|---|---|
| Appreciating and respecting diversity. | |
| Being conscious of the cultural dynamics during cultural interactions. | |
| Having the ability to perform cultural self-assessment. | |
| Developing adaptations to service delivery reflecting a deep understanding of diversity within cultures and between cultures. | |
| Integrating cultural knowledge in daily activities. | |

Cultural competence is also an essential component of delivering effective and culturally responsive health care services to culturally and ethnically diverse patients or clients.[60] Cultural competence is a process, not an event. To achieve cultural competence in physical therapy, the American Physical Therapy Association (APTA) suggests a holistic cultural pattern that includes the following steps: (1) the therapist's self-examination and self-reflection; (2) the therapist's learning about the diversity dimensions influencing health outcomes and affecting human experience in positive and negative ways; (3) the therapist's understanding the need for a patient-centered approach to delivery of culturally competent physical therapy services; (4) the therapist's use of effective communication with the patient as a fundamental means of delivery of culturally competent care; and (5) the therapist's application in all clinical settings of knowledge about culture, belief systems, and traditions to enhance their patient interactions.[57]

## CONSTRUCTS OF CULTURAL COMPETENCE

In nursing, cultural competence consists of five constructs: cultural awareness, cultural knowledge, cultural skills, cultural encounters, and cultural desires (**Table 16.6**).[60] These five nursing constructs or concepts can also be applied to physical and occupational therapy to enhance therapists' cultural competence. The implications of cultural competence in patient teaching and learning are important. Therapists should be able to use materials and teaching and learning techniques that are culturally relevant for the patient and family. Adherence with interventions and prevention techniques will also be greatly enhanced when the therapist's plan of care incorporates the patient's cultural values and beliefs.

The first construct or concept for achieving cultural competence is *cultural awareness*.[60] This concept means the therapist's self-examination and in-depth exploration of their own cultural and professional backgrounds. Cultural awareness is the foundation of communication, involving the ability to become aware of personal cultural values, beliefs, and

| Table 16.6 | Five Constructs to Achieve Cultural Competence[60] |
|---|---|
| 1. Cultural awareness. | |
| 2. Cultural knowledge. | |
| 3. Cultural skills. | |
| 4. Cultural encounter. | |
| 5. Cultural desire. | |

perceptions.[66] Cultural awareness includes the recognition of the therapist's biases, stereotypes, prejudices, and assumptions in regard to patients or clients who are different. What is considered appropriate in one culture may be inappropriate in another.[66] Patient interaction can be affected by the therapist's stereotyping by using social categories such as race or gender. Even well-intentioned therapists who are not overtly biased may demonstrate unconscious negative attitudes and stereotypes. It is easy to stereotype someone, not on purpose, but out of ignorance. The therapist's self-assessment can reveal many gaps and help him or her to avoid wrongly categorizing patients or clients during teaching and learning (**Table 16.7**).

Misunderstandings may also arise when the therapist uses his or her own cultural background to make sense of the patient's reality. It is important to minimize imposing the therapist's values and beliefs on patients from another culture and to avoid ethnocentrism. Ethnocentrism is judging other people's culture by the standards of an individual's own culture.[67] Ethnocentrism is also wrongly perceiving one's own culture as superior. Ethnocentrism is closely related to the concept of cultural bias regarding that the beliefs and values of a specific group "must guide the situation or decisions."[67(p.5)]

Cultural awareness in physical and occupational therapy makes therapists accountable to acquire the most current information about various gender attributes, socioeconomic influences, and cultural traditions that can affect their interventions including teaching and learning.[57] Every day, research in health care, social science, psychology, and medicine is yielding information that will assist in planning and revising appropriate rehabilitative interventions to meet the needs of the diverse patient or client population. Becoming aware of cultural dynamics may be difficult because culture is an unconscious, automatic concept. People are born and learn to see and do things at an unconscious level. People's experiences, values, and cultural background make up their culture. In order to experience awareness, therapists need to first know the impact of their culture on their behavior. Projecting similarities onto other people can cause misinterpretations. In patient education, the safest path for the therapist is to assume differences until similarity is demonstrated. Cultural

| Table 16.7 | *Self-Assessment Questions to Avoid Stereotyping in Teaching and Learning*[57,65] |
|---|---|

1. Do I use neutral language when teaching patients and families?

2. Do I confront bias when evidenced by other health care professionals?

3. Do I request information equally from patients regardless of gender, socioeconomic status, age, or culture?

4. Are my instructional materials free of stereotypical terminology and expressions?

5. Am I an effective role model of equality for my colleagues?

6. Do I treat all patients with fairness, respect, and dignity?

7. Does someone's appearance raise or lower my expectations of that person's abilities?

8. Do I routinely assess the educational and experiential backgrounds, personal attributes, and economic resources of patients to ensure appropriate health teaching?

9. Am I knowledgeable enough of the cultural traditions of various groups to provide sensitive care?

awareness can be divided into four levels: the parochial stage, ethnocentric stage, synergistic stage, and participatory stage (**Table 16.8**).[66]

In the parochial stage (simply explained as "my way is the only way"), individuals ignore cultural differences and the impact of their ways of life on other people.[66] The second level is the ethnocentric stage (simply explained as "I know their way, but my way is better"), which is characterized by individuals perceiving the sources of cultural misunderstandings but ignoring and reducing their significance.[66] In the synergistic stage (simply explained as "my way and their way"), individuals are very much aware of cultural differences and misunderstandings and decide to use cultural diversity to create new solutions and alternatives.[66]

The participatory stage is the last stage (simply explained as "our way"); it brings people together to create a culture of shared meanings.[66] They are participating in cultural awareness by creating new rules to meet the needs of their particular situation. By increasing cultural awareness, therapists recognize that: (1) people are not all the same; (2) similarities and differences are important; (3) there are multiple different ways to reach the same goal; and (4) the best way depends on the cultural contingency, meaning that each situation is different and requires a different solution.

| Table 16.8 | *Cultural Awareness Levels*[66] | |
|---|---|
| Parochial stage | "My way is the only way." |
| Ethnocentric stage | "I know their way but my way is better." |
| Synergistic stage | "My way and their way." |
| Participatory stage | "Our way." |

The second construct of cultural competence is *cultural knowledge*.[60] It means that physical and occupational therapists and assistants should gain knowledge about the culture of various patient or client groups. Cultural knowledge requires an understanding of how patients or clients view the world, specifically related to health, illness, disease/disorder, incidence, prevalence, prevention, and behaviors related to them.[60] This understanding is a continuous learning process about other cultures. The therapist's cultural knowledge can be acquired by assessing the patient or client and learning cultural skills.

*Cultural skills* represent the third concept of cultural awareness.[60] Cultural skills are the therapist's ability to collect relevant cultural data regarding the patient's or client's problems based on a cultural physical assessment. During the assessment, the therapist can learn about the patient's native language, communication style, health practices, beliefs about the illness, relationships with other health care providers, and the influence of religion and spirituality on him or her. The cultural skills enable the therapist to understand and use specific methods to deal effectively with cultural issues in interacting with individual patients, their families, members of the health care team, and the wider community.[57,60] The following statements and questions can be used to assist therapists assessing patients and families from culturally diverse backgrounds:

- "…so that I might be aware and respect your cultural beliefs…"
- "What do you think may be the reason you have this low back pain?"
- "What do friends, family, or others say about your pain?"
- "Can you tell me what languages are spoken in your home and the languages that you understand and speak?"
- "Can you tell me about your experiences with physical therapy (or physiotherapy) in your native country?"
- "Do you use any traditional health remedies to improve your lower back pain?"

The fourth construct of cultural competence is the *cultural encounter*.[60] This important cultural concept is a process that encourages the therapist to directly engage in cross-cultural interactions with patients from diverse backgrounds.[57,60] The cross-cultural interaction can confirm or deny the therapist's already-acquired cultural knowledge and beliefs. At the same time, cross-cultural interaction decreases the possibility of stereotyping. During cross-cultural interactions, the therapist must use cross-cultural communication, which represents any communication occurring across cultures. The fundamental skills of cross-cultural communication are demonstrating interest and showing respect for patients and their beliefs.[59] The therapist's communication skills also require active listening and the ability to elicit patients' beliefs and information.

The main cross-cultural communication skills can be achieved using the Explanatory Model of Health and Illness (explanatory/social/fears/treatment).[68] This explanatory (E) model, abbreviated ESFT, can identify a patient's problems, potential social and financial (S and F) barriers, a patient's fears and concerns, and the patient's understanding of the treatment (T) regimen.[68] The model, used mostly by physicians and nurses, explores patients' meaning of illness, plans for treatment, the social context having control over the environment, social stressors and support network, literacy and language difficulties (especially when taking medications), and management options by presenting the plan of care to the patient and determining the patient's acceptance.[68]

In physical and occupational therapy, the ESFT model can help the therapist understand differences in the explanation of illness and disease based on the patient's perspective. The ESFT model of communication provides the necessary information for the patient to conceptualize his or her illness regardless of the patient's educational background.[69] The model also addresses the patient's fears or concerns in regard to interventions and helps patient teaching via a therapeutic contract or playback of information. This playback means that when the patient says he or she understands the information, the therapist asks the patient to repeat back the instructions.[69] The approach can be supplemented by providing written instructions to the patient describing the exercises or other forms of home interventions.

The cross-cultural communication assessment of the ESFT model can be applied to physical and occupational therapy to elicit patient or family views about the illness experience including etiology, time and mode of onset, pathophysiology, prognosis, and treatment (**Table 16.9**).

The final, fifth construct of cultural competence is *cultural desire*.[60] This concept focuses on the therapist's motivation to become more culturally involved with his or her patients or clients.[60] Cultural desire has to do with the therapist's caring, being flexible when working with the patients, accepting their differences, promoting similarities, and learning all that is possible about the patients. When teaching patients in a cross-cultural situation, many options are available to the therapist. Prior to the initial examination and evaluation, the first step in any interaction with the patient is to establish effective communication. The model using the acronym LEARN can be very useful (**Table 16.10**).[57,60]

In regard to verbal communication, language barriers require interpreter services. The interpreter must be trained and certified.[35] The physical presence of the interpreter for

| Table 16.9 | *Modified ESFT Model in Physical and Occupational Therapy*[69] |
|---|---|

**Explanatory Model of Health and Illness**

- What do you think caused your problem?
- Why do you think it started when it did?
- Why do you think this illness or problem has occurred?
- How does it affect you?
- What do you think the natural course of illness is?
- How do you think the sickness should be treated?

**Social and Environmental Factors**

- How did you get here? Did you drive? Did you take the bus?
- Did you get help getting here?
- How often are you able to come here for treatment?
- How do you want to be helped?

**Fears and Concerns**

- What do you fear?
- What worries you the most?
- Have your heard about this type of treatment?
- Do you think you will be able to do that?

**Therapeutic Contracting (Treatment)**

- Do you understand how to perform this exercise (or walk) at home?
- Is your family helping you?
- Who should be involved in this decision?
- Can you tell me how you will do this exercise?

| Table 16.10 | **Modified LEARN Model for Effective Communication[57,60]** | |
|---|---|---|
| **Listen** | Identify and greet family or friends of the patient. If there is a language barrier, obtain interpreter services. The interpreter should be trained and certified. Start the interview with an open-ended question. Do not interrupt the patient as he or she speaks. |
| **Elicit** | Obtain information about the patient's health beliefs pertaining to the health condition and the reason for the visit as well as his or her expectations. |
| **Assess** | Make an assessment of potential attributes and problems relative to the patient's life that may impact his or her health behavior. |
| **Recommend** | Make recommendations for a patient-centered plan of care including a patient teaching plan. Explain to the patient and family the rationale behind the plan. |
| **Negotiate** | Negotiate an action plan with the patient and family (as necessary). |

patient education allows the patient and the therapist to visually communicate through body language and gestures.[35] If an interpreter is not available to be physically present, the next best situation is to have a trained and certified interpreter through the phone system. There are several types of phone interpreter systems available. In physical and occupational therapy, every effort should be made to obtain the help of a trained and certified interpreter. Using the patient's family or friends for interpreter services should be strongly discouraged for important reasons. Most of the time, the family member who is used for this process is a younger individual who has been educated in the American educational system and speaks English. In many cultures, it is a form of disrespect for the younger family member to be communicating for an older family member. Also, the health care information may be of a sensitive nature or the patient may need to disrobe for an evaluation. This would be totally unacceptable. Additionally, trained and certified interpreters are able to enter a conversation with the patient and family without any bias.[35] Family members or friends may incorporate their bias or feelings into the interpretation.

# The Process for Developing Cultural Competence

When moving toward cultural competence, there is an ongoing developmental process. Individuals or organizations participating in this development may go through specific stages called cultural destructiveness, cultural incapacity, cultural blindness, cultural precompetence, cultural competence, and finally cultural proficiency.[70] Cultural destructiveness acknowledges only one way of being and purposefully denies or outlaws any other cultural approaches. Cultural destructiveness means attitudes, policies, and practices that are damaging to other cultures.[70] It may include humiliating other people and assuming superiority. Today, cultural destructiveness reminds people of appalling events of the past such as the abuses during the Nazi's atrocities of World War II or the Tuskegee syphilis experiments. Hopefully such destructive and dehumanizing practices will never take place again. Cultural destructiveness is definitely a thing of the past for the American culture.

Cultural incapacity includes unintentional cultural destructiveness, bias, paternalism, ignorance, and/or fear.[70] Cultural incapacity believes in concepts such as "separate but equal." The individual or the organization going through this process exhibits the inability to deal personally with multiple approaches but has the willingness to accept their existence somewhere else.[70] Cultural blindness is a philosophy of being unbiased because culture, class, or color makes no difference.[70] However, the individual in this stage who is moving toward cultural competence can be well intentioned but still ethnocentric. Another view of cultural blindness is the assumption that people are all basically alike and what works with members of one culture should work within all cultures.[70]

Cultural precompetence is the realization of weaknesses and gaps in understanding when working with other cultures.[70] This stage toward cultural competence encourages learning and understanding of new ideas and solutions to improve cultural performance or services. The next phase, cultural competence, involves actively seeking advice and consultation and a commitment to incorporate new knowledge and experiences into a wider range of cultural practice.[70]

The final stage of cultural proficiency involves holding cultural differences and diversity in the highest esteem, proactively regarding cultural differences, and promoting improved cultural relations among diverse groups.[70] In cultural proficiency, individuals take responsibility for constant development of cultural knowledge and assume responsibility to transfer cultural skills to others.[70]

Although physical and occupational therapists and assistants do not engage in overt or covert culturally destructive relationships with their patients, they should be aware that every individual has a culture. The acronym ETHNIC emphasizes cultural collaboration with the patient during teaching and learning and the therapist's engagement toward cultural proficiency (**Table 16.11**).[71] Therapists and patients represent different segments of the population bringing in different world views, values, and beliefs. The United States' culturally pluralistic society provides opportunities and challenges for therapists.[71] The therapist's cultural competence is reflected not only through his or her culturally competent communication skills, but also through inner self-examination of the therapist's attitudes

| Table 16.11 | *Culturally Competent Concepts for Teaching and Learning Using ETHNIC[71]* |
|---|---|
| **E**veryone has a culture. |
| **T**ake time to collect relevant cultural information. |
| **H**old all judgments. Be careful about interpreting the culturally different patient's behavior, especially if unfamiliar with the culture. |
| **N**otice and negotiate differences in understanding of teaching and learning. |
| **I**nvolve cultural resources as appropriate. |
| **C**ollaborate with patients to develop educational objectives and teaching and learning strategies. |

and experiences. As a teacher and learner, the therapist needs time to collect the patient's relevant cultural information. Cultural proficiency is an evolving process and never an outcome. The therapist may not be able to reach the goal of cultural proficiency, but must strive to understand and appreciate cultures. During this process, the therapist should not make incorrect judgments about a patient's culture but keep learning about it for better understanding. In this lifelong learning process toward cultural competence, the therapist should collaborate with patients and develop teaching and learning strategies with them using the patient-centered care model.

# Guidelines for Teaching and Learning with Diverse Populations

Prior to the teaching and learning process, physical and occupational therapists and assistants can establish a concise cultural assessment of patients or clients. Such an assessment may require cultural guidelines associated with the patient-centered plan of care. The cultural strategies may include the following: (1) observing the interactions between the patient and family members and among family members, (2) determining the person making decisions (either the patient or a member of the family), (3) considering how decisions are made, (4) identifying the primary caregiver, and (5) planning the most appropriate teaching and learning plan that integrates the patient's and family's most significant needs. Achieving a teaching and learning plan of care requires the therapist to listen to the patient and family using active and reflective listening skills (**Table 16.12**).[35,71]

Table
16.12

### Culturally Competent Active Listening Skills[35,71]

Focus attention on the patient.

Give the patient time to deliver the entire message (especially if there are language barriers) and do not abruptly interrupt the patient.

Help the patient feel free to talk (by smiling and looking directly at the patient even when communicating through a translator).

Use culturally appropriate nonverbal communication skills (such as appropriate eye contact, depending on the patient's culture; slightly leaning toward the patient; keeping your hands at your side; nodding your head; varying your tone of voice; and making encouraging hand gestures as appropriate).

Ask the patient to clarify the meaning of words and/or to enlarge the statement.

Be attentive to the patient's and family's nonverbal communication.

Show empathy.

Repeat the patient's message by looking directly at the patient (even when communicating through a translator).

## CULTURALLY COMPETENT LISTENING SKILLS

Culturally competent active listening skills are more intense than general listening skills because they require cultural awareness and sensitivity.[72] Active listening requires the therapist to focus on the patient (and family) and show readiness to engage in a culturally competent therapeutic relationship with the patient. Additionally, active and reflective listening builds trust and fosters the patient's and family's cooperation.[72] Active listening requires the therapist's undivided attention, avoidance of interruptions and misinterpretation of the patient's message, and judicious use of verbal and nonverbal prompts to clarify meanings.

When the therapist listens quietly without interruption, the patient is encouraged to speak. The therapist accepting the message by nodding the head or saying "Yes," "I see what you mean," or "Go on, please" indicates consideration of the patient's message. It convinces the patient to elaborate on their statement. From time to time, the therapist can restate the patient's message by saying, "So you are saying that . . ." Clarifying the message by using questions is also important. The therapist may say, "Let me see if I understand. Do you mean ...?" Summarizing when the patient has completed the entire message may include: "In the last few minutes you have been saying that you believe..." This summary restates briefly the patient's point of view. During active listening, therapists should not make personal judgments about the patient's message and avoid reassurances or offering advice.

Additionally, active and reflective listening helps the therapist understand the patient's/family's cultural needs.[72] For example, cultural awareness regarding the patient's primary language (which may be different from the therapist's) is an important requirement. Observing the patient's rate of speech, verbal expressions, customs, or taboos can increase the therapist's knowledge of the patient's cultural beliefs and practices[72] that may interfere with interventions and modes of teaching and learning. Other cultural variables for patient-therapist interaction may include the patient's notion of time and symbolic objects and traditions that provide comfort and security for the patient. The information acquired through active listening can facilitate the patient-therapist relationship in which the therapist and the patient are both learners and teachers. The purpose of active listening is for the therapist to involve the patient or client in a patient-centered approach to care while trying to solve problems and also determine teaching and learning goals together.

# Teaching and Learning Strategies for Diverse Patient Populations

Teaching patients from different cultural groups can be challenging for physical and occupational therapists and assistants. The therapists need to incorporate culture-specific attitudes and values into their teaching and learning techniques. These culturally competent approaches can be acquired slowly by gradually understanding cultural differences and forming various strategies.

## HISPANIC AMERICAN PATIENTS

When teaching and learning from Hispanic American patients, the therapist can first identify the patient's cultural subgroup(s) (such as Mexican, Cuban, or Puerto Rican). This classification can target the patient's specific community needs and also his or her beliefs and values regarding language, illness, and disease prevention and health promotion.[73] Accounting for incidences of illness or risk factors such as diabetes, obesity, homicide, or accidental injuries can assist with specificity and adaptations of interventions and teaching and learning strategies.

When providing patient education for Hispanic Americans, the therapist may need to consider the following significant variables: (1) nonverbal communication, (2) language barriers, (3) polychronic time (time-orientation factors), and (4) the practice of folk remedies. Hispanic Americans often believe in luck, fate, or other powers beyond their control.[74] They also may consider an admiring or envious look from a person (such as a health care provider) to be the "evil eye" (*mal de ojo*).[74] This evil eye is said to cause sudden and unexplainable symptoms of illness such as fever, vomiting, restlessness, and even suicidal thoughts.[74] Children and young women are believed to be the most susceptible to the evil eye.[75] The prevention is to wear a particular type of religious jewelry.[75]

Exercise is discouraged during illness. In general, Hispanic American patients may distrust the health care system because of prior experiences with involuntary medical procedures (such as sterilization) performed in their country of origin. Also, when visiting a health care provider, some patients may be confused and associate providers and the health care system (especially the hospitals) with government, repression, or immigration.[74]

Families of Hispanic American patients should be involved in the teaching and learning process from the beginning of therapy. The family members provide support to each other, and decision making is usually done by the oldest male adult authority figure in the family.

An important part of cross-cultural teaching and learning for Hispanic Americans are the community health workers (CHWs), also called *promotoras*.[75] CHWs are lay members of their communities who work for pay or as volunteers in association with the local health care system in urban and rural environments.[75] CHWs usually share ethnicity, language, socioeconomic status, and life experiences with the community members they serve. They offer interpretation and translation services, assist people in receiving the care they need, give informal counseling and guidance on health behaviors, and advocate for individual and community health needs. For example, CHWs or *promotoras* could be older respected women from the community who assess and help Latino families who are fearful of seeking assistance from mainstream agencies.[75] CHWs are trained to provide culturally appropriate health information and distribute nonprescription birth control upon request, conduct street outreach, and arrange and conduct talks with their peers. For example in Texas *promotoras* were able to help Hispanic American patients manage their diabetes and also offered diabetes prevention education.[76] Similar to in Texas, in Arizona, *promotoras* helped Mexican Americans in a farm worker community by providing and facilitating culturally relevant support for diabetes self-management practices.[77] They implemented a community-based intervention program that included telephone support, home and hospital visits, support groups, and informal patient education by speaking with patients and their families about diabetes.[77]

In physical and occupational therapy, adequate physical space is necessary to accommodate the Hispanic American family members who typically accompany patients seeking care. Issues such as contraception, abortion, and family planning should be avoided by the therapist because of the importance of the Roman Catholic religion in the lives of many Hispanic Americans. Folk remedies such as herbs, potions, ointments, amulets, candles, medals, relics, and religious statues are commonly used by Hispanic American patients[69] and should be included in rehabilitation as long as they are not antagonistic to regular interventions. The language barrier can be remedied by use of certified interpreters and/or the *promotoras*. Time orientation related to polychronicity can be accommodated by an open or "walk-in" schedule.

Establishing a therapeutic relationship requires the therapist to display friendliness and tactfulness. In the Hispanic American culture health care providers are viewed as being informal and showing interest in their patients' lives. Communication strategies may include smiling that expresses warmth and concern, good eye contact (but not to members of the opposite sex), shaking hands, and first speaking with the male patient or caregiver.[73] The therapist should not assume total understanding of information if the patient nods his or her head or smiles. Patients from Hispanic backgrounds respect authority, and nodding the head or smiling may actually show consideration and genuine friendliness toward the therapist. The therapist must ask the patient to repeat the information in his or her own words to determine comprehension of the material. If interpreters are used, they should be able to speak the learner's dialect and translate the meaning (but not interpret the meaning). The therapist must talk directly to the patient as the learner and not talk to the translator.[73] Written material must also reflect cultural appropriateness.

## AFRICAN AMERICAN PATIENTS

Communication plays a central role when providing patient education for African American patients.[78] Establishing a relationship with the patient and inviting the patient and his or her family in the decision making aspect of care and interventions is very important. African Americans tend to be very verbal and express feelings openly to family and friends.[73] However, they are much more private about family matters when in the company of strangers. The volume of their voices tends to be louder than in other cultures and they express their thoughts in a more dynamic manner; however, these types of behaviors should not be perceived as necessarily reflecting anger or frustration.[73] The therapist must keep an open line of communication and be sensitive to the needs of African American patients to operate in a family unit. Because there is a history of poor or nonexistent access to health care, some African American patients may be reluctant to take part in rehabilitation interventions.[78] They also may appear to be overvigilant or asking too many questions.[78] Therapists should acknowledge and understand the questioning and be very clear in their communication.

The patient's teaching and learning must also concentrate on disease prevention measures for hypertension and diabetes. African Americans are likely to have less access to health care services because of economic hardship.[78] Other barriers to care are perceived as lack of culturally sensitive care, sensitivity to racial discrimination, and a general distrust of health professionals and the health care system.[78] As a result, the first step toward a therapeutic relationship is establishing a trusting rapport and recognizing the African American patients' unique responses to health and illness based on their spiritual and religious foundations, their strong family ties, and other essential traditional beliefs and cultural values.[73] Religion and spirituality are deep-seated in traditional African American culture.[79] Many patients express beliefs, values, and judgments based on their religion and spirituality being in close connection with God and spiritual existential forces.[79] Spirituality has helped African Americans to bond with each other and overcome social injustice, racism, or discrimination.[79] When illness is present, the patient's spirituality brings hope, comfort, and support. Physical and occupational rehabilitation should combine patient's practice of folk medicine with therapeutic interventions as long as they are not antagonistic to each other.[73] Any folk practices or traditional beliefs should be respected, allowed, and included in the recommended treatments.[73] Patient education should be connected to family, the community and church, spiritual beliefs, and patient's convictions. The therapists should also explore the patient's accessibility to the community's health resources and their values related to disease prevention and health promotion.

Furthermore, African American patients feel comfortable with less personal space than do some other ethnic groups. Nevertheless, direct eye contact by others outside of their culture can be misinterpreted as aggressive behavior. Therapists must be careful not to misinterpret nonverbal and verbal behaviors when delivering interventions, including patient education.[35,73] Patients of African American background are more oriented to the present than to the past or future. Thus, they tend to be more relaxed about specific time frames. Consequently, therapists must be flexible in the timing of appointments, because African Americans, the same as Hispanic Americans, have a polychronic time orientation and may not be on schedule.[75] Even though African American patients and family are very informal when they interact among themselves, they prefer to be greeted in a formal manner by health care providers.[35] Addressing them by their last name demonstrates the respect and pride they have in their family heritage.

Traditionally, the family structure has been matriarchal. This pattern persists to the present day due to a high percentage of households run by a female single parent. It is important that health care providers acknowledge the dominant role that African American women play in decision making and the need to share all teaching and learning information directly with them in addition to the patient. African American patients rely on home remedies and advice from older female family members.[73] They believe that maintaining a warm environment prevents suffering from muscle or bone aches. Exercise is not a regular part of daily activities. Also, Western medicine may be considered harsh and dangerous for some patients from an African American background.

## ASIAN AMERICAN PATIENTS

Asian American patients came to the United States from the Far East, Southeast Asia, or the Indian subcontinent. Asian Americans include people who indicate their ethnic background as Asian Indian, Vietnamese, Chinese, Filipino, Japanese, Korean, or from another Asian country (which may include people whose origins are from Burma, Pakistan, or Thailand). Another group of Asian American patients or clients are called Asian/Pacific Islanders. They are born in the east-central islands of the Pacific Ocean that include Polynesia (with the Hawaiian Islands), Micronesia and Melanesia. This vast region is called Oceania. When related to specific American states, Pacific Islanders are residents of Hawaii, Alaska and parts of California.

Most of the East and Southeast Asian cultures emphasize respect and high consideration for authority.[74] As a result, in regard to patient education in physical and occupational therapy, patients or clients will not disagree or contradict therapists. This makes it seem like patients agree, when in reality they may disagree. Also, because they want to show respect for the therapist, they may avoid eye contact.[74] As with any patient first encounter, the therapists must introduce him- or herself by last name and title and refer to the patient by his or her last name and title (such as Mr. or Mrs.). Asian Americans would consider it offensive to be addressed by their first name.

During teaching and learning with patients from Asian backgrounds it is important to remember that Asian Americans are sensitive and formal people.[73] Because they are very conventional in relation to others, they must be given permission to ask questions. Nevertheless, Asian Americans are not offended by questions from others. Respect is automatically given to most health care providers and teachers because they are seen as knowledgeable individuals.

Language barriers are usually the first and biggest obstacle to overcome, especially when providing rehabilitation to patients from the Asian/Pacific Islander backgrounds. Translators can be used to facilitate interactions. The learning style of Asian American patients is essentially passive with no personal opinions, no confrontations, no challenges, and no outward disagreements. Decision making is a family affair. Because of cultural beliefs in regard to incurable diseases, the patient's family may not want the patient to know about a negative diagnosis. Family members (especially the male authority figure) need to be included in the decision making and plan of interventions.

Therapists should be aware that Asian Americans wish to "save face" for themselves and others.[75] They avoid being disruptive and will agree to what is said so as not to be offensive. They are easily shamed, so patients must be reassured and told what is considered acceptable behavior by Western moral and legal standards. Nods of the head do not necessarily mean agreement or understanding. Questions directed to Asian American patients need to be asked in several ways to confirm that the patients understand the instructional messages. In regard to adherence to therapy, Asian Americans may abandon interventions when the symptoms subside. Therapists need to carefully explain the importance of continuing interventions to the patient or family.

Additionally, Asian Americans have a diversity of religious practices. Therapists should try to discuss these practices with the patient or family to integrate them in their rehabilitative care.[73] In some situations, they may need to invite the spiritual guide or the faith healer to the therapy session. Also, incorporating alternative medicine into physical and occupational therapy interventions may enhance the relationship with the patient and the teaching and learning aspect of care. This patient-therapist rapport can alert the rehabilitation provider of any negative effects with interventions as well as medications.

In regard to illness, Asian American patients may believe that disease is an imbalance in "yin and yang" or hot and cold.[80] Yin represents the negative, dark, cool, and diminishing force whereas yang is a positive, bright, warm, and expanding force.[80] The human body also has yang and yin. The outside of the body is considered active, light, and positive (yang) whereas the inside is thought to be passive, dark, and negative (yin).[80] These forces need to balance each other for a person to feel well. Diseases may be believed to be caused by an imbalance in these forces.

When practicing folk remedies, Asian Americans may use "cupping" and "coining" to address hot and cold imbalances.[80] During cupping, a cup is applied to the person's skin and the pressure in the cup is reduced by applying heat or by suctioning out air.[80] In this way, the skin and superficial muscle layer is drawn into and held in the cup. This form of folk remedy can be used to treat pain, as can acupuncture techniques. During coining, the side of a coin is rubbed firmly along the patient's spine and ribs, which causes red skin abrasions (scraping). Prior to coining, patient's skin is lubricated with oils such as camphor, eucalyptus, winter green, or peppermint oil. Coining is believed to help a variety of illnesses such as aches, pains, fevers, colds, abdominal pain, cough, or nausea.[74] The technique is considered effective when it produces prominent marks that last a few days. This technique is believed to draw out "cold illness from the patient."[74(p.2270)]

## NATIVE AMERICAN PATIENTS

In the past several decades, the health outcomes for Native Americans have improved. However, there are still serious health disparities among Native Americans that affect their lifestyles and behavioral choices.[81] These are diabetes, tuberculosis, mental health disorders, cardiovascular disease, cancer, pneumonia, influenza, and injuries. A large percentage (63.7% of men and 61.4% of women) of Native Americans reported having one or more of the following risk factors for heart disease or stroke: high blood pressure, smoking cigarettes and high cholesterol.[81] These factors were more common in older men and women, the unemployed and those with less education. Social, cultural, structural, and financial barriers to health disparities are: (1) limited access to appropriate health services; (2) poor access to health insurance (including Medicare, Medicaid and private); (3) inadequate quality of care; (4) insufficient federal subsidy; (5) inadequate and insufficient availability of culturally competent health services; (6) harmful behaviors or lifestyle choices; and (7) disproportionately high levels of poverty and poor education.[81] An example in regard to insufficient funding shows that in one Indian tribe, they had the best rehabilitation centers in the region concerning equipment.[61] However, they could not operate the center because of insufficient funding to properly staff the facility. Other health disparities, especially from the perspective of patient education, are Native Americans' accessibility to culturally competent health services that recognize patient's values, beliefs, and traditions in order to provide "acceptable services for specific populations."[81(p.33)] Health care providers need to increase their cultural competence and decrease their biases toward Native American patient encounters to be able to meet the patient's own cultural ground. They should take into consideration patient's attitudes about health, religious views, and concept of death to understand compliance and disease management. For example, an important factor for Native Americans is to incorporate their traditional healing and medicines into the contemporary health care interventions. Working collaboratively with traditional healers can be very beneficial for Native American patients.

In physical and occupational therapy, the therapists should consider the patient's beliefs that:[82]

- Health reflects living in harmony with nature

- Earth is a living organism

- One must maintain a continuous relationship with nature

Disease for Native Americans means that some material object invaded the body (due to witchcraft and evil spirits), the individual did not wear or use charms, or he or she lost their spirit or soul.[82] Also, illness may be a cause for something that was not paid for in the past or even in the future.[82] The therapist should work together with the medicine-man (medicine-woman) to make the diagnosis and apply the treatment. Chanting or singing are important rituals to be considered because psychologically are significant for the patient.

Teaching and learning for Native American patients need to focus on giving information about diseases and risk factors and also emphasizing skills related to the importance of exercises. Additionally, building positive coping mechanisms for emotional problems can be another priority for referral to counselors or psychologists. Although all Native Americans share some of the core beliefs and practices of their culture, each tribe is unique in its customs and language. For example, Navajo Native Americans believe that sustained eye contact when speaking directly is rude and possibly confrontational, whereas avoiding eye contact is respectful.[35]

Native American patients expect the therapist to figure out their health problem through instinct rather than asking questions. During the initial examination and evaluation, the therapist should speak with the patient and the oldest member of the family.[83] Note taking is not acceptable. Patient history can be acquired using a conversational communication style.[83] Native Americans believe that health and wellness exist in harmony with other living things such as spirits. Problem solving and decision making are achieved by the group, specifically the respected elders. Because decision making is a group experience, respected elders or the family are the individuals who often make decisions on behalf of the patient.[83]

Community health representatives (CHRs) must be considered when teaching and learning with Native American patients, especially during prevention and health promotion education.[81] CHRs, similar to the CHWs, are Native American outreach workers who live and work in the community.[81] They play a significant role in case finding, early diagnosis, and reinforcement of patient and other health education recommendations. Involving the CHR in patient teaching and learning is an important way to reinforce behavior changes with the community and home. The Indian Health Service's CHRs provide a wide array of services in their individual communities.[81] Because needs vary tremendously among the tribes, no single job description can account for the multiplicity of duties and responsibilities that these important paraprofessionals can offer.[81] For example, CHRs can provide prenatal education in the home of a mother-to-be who is afraid to visit the clinic. They can make available regular home visits and a listening ear to elders, ensure medications are taken properly, and assess the home environment for adequate care and risks such as loose carpet or frayed electrical cords.[81]

# CONCLUSIONS

## Section IV Summary

This section identified the major ethical systems and theories used in physical and occupational rehabilitation as well as the legal principles of care, such as negligence and malpractice, confidentiality, and informed consent. Ethical dilemmas and conflict resolution skills were explained, emphasizing the importance of assertiveness in verbal and nonverbal communication. The role of the therapist's professional values was highlighted as an affective component of human behavior during patient education. Cultural factors of teaching and learning were described by explaining the important characteristics of culture and cultural dimensions. Issues such as individualism and collectivism, egalitarianism and hierarchy, monochronic and polychronic time, proxemics, the roles of men and women across cultures, and communication play a large part in therapists' cultural deliberations to create and support positive relationships with their patients. Section IV concluded with a description of constructs to achieve cultural competence and specific strategies for culturally appropriate teaching with diverse patient populations.

**Section IV Case Study**

## CULTURALLY COMPETENT PATIENT EDUCATION USING THE LEARN MODEL

Per the APTA's *Guide to Physical Therapist Practice*,[84] the patient physical therapy diagnostic classification pattern is:

Impaired motor function and sensory integrity associated with acute or chronic polyneuropathies

ICD-9-CM Codes: 250.6 Diabetes with neurological manifestations

APTA's *Guide to Physical Therapist Practice*[84] recommendations for patient-related instruction:

Instruction, education, and training of patient and caregiver regarding:

- Current condition (pathology/pathophysiology, impairments, functional limitations, or disabilities)
- Enhancement of performance
- Health, wellness, and fitness programs
- Plan of care
- Risk factors (pathology/pathophysiology, impairments, functional limitations, or disabilities)
- Transitions across settings
- Transitions to new roles

### Patient Description

Patient is a 43-year-old man with a medical diagnosis of polyneuropathy secondary to diabetes mellitus. He has a 12-year history of impaired glucose tolerance. Medically, he also has hypertension. He complains of severe pain and sensations of "pins and needles" in his right ankle and foot. The patient works for a landscape company. The patient is fluent in Spanish and speaks no English. He smokes and uses alcohol regularly. He is more than 50 pounds overweight. He has pain in his right foot and leg and walks holding onto his son's arm. His son is 20 years old and translates for his father. He told the physical therapist that his father cannot go to work anymore, is sad and tired all the time, smokes, and lies in bed all day. Almost 3 weeks ago, he took his father to the emergency room because he was dizzy and vomiting. In the emergency room, the doctor told him his sugar was very high. He was in the hospital for 3 days and sent home with a prescription for medications and physical therapy. The medications have been helping him but not enough to be able to get rid of his pain in his right foot and leg or his tiredness.

The emergency room report described that the patient had double vision, severe pain in his lower back, and pain in his chest and stomach. His blood glucose level was 300 mg/dl. His blood pressure was 190/115. His complete blood count and lipid panel were abnormal. EMG and nerve conduction studies performed in the hospital showed focal neuropathy. During the hospital stay the patient's blood glucose level was stabilized. The neuropathy started to improve but his main problem now is tarsal tunnel entrapment in his right foot. At discharge from the hospital, the patient received information about diabetes and the importance of being physically active.

In physical therapy, patient presents with a burning type of pain and paresthesia of his right foot and lower leg. He also has weakness of the bilateral lower extremities, but it is worse on the right. He has no open lesions on either foot and has intact protective sensation for both feet. His reflexes are normal and pedal pulses are palpable. He has equinus gait on the right. His blood pressure is 150/95. The patient's son stated his father took his medications in the morning.

## *Guiding Ideas for Culturally Competent Interventions*

Use the LEARN model to create a culturally competent patient education plan of care:

- **Listen:** Identify and greet family or friends of the patient. If there is a language barrier, obtain interpreter services. The interpreter should be trained and certified. Start the interview with an open-ended question. Do not interrupt the patient as he speaks.

- **Elicit:** Obtain the patient's health beliefs pertaining to the health condition and the reason for the visit, as well as his expectations.

- **Assess:** Make an assessment of potential attributes and problems relative to the patient's life that may impact his health behavior.

- **Recommend:** Make recommendations for a patient-centered plan of care including a patient teaching plan. Explain to the patient and family the rationale behind the plan.

- **Negotiate:** Negotiate an action plan with the patient and family (as necessary).

## *Examples of Culturally Appropriate Strategies*

1. Use positive facial expressions and avoid neutral and negative facial expressions (such as flat affect and frowning). Smile expressing warmth and concern.

2. Keep arms relaxed at your sides and maintain good eye contact. A female therapist may need to avoid intensive eye contact with this male patient.

3. Shake hands and speak first with the patient (because he is the older male).

4. Use an interpreter (instead of the patient's son). Begin each contact with small talk. If the interpreter is not available, focus on the patient and use the son as a translator. When using the son as a translator, do not ask any intimate questions. Ask the son to translate the exact meaning without interpretations. Look at the patient's

nonverbal behavior to indicate his understanding. Make sure the son translates after each small bit of information.

5. Do not rush or give the impression of being in a hurry.

6. Speak slowly and clearly without being condescending. Repeat important concepts and ideas. Present one idea at a time.

7. Use anatomical models, photographs, or drawings to describe and explain the pathology/pathophysiology, impairments, functional limitations, and disabilities.

8. Remember that shaking the head up and down and saying "yes" and "si" do not reflect a true positive answer or understanding of an explanation (or question).

9. Ask questions at least two times, especially to find out information related to alternative health care interventions. Also, some families are afraid to discuss private family information because of fear of immigration or funding services.

10. Ask questions for which "No" will be a positive answer, such as: "Do you have burning pain in your left foot?" The doctor reported the patient has pain in his right foot.

11. Encourage the patient to discuss his pain. Occasionally people, especially men, are reluctant to discuss pain if asked, "Do you have pain?" It is better to ask, "Where does it bother you?"

12. Encourage the patient to ask questions. Some people think that questioning medical personnel is offensive. State that medical people are happy to answer questions. This also can decrease the son's discomfort.

13. Involve the patient's son in physical therapy interventions including balance training, activities of daily living, and a home exercise program. Teach the son and family to allow the patient to do the exercises independently. Teach the son how to spot his father during ambulation and exercises. Show the patient and the son techniques to stand up from sitting by performing weight shifting.

# *Section IV References*

1. Singer PA. Medical ethics. *Brit Med J.* 2000; 321:282–285.
2. Davis CM. *Patient Practitioner Interaction: An Experiential Manual for Developing the Art of Health Care.* Thorofare, NJ: SLACK; 2006.
3. Ridley A. *Beginning Bioethics.* New York: St. Martin's Press; 1998.
4. Keller J. Care ethics as a health care ethic. *Contexts.* 1996;4(4). Available at: http://www.uhmc .sunysb.edu/prevmed/mns/imcs/contexts/care/carejean.html. Accessed May 2008.
5. Romanello M. The "ethic of care" in physical therapy practice and education: challenges and opportunities. *J Phys Ther Ed.* 2000;14(5):1–15. Available at: http://findarticles.com. Accessed May 2008.

6. Jecker NS, Jonsen AR, Pearlman RA. *Bioethics: An Introduction to the History, Methods, and Practice.* 2nd ed. Sudbury, MA: Jones and Bartlett; 2007.

7. Baker RB, Caplan AL, Emanuel LL, Latham SR, eds. *The American Medical Ethics Revolution: How the AMA's Code of Ethics Has Transformed Physicians' Relationships to Patients, Professionals and Society.* Baltimore, MD: The Johns Hopkins University Press; 1999.

8. Pellegrino ED. The metamorphosis of medical ethics: a 30-year retrospective. JAMA. 1993;269(9):1158–1162.

9. Von Englehardt D, Spinsanti S. Medical ethics, history of: Europe: contemporary period: introduction. In: Reich WT, ed. *Encyclopedia of Bioethics.* New York: Simon & Schuster; 1995:1554–1556.

10. Rothman DJ. Were Tuskegee and Willowbrook "studies in nature"? *Hastings Cent Rep.* 1982;12:5–7.

11. National Institutes of Health. Regulations and ethical guidelines. The Belmont Report: ethical principles and guidelines for the protection of human subjects of research. Available at: http://www.ohsr.od.nih.gov/guidelines/belmont.html. Accessed May 2008.

12. Beauchamp TL, Childress JF. *Principles of Biomedical Ethics.* New York: Oxford University Press; 1994.

13. Cascais F. Bioethics: from the early days to the present. *Bioethics J.* 2001;3:1–49. Available at: http://www.utopia.duth.gr. Accessed May 2008.

14. Grodin MA, ed. *Meta Medical Ethics: The Philosophical Foundations of Bioethics.* Boston, MA: Kluwer Academic Publishers; 2001.

15. Pellegrino ED. The origins and evolution of bioethics: some personal reflections. *Kennedy Inst Ethics J.* 1999;9(1):73–88.

16. Falvo DR. *Effective Patient Education: A Guide to Increased Compliance.* Sudbury, MA: Jones and Bartlett; 2004.

17. Levy N. *Neuroethics: Challenges for the 21st Century.* New York: Cambridge University Press; 2007.

18. Fins JJ, Bernat JL, Hirsch J, et al. Neuroimaging and disorders of consciousness: envisioning an ethical research agenda. *Am J Bioeth.* 2008;8(9):3–12.

19. Swisher LL. A retrospective analysis of ethics knowledge in physical therapy (1970–2000). *Phys Ther.* 2002;82(7):692–706.

20. American Physical Therapy Association. APTA Professional Ethics—Overview. Available at: http://www.apta.org. Accessed May 2008.

21. American Occupational Therapy Association. Occupational Therapy Code of Ethics; 2005. Available at: http://www.aota.org. Accessed May 2008.

22. Hope T, Savulescu J, Hendrick J. *Medical Ethics and Law: The Core Curriculum.* London, United Kingdon: Churchill Livingstone; 2003.

23. McCullough LB. Ethics in the management of health care organizations. *Phys Exece.* 1993;Nov/Dec:1–6. Available at: http://findarticles.com/p/articles/mi_m0843/is_/ai_14686674. Accessed December 2008.

24. Katsuhara Y. What moral requirements cause ethical dilemmas among nurse executives? *J Jpn Acad Nurs Sci.* 2003;23(3):1–10.

25. Greenfield B. The role of emotions in ethical decision making: implications for physical therapist education. *J Phys Ther Ed.* 2007;21(1):14–21.

26. Lo B. *Resolving Ethical Dilemmas: A Guide for Clinicians.* Baltimore, MD: Lippincott Williams & Wilkins; 2005.

27. Layon AJ, Amico RD, Caton D, et al. And the patient chose: medical ethics and the case of the Jehovah's witness. *Anesthesiology*. 1990;73:1258–1262.

28. Rest JR, Narvaez D, eds. *Moral Development in the Professions: Psychology and Applied Ethics*. Hillsdale, NJ: Lawrence Erlbaum Associates; 1994.

29. Farah MJ. Neuroethics: the practical and the philosophical. *Trends Cogn Sci*. 2005;9(1):34–40.

30. Nosse LJ, Sagiv L. Theory-based study of the basic values of 565 physical therapists. *Phys Ther*. 2005;85(9):834–850.

31. Haidt J. The moral emotions. In: Davidson RJ, Scherer KR, Goldsmith HH, eds. *The Handbook of Affective Sciences*. Oxford, United Kingdom: Oxford University Press; 2003:852–870.

32. Milliken ME, Honeycutt A. *Understanding Human Behavior: A Guide for Health Care Providers*. 7th ed. Clifton Park, NY: Delmar Cengage Learning; 2004.

33. Drench ME, Noonan AC, Sharby N, Ventura SH. *Psychosocial Aspects of Health Care*. Upper Saddle River, NJ: Pearson Education; 2007.

34. Alberti RE, Emmons ML. *Your Perfect Right: A Guide to Assertive Living*. 7th ed. San Luis Obispo, CA: 1995.

35. Dreeben O. *Introduction to Physical Therapy for PTAs*. Sudbury, MA: Jones and Bartlett; 2007.

36. Masin HL. Education in the affective domain: a method/model for teaching professional behaviors in the classroom and during advisory sessions. *J Phys Ther Ed*. 2002;16(1):1–10. Available at: http://findarticles.com. Accessed May 2008.

37. May WW, Morgan BJ, Lemke JC, et al. Model for ability-based assessment in physical therapy education. *J Phys Ther Ed*. 1995;9(1):3–6.

38. Boyle AP, Maguire S, Martin A, et al. Fieldwork is good: the student perception and the affective domain. *J Geogr Higher Ed*. 2007;31:299–317.

39. Reed KL, Sanderson SN. *Concepts of Occupational Therapy*. 4th ed. Philadelphia: Wolters Kluwer/Lippincott Williams & Wilkins; 1999.

40. Gleeson PB. Understanding generational competence related to professionalism: misunderstandings that lead to a perception of unprofessional behavior. *J Phys Ther Educ*. 2007; 21(3):23–28.

41. Spielman BJ. *Bioethics in Law*. Totowa, NJ: Human Press; 2007.

42. Redman BK. *Advances in Patient Education*. New York: Springer Publishing Company; 2004.

43. Vatz RE, Weinberg LS. Dr. Kevorkian on the air: CBS and *60 Minutes*: dropped the ball. *USA Today*. May 1,1999; Society for the Advancement of Education:1–4. Available at: http://find articles.com. Accessed May 2008.

44. WebMD. *Webster's New World Medical Dictionary: Fully Revised and Updated*. 3rd ed. Hoboken, NJ: Wiley Publishing; 2008.

45. Parker JS, Waichman HL. Nursing home problems missed in inspections, GAO says. May 2008. Available at: http://www.yourlawyer.com. Accessed May 2008.

46. Nicholson SK. *The Physical Therapist's Business Practice and Legal Guide*. Sudbury, MA: Jones and Bartlett; 2007.

47. American Physical Therapy Association. Guidelines: Physical Therapist in Occupational Health BOD. Available at: http://www.apta.org. Accessed June 2008.

48. Snyder L. *Ethics and Professionalism*. 2000. American College of Physicians: Internal Medicine/ Doctors for Adults. International Medical Graduates. Available at: http://www.acponline .org/about_acp/international/graduates/practicing_in_us/snyder.htm. Accessed March 2008.

49. Christiansen CH, Baum CM, Haugen JB, eds. *Occupational Therapy: Performance, Participation, and Well-Being*. Thorofare, NJ: SLACK; 2004.

50. Simon RI. The law and psychiatry. *Focus*. 2003;1(4):349–372

51. Bennett J, American Physical Therapy Association. Informed Consent: Tips and Caveats for PTs: Liability Awareness. Available at: http://www.apta.org. Accessed December 2008.

52. Bastable SB. *Essentials of Patient Education*. Sudbury, MA: Jones and Bartlett; 2006.

53. Leininger M. Culture care theory: a major contribution to advance transcultural nursing knowledge and practice. *J Transcultural Nurs*. 2002;13(3):189–192.

54. Leininger M, McFarland MR. *Transcultural Nursing Concepts, Theories, Research and Practice*. New York: McGraw-Hill; 2002.

55. Carillo JE, Green AR, Betancourt JR. Cross cultural primary care: a patient-based approach. *Ann Intern Med*. 1999;130:829–834.

56. Ekelman B. Developing cultural competence in occupational therapy and physical therapy education: a field immersed approach. *J Allied Health*. 2003;32(2):1–12. Available at: http://findarticles.com. Accessed June 2008.

57. American Physical Therapy Association. Cultural Competence: Major Values and Principles Integral to a Culturally Competent System of Education and Service Provision. Available at: http://www.apta.org. Accessed December 2008.

58. Padilla R. Culture and patient education: challenges and opportunities. *J Phys Ther Educ*. 1999;13:1–16. Available at: http://findarticles.com. Accessed June 2008.

59. Andrews MM, Boyle JS. *Transcultural Concepts in Nursing Care*. Philadelphia: Lippincott Williams & Wilkins; 2007.

60. Campinha-Bacote J. The process of cultural competence in the delivery of healthcare services: a model of care. *J Transcultural Nurs*. 2002;13(3):181–184.

61. Battle DE. *Communication Disorders in Multicultural Populations*. Boston, MA: Butterworth Heinemann; 2002.

62. Kim U, Triandis HC, Kagitcibasi C, Sang-Chin C, Yoon G, eds. *Individualism and Collectivism: Theory, Method, and Applications*. Thousand Oaks, CA: Sage Publishing; 1994.

63. Costa PT, Terracciano A, McCrae RR. Gender differences in personality traits across cultures: robust and surprising findings. *J Pers Soc Psych*. 2001;81(2):322–331.

64. Roberts L, Bucksey SJ. Communicating with patients: what happens in practice? *Phys Ther*. 2007;87(5):586–594.

65. Cross TL. *Towards a Culturally Competent System of Care: A Monograph on Effective Services for Minority Children Who Are Severely Emotionally Disturbed*. Vol. 1. Washington, DC: CASSP Technical Assistance Center, Georgetown University Child Development Training Center; 1989.

66. Quappe S, Cantatore G. What is Cultural Awareness, Anyway? How Do I Build It? Available at: http://www.culturosity.com/articles.htm. Accessed June 2008.

67. Srivastava RH. *The Healthcare Professional's Guide to Clinical Cultural Competence*. Toronto, Canada: Elsevier; 2007.

68. Betancourt JR, Carrillo JE, Green AR. Hypertension in multicultural and minority populations: linking communication to compliance. *Curr Hypertens Rep*. 1999;1(6):482–488.

69. Betancourt JR. Cultural competency: providing quality care to diverse populations. *Consultant Pharm*. 2006;21(12):988–995.

70. Cuéllar I, Paniagua FA. *Handbook of Multicultural Mental Health*. San Diego, CA: Academic Press; 2000.

71. Royeen M, Crabtree JL. *Culture in Rehabilitation: From Competency to Proficiency*. Upper Saddle River, NJ: Prentice-Hall; 2006.

72. Jandt FE. *An Introduction to Intercultural Communication: Identities in a Global Community.* London, England: Sage Publishing; 2007.
73. Dreeben O. *Physical Therapy Clinical Handbook for PTAs.* Sudbury, MA: Jones and Bartlett; 2008.
74. Juckett G. Cross-Cultural Medicine. *Am Fam Physician.* 2005;72:2267–2274.
75. Fong R, ed. *Culturally Competent Practice with Immigrant and Refugee Children and Families.* New York: The Guilford Press; 2004.
76. University of Arizona, Rural Health Office. Community Health Worker Evaluation Toolkit; 2002. Available at: http://www.publichealth.arizona.edu/CHWtoolkit. Accessed June 2008.
77. Ingram M, Torres E, Redondo F, et al. The impact of promotoras on social support and glycemic control among members of a farmworker community on the U.S.–Mexico border. *Diab Educ.* 2007;33(6):172–178.
78. Ashton CM, Haidet P, Paterniti DA, et al. Racial and ethnic disparities in the use of health services: bias, preferences, or poor communication? *J Gen Intern Med.* 2003;18(2):146–152.
79. Moore-Thomas C, Day-Vines NL. Culturally competent counseling for religious and spiritual African American adolescents. *Prof School Couns.* 2008;11(3):159–165.
80. Cassileth B. *The Alternative Medicine Handbook.* New York: W.W. Norton & Co.; 1998.
81. U.S. Commission on Civil Rights. Broken Promises: Evaluating the Native America Health Care System; September 2004. Available at: http://www.usccr.gov/pubs/nahealth/nabroken.pdf. Accessed September 2008.
82. Spector RE. *Cultural Diversity in Health and Illness.* 7th ed. Upper Saddle River, NJ: Pearson/Prentice-Hall; 2008.
83. U.S. Department of Health and Human Services, Indian Health Service. The Federal Health Program for American Indians and Alaska Natives: Community Health Representative. Available at: http://www.ihs.gov/NonMedicalPrograms/chr. Accessed September 2008.
84. American Physical Therapy Association. *Guide to Physical Therapist Practice.* 2nd ed. Alexandria, VA: APTA; 2001.

# Selected Topics in Patient Education: Examples in Rehabilitation

Section V of this book, "Selected Topics in Patient Education: Examples in Rehabilitation," describes specific motor learning approaches and patient instruction related to older adults' knowledge of exercises/activities and use of the Internet. Section V concludes with patient education related to wellness, health promotion, and disease prevention. Section V is divided into the following three chapters:

Chapter 17: Teaching and Learning Strategies for Motor Performances

Chapter 18: Patient Education for Older Adults Related to Exercises/Activities and Internet Utilization

Chapter 19: Teaching and Learning Considerations for Wellness, Health Promotion, and Disease Prevention

# TEACHING AND LEARNING STRATEGIES FOR MOTOR PERFORMANCES

## Objectives

After completing Chapter 17, the reader will be able to:

- Describe terminology related to motor control and motor skills.
- Explain the difference between motor learning and motor performance.
- Describe learning modes for motor performance.
- List motor learning theories.
- Identify practice and feedback variables.
- Describe the stages of motor learning and their characteristics.
- Appreciate teaching and learning strategies used in motor learning.
- Discuss the importance of practice and feedback when teaching motor skills.
- Apply Bloom's taxonomy to motor learning.

## The Significance of Motor Learning and Motor Performance

In physical and occupational therapy, movement is an intrinsic part of patient or client rehabilitation. Most rehabilitative interventions include training and retraining patients to perform particular movements. These movements are initiated and controlled by mechanisms that involve several variables, from the brain and spinal cord to the individual and the environment.

## MOTOR CONTROL AND MOTOR SKILLS

A person's ability to regulate or direct the mechanisms needed for movement to occur is called *motor control*. It means that brain structures and complex processes of cognition, perception, and environment must harmoniously work together to produce smooth movements and actions for a particular task.[1] Controlled movements needed for specific actions or activities emerge from an interaction among the individual, the task, and the environment.[1] Understanding all aspects of movement or motor control can help therapists apply teaching techniques for motor learning.

Acquiring knowledge and permanently changing a behavior is part of the learning process. In motor learning, the teaching process is associated with practice or experience. Motor learning leads to "relatively permanent changes in the capability"[1(p22)] to generate skilled actions. During motor learning, patients acquire *motor skills*. These skills can be defined as tasks individuals demonstrate when performing movements. The basic characteristics of motor skills are: (1) there must be an achievable goal; (2) the skill must be voluntarily performed; and (3) body movements must take place to achieve the goal.[2]

## MOTOR LEARNING VERSUS MOTOR PERFORMANCE

*Motor performance* and *motor learning* are two processes that complement each other and cannot be separated.[2] Motor learning is the interval process or state reflecting a person's current capability for producing a particular movement.[2] The only differentiation between motor learning and motor performance is that motor learning includes both acquiring and retaining the new skilled movement whereas motor performance includes only acquiring the skill and performing it at any given moment.[3] Motor learning has to *effect a relatively permanent change* to enhance a person's motor performance. Short-term changes are not considered motor learning.

In physical and occupational therapy, the therapist has to observe the patient's motor performance in order to determine his or her motor learning capability for producing a motor skill. During motor performance assessment, the therapist can note changes related to skill practice and/or the patient's experience. For example, during the early learning of ambulation with crutches, the patient needs to generate an idea of movement or understand the pattern of coordination. The patient must problem-solve involving cognitive activities related to stepping and use of crutches. In the beginning of learning, the patient's motor performance may be slow and inconsistent. Leg and arm movements may be stiff and inaccurate. After practice, the patient will execute more accurate and consistent movements. For the performance to become consistent, the patient must be able to modify and adapt the movements. This process of modification and adaptation is dependent on the type of skill and the environment. Finally, after sufficient practice of the skill, the patient will be able to perform the skill automatically.

Application of motor performance to function requires physical and occupational therapists and assistants to become skilled teachers and trainers. Although called "motor learning," the learning of motor tasks always involves both motor and sensory systems. Motor learning is a process that includes teaching and learning new skills or tasks to improve a person's ability to effectively use the skeletal muscles and perform functional activities. Motor learning engages the whole organism and the environment in which the organism functions, leading to a new learned behavior.[1] The process of teaching and learning typically involves the development of a social relationship between the teacher and the learner. This relationship also is based on the patient's motivation and self-esteem. Additionally, motor learning can be regarded as:

- Functional motor-sensory learning

- Learning of new motor actions

- Learning to achieve specific results

Learning a motor skill is dependent on sensory information and feedback processes. The central nervous system (especially the basal ganglia and cerebellum) is considered critical to motor learning. Motor skills and motor control also depend on the proper functioning of the skeleton, muscles, and joints. Accurate functioning of the central nervous system and musculoskeletal system allows an individual to perform a skilled motor task. This performance involves, among others, a combination of four elements: force, velocity, accuracy, and purposefulness. All these elements must function at the same time in exactly the right combination and amount. Force reflects how an individual's body acts to initiate, change, or stop motion during an activity.[4] Velocity describes displacement of a body in a certain direction.[4] The magnitude of velocity is speed (amount of distance per time).[4] Accuracy can be characterized by the smoothness and precision of movement while performing the activity. Purposefulness can be associated with emotional and behavioral involvement for learning to occur. Other elements that influence an individual's motor performance may include age, motivation, assistance, fatigue, anxiety, boredom, the amount of learning and practice, and pharmacologic agents.[5] In addition, most motor skills are learned throughout the lifespan and can be affected by disabilities. During motor performance an individual also requires action and coordination of limbs and the development of strength, posture control, balance, and perceptual skills (visual, auditory, and tactile or kinesthetic).

Motor learning can be measured using four variables: motor performance, retention, transfer, and generalizability.[6] Motor performance, previously discussed, is the most frequent measure of learning, and assesses temporary acquisition of a skill. Motor performance is a complex variable to evaluate because it involves other variables related to the learner's motivation, anxiety, or fatigue. Because of its relationship with other variables, motor performance is not "solely a measure of absolute learning."[1] Consequently, the individual's motor learning may be better estimated by the amount of material that was retained or was transferred from one environment to another. Retention is considered a better measure of motor learning because it can assess acquisition and preservation of the motor skill.[1] During practice, the evaluation of motor performance in the same environment in which training occurred is called a *retention test*. The evaluation of motor performance in a different environment than where practice occurred is called a *transfer test*. As an example of retention, a patient with a stroke was able to learn to walk with a walker on tiles while he was hospitalized for 4 days. After discharge from the hospital, the patient spent his time at home sitting in a wheelchair. One month later, when the patient was approved for physical therapy at home, he was not able to use the walker anymore. The patient had to learn the skill again. This happened because the patient did not practice enough to *retain* the learning. At the same time, the patient was not able to *transfer* the motor task that he learned on the hospital's tiled floor to his carpeted-floor home environment. This transfer of learning is called *generalizability*. It is used to examine the application of a learned skill to other similar tasks without practice.[6] In this situation, to generalize what he has learned, the patient would need to practice walking inside his home on the carpet and apply (without practice) the skill of ambulation with the walker to outside his home on the grass. The patient would transfer the learned information from one environment to another.

# *Learning Methods for Motor Performance*

Motor learning involves simple and complex methods of learning. These methods include classical and operant conditioning, associative and nonassociative learning, and implicit (procedural) and declarative (explicit) learning (**Table 17.1**).[1]

   *Classical conditioning* (mentioned in Chapter 9) is a form of *associative learning*. The individual learns that certain things go together. Pavlov's experiments demonstrated this form of learning by creating an unrelated stimulus (the bell) and "conditioning" the dogs to salivate when they anticipated food. Classical conditioning is a form of respondent conditioning. The first step in changing a behavior requires an involuntary or reflexive behavior. Associating a conditioning stimulus to a person can produce a conditioned behavioral response. An example of classical conditioning applied to motor learning would be when a therapist repeatedly gives a patient a verbal cue and physical assistance to perform a movement. After practice, the patient would perform the movement with only a verbal cue, and finally would be "conditioned" to perform the movement independently. For a patient who had a stroke, an example of conditioned motor performance could be the association of the motor task of walking with the therapist coming into the room and holding a walker. As a result, the patient knows that when the therapist shows up in their room holding a walker it is time to perform gait training. Also during the motor task, if the patient has difficulty with balance, the therapist can associate a sentence such as "Watch your step" with the patient's impairments. After repeated practice and associating the sentence with instability in movement, the patient will learn that their stability is affected[1] and they cannot put too much weight on the involved leg. This form of associative learning also has proven successful with individuals who have sensory and motor as well as developmental disabilities; for example, children with autism who have cognitive difficulties understanding new words are able to associate a novel word with a picture.[7]

| Table 17.1 | Summary of Learning Methods for Motor Performance[1] |
|---|---|
| Classical conditioning | Learning to associate two kinds of stimuli. |
| Operant conditioning | A form of trial and error learning. |
| Nonassociative learning | Can cause habituation and sensitization. |
| Procedural learning | Learning to perform tasks automatically (can be reflexive, automatic, and habitual). |
| Declarative learning | Learning that results in knowledge that can be consciously recalled (requires attention, awareness, and reflection; includes four processes called encoding, consolidation, storage, and retrieval). |

*Operant conditioning* is characterized as an associative and trial-and-error type of learning.[1] Operant conditioning requires a voluntary behavior (whereas classical conditioning involves innate reflexes). In operant conditioning, a behavior produces events. The events can be rewarding experiences or negative experiences. The behavior changes as a result of such events. If the consequences of a behavior are pleasant, the preceding behavior becomes more frequent; if the consequences are unpleasant, the behavior will diminish and in some cases will become extinct.[1] An intermittent reward is necessary to reinforce learning, whereas discontinuing the use of reinforcement tends to extinguish the learned behavior.

Accordingly, behaviors that are rewarded are typically repeated. Behaviors that receive aversive stimuli are usually not repeated.[1] Operant conditioning can be used in physical and occupational therapy for behavioral reinforcement of a motor skill. For correct motor performances to be repeated, the therapist can praise the patient or client for his or her motor actions.

*Nonassociative learning* is one of the most basic forms of learning. It is also called single event learning because it requires a single stimulus (repeated frequently) for the learning to take place.[1] Nonassociative learning involves learning that some events are unrelated and irrelevant. There are two simple forms of nonassociative learning, habituation and sensitization.[1] Habituation causes a decrease in response due to a harmful or noxious stimulus. In physical therapy, habituation training can be used as an intervention for certain cases of dizziness and balance impairments caused by benign paroxysmal positional vertigo (BPPV).[1] During habituation training, patients or clients are asked to repeatedly move in ways that provoke their symptoms. Repetition of the movements results in "habituation of the dizziness response."[1(p24)] Sensitization is a form of training totally opposite to habituation. It causes an increased response due to a harmful or a noxious stimulus.[1] In physical therapy, sensitization may be used to increase a patient's sensitivity to a threatening stimulus in order to enhance their awareness of the stimulus.[1] This form of training may be necessary to reduce the possibility of accidental falls in older individuals.[1]

*Procedural or implicit learning* means learning tasks that can be performed automatically (without conscious thinking).[1] Procedural learning is characterized as a passive process, where people are exposed to information and acquire knowledge of that information simply through that exposure.[1] Examples of motor activities that can be accomplished through procedural learning are riding a bike, swimming, touch typing, or playing a musical instrument. Generally, individuals can learn to do these activities but cannot explain how they do it. Procedural or implicit learning can be acquired gradually through repetition of motor tasks.[1] This form of learning does not require awareness, attention, and higher order cognitive processes.[1] Most of the learning of motor tasks related to movement and force production uses procedural learning.[1] Procedural learning of motor tasks can last longer than declarative (explicit) learning (discussed next), to the point where the individual loses the ability to explain how to perform the task. Procedural learning is dependent on the therapist's structuring the environment and providing consistent cues and necessary task practice.[8]

In physical and occupational therapy, procedural learning can be used to teach patients motor skills such as transfers,[1] bed mobility activities, gait training, and balance and coordination skills. For example, when teaching transfers, to help the patient form certain rules associated with the task, the therapist needs to continuously change and structure the environment. The transfers should take place from different surfaces and elevations and in various situations and contexts. Consequently, effective procedural learning needs environmental structure, continuous practice, frequent repetitions, and constant and reliable feedback.

*Declarative or explicit learning* is characterized as an active process where people seek out the structure of any information that is presented to them. Declarative learning requires attention, awareness, and reflection.[1] Declarative or explicit learning is considered an analytical, language-based, and memory-dependent approach to acquiring and retaining knowledge. Declarative learning includes four different types of information processing developments (described in Chapter 9) called encoding, consolidation, storage, and retrieval. Encoding requires attention and the association of new information with knowledge already stored in long-term memory.[1] Consolidation and storage are two processes that secure and hold the new data in long-term memory. The retrieval process facilitates data recall by accessing stored memories.

As mentioned in Chapter 9, information processing involves four major learning phases: attention, processing, memory storage, and action. During encoding, the therapist has to acquire the patient's attention and orient him or her toward the motor skill. When there is extensive damage to the patient's perceptual system, it may be very difficult for declarative learning to take place.[1] During consolidation, learning occurs through information processing. It means the patient's senses must process the data.[1] The therapist may need to consider the patient's sensory and motor impairments that interfere with learning and use the patient's uninvolved functions; for example, if the patient has visual impairments, he or she may need verbal and kinesthetic instruction to consolidate the material in the long-term memory. During storage, the information is stored in short-term memory (for less than 30 seconds).[1] To add new data to long-term memory requires practice and reinforcement. During retrieval, the patient has to act to be able to recall the learned material. Using feedback mechanisms, the memory recall process also addresses the necessary corrections for accuracy and safety.[1]

Typically, data recalling (retrieving) from long-term memory requires four action steps called recall, recollection, recognition, and relearning.[9] During the retrieval process, the learner must use a retrieval cue or a prompt to trigger the action. In the recall step, the retrieval involves only accessing the information without being cued with any part of the memory.[9] A classroom example could be answering a question on a fill-in-the-blank test. Recollection involves a more complex process of reconstructing memory. The learner can use partial memories, narratives, or prompts.[9] A classroom example could be answering a question on an essay exam that involves remembering small pieces of information and restructuring the remaining data based on partial memories. Recognition is a type of memory that requires identifying the information when seeing that information again in a new context.[9] A classroom example could be recognizing the correct answer from a group of available answers in a multiple choice exam. Relearning is a form of memory that involves relearning information that has been learned in the past.[9] The process of relearning can improve the strength of memories. Consequently, in rehabilitation, connecting new motor tasks with the patient's already known activities engages the relearning process. This can enhance information retrieval and improve the patient's learning.

Declarative learning, as with procedural learning, can be used in physical and occupational therapy when teaching patients and clients motor skills. Typically, declarative learning can change after practice into procedural learning. As an example, when learning activities of daily living, patients need to remember factual information regarding functional activities such as washing, dressing, or eating. A therapist can teach a patient who had an amputation of his dominant hand and forearm to put his shirt on using a one-handed dressing technique. The teaching process will consist of the patient acquiring knowledge of the technique one step at a time. In the beginning, using declarative learning, the patient will verbally describe each step as he is performing the skill. After several practice sessions, the patient will be able to automatically dress himself without paying attention to the practiced steps or being supervised by the therapist. This means declarative learning has changed into procedural learning through constant and recurring practice of the skill. Declarative learning can also take place when individuals mentally rehearse the necessary steps for an activity.[1] An example could be a figure skater rehearsing in her mind the skating sequence prior to her performance.[1]

In physical and occupational therapy, declarative and procedural learning can be applied to developmentally disabled patients' motor learning. However, the therapist must consider the anatomical location of the lesion in the central nervous system. For example, research shows that declarative or explicit learning is appropriate mostly for patients who have an intact medial temporal lobe and diencephalic structure, especially the hippocampus.[10] Procedural or implicit learning generally requires intact basal ganglia.[10] For example, patients with Alzheimer's disease with intact basal ganglia are able to learn motor tasks using procedural learning.[10]

Although procedural learning is thought to require an intact basal ganglia, it can work with patients who are in the early stages of Parkinson's disease (PD).[11,12] The reason may be that procedural learning involves complex brain mechanisms that are not associated with only one structure (basal ganglia) but with many other neuroanatomical components.[11,12] Procedural learning is "an aggregate of heterogeneous skill learning processes,"[11(p.2887)] allowing patients with PD to learn a motor sequence in the same amount of time as a control group. One study found the serial reaction time task (SRTT) is the same in patients with PD (in the early stages and nonmedicated) as in the control group.[11] Additionally, neuropsychological testing of patients with PD showed no impairments in their cognitive measures.[11] The only impairments were related to attention and executive functions, visuospatial skills, and immediate and delayed explicit memory (associated with declarative learning).[11]

In healthy subjects, a manual procedural skill can be learned in four specific steps: (1) demonstration, (2) deconstruction, (3) formulation, and (4) performance.[13] During demonstration the therapist can show the task to the patient by performing it at the normal speed. In the deconstruction stage, the therapist still continues to demonstrate the task to the patient but at a slower pace while verbally breaking it down into simple steps or components.[13] In the third stage of manual procedural skill learning (formulation) the therapist performs the task at the same slower pace while it is being "talked through"[13(p.1358)] for each step by the patient. Finally, in the performance phase, the patient performs the task slowly while talking him- or herself through it. This form of procedural skill learning can help therapists develop objective methods to measure and document their teaching skills with patients. For example, if the patient needs more cognitive knowledge prior to skill performance, the therapist would be able to recognize this without the patient having to go through trial and error. This can be important for the patient's safety as well as motivation when learning novel motor skills that cannot be related to the patient's prior experiences. Also, trial and error may be best suited for later motor training.

## Theories of Motor Learning

Motor learning theorists have long been researching the best methods for integrating educational techniques to acquire the necessary knowledge to produce skilled actions. These theorists' contributions to physical and occupational rehabilitation are important for the application of training and retraining strategies in clinical practices. Principles of motor learning used mostly in rehabilitation are attributed to the following motor learning theorists: Fitts and Posner (1967), Adams (1971), Gentile (1972), Schmidt (1975), and Newell

(1991). Fitts and Posner's Three-Stage Model proposed a classical theory of motor learning that includes three sequential stages of learning: cognitive, associative, and autonomous.[1] Adams's Two-Stage Model combines Fitts and Posner's cognitive and associative stages to achieve the autonomous stage. Adams's theory, also called closed loop, emphasizes the role of sensory feedback for learning.[1] Gentile's Two-Stage Model is based on the premise that tasks are dependent on goals, environment, and the individual's neuromotor processes.[14] Schmidt's theory states that individuals do not learn specific movements[1] but construct a generalized motor program for themselves called a schema. Newell's theory emphasizes the relationship among the individual, the task, and the environment.[1]

## FITTS AND POSNER'S STAGES OF MOTOR LEARNING

The Three-Stage Model created by Fitts and Posner is considered to be the classical representation of motor learning.[5] These two theorists suggested that the learning process is sequential and that individuals move through specific phases when they learn. The model describes three stages involved in skill learning: cognitive, associative, and autonomous (**Table 17.2**).[5]

Fitts and Posner indicated that the learning process is sequential, moving from one stage to another.[5] In the cognitive stage, learners try to form an overall concept (such as a mental concept) of a motor skill.[5] Learners gather the information through observation, through verbal feedback from others, and kinesthetically through the muscle spindles. In this stage, the learner attempts to define his or her goal and the general methods for achievement. In regard to practicing the skill, this stage represents trial and error.[5] When performing the motor skill, the learner knows that his or her movement is not sufficiently accurate and needs help to correct it.

In physical and occupational therapy, the cognitive stage of motor learning requires the learner to develop a general understanding of the task. This stage represents the beginner level of ability when the patient is first introduced to basic concepts and ideas. The patient as the learner must learn "what to do" in order to be able to perform the task correctly and in a safe manner.[6] The learner has to think continuously about the task and the sequence of movements. Also, the learner has to practice the task many times. In the cognitive stage,

| Table 17.2 | **Fitts and Posner's Stages of Motor Learning[5]** |
|---|---|
| | 1. Cognitive stage: Developing a general understanding of the motor task. |
| | 2. Associative stage: Practicing and perfecting the motor task. |
| | 3. Autonomous stage: Performing highly organized and coordinated patterns of the motor task. |

errors are normal and corrections of mistakes can improve the learner's performance. The learner bases his or her knowledge on visual practice and feedback from the therapist. The environment must be controlled for noise or any distractions or interruptions that may disturb the learner's concentration. Toward the end of the cognitive stage, the learner is able to self-correct his or her errors and find a reasonable motor strategy sequence.

Fitts and Posner's second stage is called the associative stage. In this stage, the performance becomes more consistent. The learner understands how parts of the movement relate to each other and links the component parts of the motor skill into a smooth action. The learner practices the skill and uses feedback to perfect the skill.[5] In the associative stage, errors are fewer because the learner can recognize and correct inaccuracies in the performance. In physical and occupational therapy, the associative stage of motor learning is characterized by modifications and refinement of learning. This stage represents the intermediate level of ability. The patient as the learner must learn "how to do" the task in order to perform it correctly and safely with the least amount of errors and inappropriate movements.[6] In the associative stage, the patient bases learning achievement on continuous practice and kinesthetic (proprioceptive) cues. The patient is less dependent on visual learning.[6] The patient explores various self-modifications of the task based on environment and innovative motor strategies. The learning process includes decreased therapist feedback. Learning a task in the associative stage is dependent on the type of motor task and the learner's prior learning experience and intrinsic motivation.

The third and last stage is the autonomous stage. This stage is characterized by the learner's ability to focus attention on other details of the environment and make immediate corrections.[6] In the autonomous stage, the skill becomes automatic. Not all individuals reach this stage. In physical and occupational therapy, this final stage is characterized by motor performances that are automatic. The autonomous stage represents the advanced level of skill. During this stage, the patient as the learner must learn "how to succeed" at something competitive (such as sports). Typically, in physical and occupational therapy, patients are discharged prior to this stage, except for athletes. The learner does not require continuous attention to movement (as in the cognitive stage) and is able to perform different tasks simultaneously. The learner's cognitive self-monitoring is substantially decreased. The learner is able to execute motor tasks in highly organized and coordinated patterns without any interference from the environment. During this autonomous stage of motor learning, the learner is able to perform high-level motor tasks in conventional or changeable environments.

## ADAMS'S TWO-STAGE MODEL

In 1971 Adams created a comprehensive theory of motor learning also called the closed-loop theory. It is based on verbal and motor stages. To increase the learning process, Adams's theory emphasizes the role of sensory feedback and "specificity of practice and learning."[5(p.419)] Specificity of practice means that previously practiced skills are performed better than new skills. Also, actions must be performed slowly to be guided by sensory signals. The biggest criticism of Adams's theory is that it is not always necessary for individuals to learn movements based on sensory feedback.[1] Also, some individuals can accurately perform new tasks without any prior practice. Animals and humans are able to accurately perform movements even if they do not have sensory feedback.[1]

In physical and occupational therapy, Adams's model is important when teaching patients to perform slow actions.[5] These slow movements need constant regulation for accuracy. An application could be neurological interventions using neurodevelopmental treatment (NDT) to recover function of patients with hemiplegia.[5] Because the movements are slow, patients have time to receive feedback and make the necessary corrections. The feedback can come from vision, hearing, or proprioception.[5] The advantage is correctness because the movements can be controlled as they are happening. The disadvantage is that feedback takes time and fast movements are not possible.[5]

Biofeedback is another form of intervention in physical and occupational therapy that applies the closed-loop principle to effect changes in motor performance due to sensory feedback. As an example, motor imagery as a form of biofeedback interventional technique can complement physical therapy treatments for patients with neurologic conditions.[15] Learners can use mental practice (mental rehearsal) as a form of cognitive practice. It means that mentally, learners rehearse the necessary steps of the motor skills. The mental practice of motor imagery by using voluntary mental rehearsal of motor tasks is strongly correlated with patients' executed movements.[15] This form of biofeedback can improve motor performance and assist patients to learn motor skills.[15]

## GENTILE'S TWO-STAGE MODEL

Gentile's Two-Stage Model includes two stages called "getting the idea" and "fixation/diversification."[14] For each stage, this model takes into consideration the goals of the learner.[14] The goal of the first stage is to develop an understanding of the overall movement pattern. The characteristics of the first stage are problem-solving and trial and error.[14] In the getting the idea stage, the following variables are emphasized:[1]

- The goal of the task

- The development of basic movement to accomplish the goal

- The environmental elements contributing to the movement

The learner must distinguish between significant and insignificant environmental conditions. These conditions can have a stable or a moving environment. The stable environment does not change and is considered closed and predictable. In a closed and predictable environment, the patient can practice closed (stable) skills. An example of a closed skill in physical therapy is practicing a three-point gait walking pattern on an even surface such as a tiled floor. Opposite to a closed environment, a moving environment changes and is considered open and unpredictable. In an open and unpredictable environment, the patient can practice open (dynamic) skills. An example of an open skill is practicing a three-point gait walking pattern on an uneven surface such as on carpet or outside on grass.

Additionally, in the first stage of Gentile's model, the individual's motor performance may be inconsistent. The person may need to concentrate on movement flaws that cause the most errors.

In the second stage of Gentile's model called fixation/diversification, the learner acquires a set movement pattern that can become habitual. This pattern must be refined.[14] However, refinement of movement is dependent on the type of skill, open versus closed.[1] Because closed skills do not offer environmental challenges, the learner needs to concentrate on skill performance. It means that for closed skills the learner must develop the ability to perform the skill efficiently and consistently. The emphasis is on success and consistency.[14] Open skills offer environmental challenges allowing the learner to adapt his or her skill to the environmental demands. Practice situations must be established.[14] The situations should vary, allowing the learner to adapt to new conditions and unique situations. Using prior experience is prohibited in this stage.

As a general rule, Gentile's second stage calls for refinement and diversification of movement. During the fixation part of the second stage, the learner performs repetitions of the same action to achieve efficiency and consistency of his or her closed motor skills[14] (in a stable and unchangeable environment). Because the environment is stable, at the end of this practice, the movement pattern is efficient and consistent but has no variability. It means that the learner who practiced three-point gait at the parallel bars achieves *movement efficiency and consistency*. During the diversification part, the individual practices in an open, moving environment to achieve variability of motor actions. It means that the learner who practices the three-point gait at the parallel bars, on carpet, on tiles, and outside on the grass achieves *movement diversification*.

## Schmidt's Schema Theory

Schmidt's schema or open-loop theory of motor learning emphasizes that an individual learns "schema and motor programs during practice."[5(p.420)] The schema is an abstract representation stored in an individual's memory.[1] There are two types of schema, recall and recognition schema. In Schmidt's theory, a schema is constructed in the individual's short-term memory. A schema consists of a generalized motor program containing four pieces of information: (1) the initial movement (the starting point of the movement), (2) the parameters necessary for the movement (certain aspects of the motor action such as duration, repetitions, or level of force), (3) the outcome of the movement (results of the action such as success or failure), and (4) the sensory consequences of the movement (how the movement felt).[1,5,6]

A schema allows an individual to connect parameters from movements to outcomes.[5] People have the movement in their short-term memory; for example, when throwing a ball, the individual knows various distances or various directions. In Schmidt's open-loop theory, the learner does not receive feedback during the movement.[5] The motor actions are preplanned in memory and controlled by the generalized motor program and its four pieces of information. Because the motor program is made up of a predefined set of information or commands, once sent out, movement is completed without feedback.[5] As a result, the movement is fast because the feedback time is eliminated.

In physical and occupational therapy, Schmidt's theory can be applied mostly to orthopedic rehabilitation of athletes using ballistic and repetitive movements for sports. After surgeries, athletes need retraining to regain speed and their athletic capabilities. For the older patient population, the therapist can use the theory to train patients or clients to practice several versions of a motor task including new and well-known actions.[5] Also, patients can be allowed to make errors in order to differentiate between correct and incorrect feedback and motor actions. Errors can enhance the learning process. The limitation of this theory is its lack of specificity regarding modes of creating the schema.[1]

## NEWELL'S THEORY

Newell's theory is also called ecological theory. Newell's motor learning is based on the relationship between the sensory and motor processes. The theory proposes that motor learning is a process that increases the coordination between perception and movement.[1] It means that during motor practice an individual searches for the best strategies to solve the motor task considering the task constraints. This search looks not only at motor responses, but also at perceptual (sensory) cues. The individual needs to integrate perceptual and motor cues to produce the action. Perceptual cues relate to understanding the goal of the motor task and the movements that need to be learned.[1] Feedback is important in this theory, especially when related to outcomes. This is a dynamic and exploratory approach to motor learning.

In physical and occupational therapy, Newell's theory may be applicable to children and younger adults. Older adults with various impairments related to the perceptual system may not be able to effectively and safely use this theory.[1] A patient would need to recognize sensory cues to be able to perform the task; for example, when the patient ambulates outside on the grass, the patient must be able to relate the perceptual cues from the grass and modify his or her gait pattern and speed of movement. However, because of impairments, the patient may not able to receive and recognize sensory cues (that the grass is slippery). As a result, the patient may be in danger of falling.

# *Variables of Motor Learning*

In regard to motor learning, patients should be direct and active participants not only in the teaching and learning process, but also in preparing their learning goals. In current patient-centered care, physical and occupational therapists are inclined to focus on goals set by their patients or clients, especially those related to functional limitations and disabilities.[16] Goals should be objective, measurable, motivating, and also challenging to the patient.[5]

From a motor learning perspective, patients and clients are learners who analyze tasks and are able to develop effective personally suited motor strategies for performing the tasks under varying environmental conditions.[16] Functional tasks are critical in motor learning. These functional skills can include the environments in which patients want to engage at the completion of rehabilitation. As a result, the patient must be able to practice different versions of the task or adapt the task to different environments. This is a significant part of *motor practice*.

## MOTOR PRACTICE VARIABLES

The amount of practice is important when teaching and learning motor tasks. Increasing the amount of practice may increase the amount of learned material.[5] Typically, during motor skill practice the learner's performance improves faster in the early part of a new task.[1] After a large amount of practice, the performance improvement increases at a slower rate. In time, the learner's performance is still improving but the "increments may be small."[1(p.35)] The amount of practice may be directly related to the type of task and its difficulty, the learner's skill level, the feedback, the effects of various practice conditions,[17] and the order in which the motor task is practiced. For example, random practice seems to have a larger influence on the learner's retention of the task than blocked practice.[17] The reason may be that random order practice requires more cognitive processing during the acquisition of the task than blocked or repetitive order practice.[17,18] In addition to random and blocked practice, other types of motor practice include massed and distributed, parts versus whole task, open and closed environments, physical and cognitive (mental), and guidance versus discovery practice (**Table 17.3**).

During motor learning, the learner can complete blocked practice by repeatedly and uninterruptedly practicing just one task. In contrast, a learner can complete random practice by practicing a variety of tasks scheduled randomly across trials. Blocked practice can increase the learner's initial performance and is suited better for patients who need a high degree of structure and consistency for learning to occur.[5] In the beginning of learning a motor task, the learner can acquire the information more easily during blocked practice. Learning different tasks in random order is more difficult in the beginning; however, the learner's performance will be enhanced through random practice. Random practice is better for skill retention because it can increase the learner's depth of cognitive processing to retrieve the information from his or her long-term memory.[6] As a result, the motor skill can be applied to other tasks and environments.

During motor learning, when high interference practice conditions are used in random order, a learning occurrence called *contextual interference* takes place. It means that during random practice the learner can better remember the movement patterns as a result of: (1) more distinctive and elaborate processing comparing multiple tasks stored in short-term memory; and (2) forgetting the processing from prior trials, requiring the learner to reconstruct an action plan for the task.[19] The reconstruction processing results in a more detailed and permanent memory representation of the task that increases retention and transfer of learning. Contextual interference has been extensively studied but its application is still controversial. The effect of contextual interference is stronger in research but weaker in its application.[20] Consideration should be given to the task and the learner; for example,

Table
17.3

## *Types of Motor Learning Practice*[1,5,6,14]

| | |
|---|---|
| Blocked practice | Continuously and uninterruptedly practicing just one task. |
| Random practice | Randomly practicing a variety of tasks across trials. |
| Massed practice | Time for the performance session is longer than for the resting session. |
| Distributed practice | Time for the performance session is the same as or less than for the resting session. |
| Practicing parts of a task | Practicing separately each part of a complex task. |
| Practicing the whole task | Practicing the entire task (at once). |
| Practice in closed environments | Practicing in a closed and structured environment. |
| Practice in open environments | Practicing in an open and challenging environment (similar to the real world). |
| Physical practice | Performing the task. |
| Mental practice | Cognitively rehearsing a motor task ("how to perform" the task). |
| Guidance practice | Also called guidance learning; practicing the motor task by physically guiding the learner through the task. |
| Discovery practice | Also called discovery learning; practicing the motor task by providing the learner with a challenging and achievable problem and encouraging them to discover and practice their solution(s). |

complex tasks may be difficult to acquire, especially for young children, possibly because they have not yet acquired problem-solving proficiency, which takes place during the motor skills stage of development. Children between 7 and 10 years old seem to have difficulties performing complex tasks in random practice.[21] Motor performance in random practice seems to be the same as for blocked practice, however.[21]

Massed practice refers to practice sessions in which the amount of practice time is greater than the amount of rest time between repetitions.[1] Massed practice seems to be less effective for skill acquisition than distributed practice. The reason may be the learner's fatigue. For continuous tasks, massed practice also may decrease the task performance.[1] When using massed practice, especially with older adults, the therapist should consider the learner's fatigue and the risk of injury. Massed practice can be unsafe[1] in cases of overfatigue; however, for individuals with chronic incomplete tetraplegia, massed practice augmented by somatosensory stimulation seems to be beneficial for task-oriented skills to improve hand and upper-extremity function.[18] Massed practice can also be suited for learners who are highly motivated and demonstrate skillful performance using good concentration and endurance.[18]

Opposite to massed practice, distributed practice requires small units of practice alternated with longer rest periods. The practice time is less than the rest time. In regard to the patient's learning process, distributed practice is more efficient,[6] especially for patients who have decreased performance capability and endurance. Also, adequate or longer rest periods are important for the patient's safety due to fatigue as well as enhancement of motivation and self-worth.[5]

During motor learning, complicated motor tasks can be broken down into parts in order to be practiced. The learner can practice each part separately before trying the whole task. Separating the performance into parts contributes to cognitively learning the necessary steps prior to executing the entire act.[6] To develop the skill completely the learner also needs to complete the whole skill after he or she has accomplished parts of the skill. Practicing parts and then the whole task is suggested for serial motor tasks that include independent movements.[5] Analyzing the task by breaking it into several components can be beneficial when training a patient in functional activities;[1] however, this type of practice is not recommended for continuous and highly integrated motor skills.[5]

Practicing in an open or closed environment are two kinds of practice related to either predictable or changeable surroundings.[5] As previously mentioned, practicing in an open, constantly changing environment requires the learner to continuously plan his or her response. The learner's success is determined by the extent to which he or she is able to adapt the skill to the changing surroundings. A closed and stable environment offers a predictable form of practice. The learner may make changes he or she already learned as a result of practice. The learner can also anticipate the behavior of the environment. In physical and occupational therapy, in the early learning stages, a closed environment is more beneficial for the learner to concentrate and be successful in their performance.[6] Later, altering the setting can mimic the real world and challenge the patient's performance. However, consideration should be given to patients with traumatic brain injury and other limitations who cannot adjust in an open, unstructured environment.

Physical and mental practices represent additional forms of motor practice. Physical practice is the learner's actual motor performance. Mental practice means having the learner cognitively rehearse the skill prior to the action. Practicing the skill mentally "can produce large positive effects on the performance of the task."[1(p.39)] Mental rehearsal (also called mental imagery and mental visualization) resembles perceptual experience except that it occurs in the absence of the appropriate stimuli for the relevant perception.[22] When comparing mental with physical practice to restore motor function of patients with hemiplegia, it seems they are equivalent.[22] Furthermore, when the task is difficult, concurrent use of mental imagery with physical practice can be beneficial for motor learning, restoring function for patients with hemiplegia.[22] Although mental practice enhances learning, physical practice still remains the best mode for motor skill practice.[1]

The last two forms of practice and learning are guidance and discovery learning. During guidance learning in physical and occupational therapy, the therapist physically guides the patient through the motor task. During discovery learning the therapist provides the patient with a challenging and achievable problem, encouraging them to discover and practice their solution(s).[5] When a patient starts to acquire a skill, guidance learning seems to be more effective than discovery learning. Consequently, it is suggested that discovery learning be used at the "outset of teaching a task."[1(p.39)] Discovery learning is a form of active learning in which the individual has to learn a new skill by actively choosing the specific components of the task on which to train.[23] However, it seems that although active learning is the best form of learning, the learner's choices in the beginning of the action are strongly influenced by motor errors.[23] If the action produces a large error, the learner repeats the wrong action. This means that, especially in rehabilitation, therapists should help and guide their patients to choose an optimal training sequence of a motor skill.

## FEEDBACK VARIABLES

When learning a motor skill, feedback is considered the second most important element after the necessary amount of practice to learn the skill.[5] Typically, the amount of practice and the amount of information learned "are directly related."[5(p.403)] The feedback presented before, during, or after performance of a skill gives the learner the needed data regarding the correctness and effectiveness of his or her action. There are numerous types of motor learning feedback (**Table 17.4**).

Feedback can be intrinsic, occurring naturally from the learner, or augmented, being provided by the therapist as the teacher. Examples of intrinsic feedback could be proprioceptive, vestibular, cutaneous, or visual signals that arise from the execution of a motor task.[6] The patient as the learner can recognize these signals when attempting to perform a task, while doing the task, and at the completion of the task. Intrinsic feedback gives the learner knowledge of performance (KP) and knowledge of results (KR).[6]

Augmented feedback provided by the therapist is typically supplemental to the learner's intrinsic feedback.[5] Augmented feedback can arise from a mechanical device (such as electromyography biofeedback) when the therapist controls the type, the timing, and the frequency of feedback. Additionally, augmented feedback could also be presented to the patient

| Table 17.4 | Types of Motor Learning Feedback[1,5,6] | |
|---|---|---|
| Intrinsic | Arising naturally from the learner's performance of the task; recognized by the learner. | |
| Augmented | Arising from mechanical (such as electromyography) feedback and external sources that are supplemental to intrinsic feedback; recognized by the teacher. | |
| Knowledge of performance (KP) | Related to the nature or quality of the performance of a motor task. | |
| Knowledge of results (KR) | Related to the end outcome of the motor performance. | |
| Immediate feedback | Occurs immediately after execution of a task. | |
| Delayed feedback | Occurs after an interval of time when the task was performed. | |
| Summed feedback | Occurs after several repetitions of a task; describes average performance. | |
| Intermittent feedback | Occurs irregularly and at random. | |
| Continuous feedback | Occurs regularly on a continuous basis. | |

verbally, visually (asking the patient to look in a mirror while performing the skill), or using tactile cues.[6] The same as intrinsic feedback, augmented feedback includes knowledge of results (KR) and knowledge of performance (KP).

KR relates to the end result or overall outcome of the movement whereas KP is relevant to the nature or quality of the movement pattern.[6] The significance of KR and KP for the patient is dependent on the variability of the task and the available intrinsic feedback. The timing of augmented feedback is also related to the teaching and learning process. In the initial stage of learning, the patient may need immediate feedback after a task is completed to allow for modifications in performance and increase the patient's skills.[5] Delayed feedback offers information to the learner at a later time, allowing the learner to reflect on his or her performance. Delayed feedback may be more beneficial than immediate feedback because it can give the learner enough time for introspection and self-assessment. Summary feedback (or summed feedback) is typically applied after several repetitions of the skill and reflects the average presentation of the skill.[5] Feedback also can be intermittent (occurring randomly) or continuous on an ongoing basis. Intermittent feedback was shown to promote effectiveness of learning whereas continuous feedback increased the time it took the learner to acquire the desired skill.[6]

Summary feedback of knowledge of results (summary KR) is considered to be the best type of feedback.[1] It is typically given after a certain amount of trials that are dependent on the type of task performance. It seems that the most effective summary KR is after five performance trials.[1]

Precise quantitative (units of measure) feedback is important to adults but may be confusing in children.[1] Also, reduced frequency of feedback in adults can increase the adults' information processing capability for permanent successful learning effects.[24] Feedback offered frequently to adults can be beneficial during practice but can interfere with problem-solving abilities.[24] In regard to retention of information, when comparing children and adults, adult learners perform better with reduced feedback whereas children show less accuracy and consistency in their skills.[24] Because children have a different information processing capability, they require more practice trials with more frequent feedback than adults.[24] For effective motor learning, children with developmental disabilities (caused by brain damage such as in cerebral palsy) may need extended practice and a gradual reduction of feedback.[1]

## Application of Motor Learning to Physical and Occupational Therapy

The motor learning theory used most often in physical and occupational therapy is Fitts and Posner's model. As previously mentioned, this model includes three phases: cognitive, associative, and autonomous.[1]

### FEEDBACK MECHANISMS APPLIED TO FITTS AND POSNER'S MODEL

In the cognitive ("what to do") stage, the patient as the learner should be able to understand the task and also attempt to perform the task.[1] The therapist's role is to explain clearly to the patient the function and importance of the task, to demonstrate the task, and to establish the most important elements of the task that need to be assessed during its performance. The assessment of task elements can help with feedback. Additionally, relating the task to the patient's prior learning of a different movement skill is important to find similarities and differences between the two skills. During the cognitive learning, the patient must use visual perception to identify, organize, and interpret sensory data received through the eyes.[5] Consequently, the therapist must have the patient watch when the therapist performs the task.

The therapist can use two types of feedback, knowledge of performance (KP) and knowledge of results (KR). KP feedback gives the patient specific information on how a movement is performed or a correction for the specific movement (such as "Your right leg must be one step forward"). KR feedback specifies how well the overall task attempt was performed (such as "Yes, you did it!"). Correct task performance requires reinforcement using praise. The therapist can use behaviorist teaching and learning principles to give prompt reinforcement with enthusiastic praise for the learner's attempting and subsequently achieving the psychomotor task.[14] Providing praise for correct performance increases patients' motivation. Additionally, feedback after every trial can improve learners' performance during the early phase of learning.[5]

In the cognitive stage of learning, the feedback can increase the depth of cognitive processes and improve retention.[6] When the patient starts to practice for the first time, he or she needs manual guidance to assist with movement and repeated practice to improve performance. Initially, complex tasks have to be broken down and taught and practiced as small components. Then, the whole task should be accomplished. The teaching and learning environment must be free of distractors, allowing the learner to concentrate and be attentive to the task.

In the associative ("how to do") stage, the patient as the learner should be able to practice the task and also refine the motor performance. The learner is less dependent on visual feedback, relying mostly on proprioceptive cues. The therapist's role is to use mostly KR feedback, emphasizing the functionality of the task.[5] The patient needs assistance to self-evaluate and improve their performance. The therapist's feedback is essential in this stage for enhancing the patient's motivation and retention.

In the associative stage, the patient's teaching and learning should be in an open environment that is changeable and increasingly challenging for learning.[6] This could prepare the patient for performing the motor task at home, at work, and in the community.

In the autonomous ("how to succeed") stage, the patient as the learner should be able to continue to refine the motor task to a level of error-free automatic movements. The therapist's feedback is minimal to none. Teaching and learning emphasizes open environments, challenges, and high levels of practice (called massed practice).[6] The learner should focus on competitive performances of the learned task.

## ESTABLISHING PATIENT GOALS/OUTCOMES FOR MOTOR LEARNING

When establishing a patient's motor learning goals, specific variables must be considered. The patient's performance of a motor task is influenced by permanent and temporary variables such as the patient's age and disorder, motivation and fatigue, medications, stress, and how much learning and practice can be applied for retention of information. The patient's age at the time of the lesson can also affect learning motor skills. For example, children and older adults demonstrate long reaction and movement times when performing motor skills.[5] Slowness in central information processing can decrease the sensory and motor control of children and older adults. Although motor performance tends to decline with age, the learning capabilities of older adults remain intact.[25] Older adult learners are able to achieve considerable performance gains. The extent to which the learning capability varies with age has to be considered very carefully. Age-related learning differences are increased in complex tasks, whereas in low-complexity tasks, the learning of younger and older adults is very similar.[25] The decline in motor learning that accompanies aging is task specific and not absolute. Other motor learning variables of the older adult may be related to muscular atrophy that can lead to decreased functional strength and the ability to perform functional tasks. Neurological changes can also affect muscular strength and coordination. As a result, when teaching and learning motor skills, patients with perceptual deficits need increased performance feedback to reinforce positive behavioral changes.[26]

Appropriate establishment of a patient's motor learning goals can increase performance by motivating and challenging the patient. Before beginning the practice of a motor task, the therapist must ensure that the patient understands the goals as outcomes and the strategies for achieving the task. When establishing teaching and learning outcomes for motor performance, therapists must communicate clearly with their patients, use simple words, and actively engage patients to participate in the motor task.[26]

An overview of the learning process must be provided from the start of the therapy session, conferring with the patient in regard to teaching objectives, the rationale, and the procedures to follow.[26] For example, considering Bloom's taxonomy of learning **(Table 17.5)**,[27] the patient education outcomes for each motor performance can be classified into three separate objectives: (1) patient knows the task procedures (cognitive), (2) patient demonstrates skillful task performance (psychomotor), and (3) patient demonstrates enthusiasm and motivation when talking about the task (attitude). The patient's knowledge can be assessed by asking the patient to verbally repeat the procedure, his or her skill can be assessed by rating the performance, and motivation can be determined by observing and questioning the patient.

Before starting the motor learning process, the therapist can select with the patient (and/or the patient's family/caregiver) specific performance outcomes that will serve as a guide for the teaching and learning process as well as the patient's own assessment of learning. When assessing the performance of the task with the patient, the therapist should use understandable and clear terms such as "follows safety procedures" instead of "being safety

| Table 17.5 | ***Examples of Basic Objectives Using Bloom's Taxonomy[27]*** |
|---|---|
| 1. | Patient demonstrates the ability to explain the procedure. |
| 2. | Patient demonstrates the ability to perform the procedure. |
| 3. | Patient demonstrates enthusiasm and motivation when talking about the procedure. |

| Table 17.6 | Examples of Specific Learning Outcomes |
|---|---|

**Objective:** "Patient knows the three-point gait with walker."

1. Patient describes which leg advances first in the three-point gait with walker.

2. Patient states which leg advances last in the three-point gait with walker.

3. Patient describes the entire procedure of three-point gait with walker.

4. Patient performs three-point gait with walker.

5. Patient distinguishes between proper and improper performance of three-point gait with walker.

conscious." Also, the outcomes must include the most important elements of the procedural task. Additionally, a simple task may include only one general objective whereas a more complex task may have several. After selecting the teaching objective with the patient, the therapist should determine specific learning outcomes for the learned task (**Table 17.6**).

The number of learning outcomes chosen depends on the type and difficulty of performance of the motor task. Complex tasks may need multipart objectives and several outcomes related to the key elements of the specific performances.

In patient education, similar to classroom teaching, preparing the instructional objectives can help the therapist select teaching and learning materials and methods. As mentioned prior, the objectives and learning materials and methods are decided with/for the patient to assist him or her the most in the learning process. In patient teaching and learning, assessing the patient's learning performance is the last part of instructional planning (**Table 17.7**), allowing the therapist to provide accurate feedback to the patient.

| Table 17.7 | Sequence of Instructional Planning |
|---|---|

1. Plan instructional objectives.

2. Select teaching methods and materials.

3. Plan assessment tools.

Additionally, the assessment helps the therapist modify teaching and learning objectives as well as his or her teaching methods to improve the instruction.

When planning instructional objectives, there are different frames of reference related to various teaching and learning styles and preferences. For example, when using Bloom's taxonomy of teaching and learning, the levels of instruction are classified as cognitive, psychomotor, and affective.[27] The cognitive domain is concerned with intellectual outcomes ranging from lower to higher level. Examples of lower-level cognitive outcomes are those using the following terms: recalling, interpreting, comparing, classifying, or applying. Higher-level cognitive outcomes may use words such as analyzing, identifying, relating, formulating, generating, judging, or inferring. The psychomotor domain is concerned with motor skills and performance outcomes.[27] These can be expressed using words such as demonstrating, performing, originating, drawing, writing, or operating. The affective domain focuses on outcomes related to appreciation, attitudes, and values.[27] The affective domain terminology of outcomes may be responding, listening, valuing, or relating.[27]

## BARRIERS TO MOTOR LEARNING

When teaching and learning motor performances, the therapist should gain the learner's attention and stimulate his or her recall of prior knowledge related to the topic. It also is important to identify and take measures in regard to any barriers the patient may have that could interfere with teaching and learning, such as vision, hearing, or cognition deficits. For example, older adults may experience normal age-related visual changes such as presbyopia.[26] This visual loss may decrease the learner's ability to focus properly and/or adapt to darkness and light. Because presbyopia is corrected by glasses or contact lenses, the therapist must make sure the patient is wearing his or her glasses (or contact lenses) during teaching and that the training room has good lighting.[26] Hearing loss as a result of aging can affect the learner's understanding of information. If the patient has a hearing aid, the therapist has to check that the hearing aid is on and working properly. If the patient reads lips, the therapist should face the patient (placing him- or herself directly in front of the patient at eye level) and talk slowly and clearly.[26] Gestures and demonstrations reinforce the information. Teaching and learning with patients who have cognitive impairments (especially with younger adults with conditions such as traumatic brain injury) can use contextual strategies related to daily activities instead of memorization.[5] Additionally, it is important to use patient education for functional skills and to add simple written instructions to the learning process.[26]

The patient's learning style, preferences, and culture should be considered. For example, patients whose predominant learning style is auditory learn best through verbal communication as they hear and remember. The therapist as the educator should speak clearly, repeat important points, and look directly at patients when speaking (because they also read lips).[26] Patients with an auditory learning style memorize best with recorded cassette tapes they can take home. When they learn, they need to hear themselves say the information to remember it. For problem solving they need to talk it through aloud to solve it. Sometimes the material can be remembered best when the specific movement is inserted into a rhythmic or musical pattern.[26] Visual learners are able to demonstrate appreciation for a drawing or an illustration of a task.[5] Videos of the movement can help patients who are pictorial learners consolidate a mental picture of the motor pattern in their long-term memory.[5] Kinesthetic learners respond best to movement. These patients are active, action-oriented individuals who enjoy movement such as ambulation and exercises. Although kinesthetic learners typically have a short attention span, they respond best by physically participating in the task performance from the beginning.[26]

Organizing the learning experiences over a period of sessions is important to break up the total information into a series of smaller components.[26] The therapist can determine with the patient the best teaching and learning sequence, such as from simple to more complex or from familiar to unfamiliar. Practicing the information is necessary, as is providing feedback. The teaching and learning environment must be controlled and monitored for the patient's physical and emotional comfort, confidence, reassurance, and satisfaction.[26]

Other recommendations for teaching and learning motor tasks are related to the learning process, which should be active and directed by the learner (**Table 17.8**).[26] Teaching and learning motor skills can be enhanced by the therapist's accurate demonstrations and the use of terminology the patient understands. The learner's full attention is necessary at all times. Consequently, learning cannot take place when the patient is uncomfortable, distracted, or fatigued. Repetition, practice, and accurate feedback are essential elements of success in motor performance.[5] Ambiguous feedback that is in conflict with other feedback can lead to confusion. Reinforcement such as praise, respect, or a smile can be used to encourage the repetition of a desired behavior.[5] The timing of reinforcement is important, especially when offered immediately after the performance or during the performance. Increasing the patient's motivation can improve the learner's desired behavior. Intrinsic motivation related to the learner's desire to accomplish the task is the most powerful force for successful performance.

## USING BLOOM'S TAXONOMY WITH MOTOR LEARNING

Bloom's taxonomy of learning can be used to teach motor performance skills to the patient. Generally, Bloom's taxonomy is applied to classroom education in medicine, nursing, and the allied health professions such as physical and occupational therapy. However, in this author's opinion, Bloom's taxonomy can be used as a functional method for teaching motor skills. From an instructional perspective, Bloom's taxonomy provides a framework that supports all levels of education.[28] It is considered a perfect tool for formative learning[28] that enables the learner's self-assessment and reflection in learning and encourages teacher–learner dialogue. Additionally, Bloom's taxonomy can provide the learner with quality information to help improve the learning process and also encourage the learner's motivation and self-confidence. Bloom's domains can also be described by categories referred to as knowledge, skills, and attitude (KSA) (as stated in Chapter 9).[27] These three categories can be considered *the goals of the motor learning process*.

The goals of the cognitive domain emphasize increasing the learner's knowledge and the development of theoretical skills.[27] This domain includes teaching the patient to describe procedural patterns and recall specific activity facts. When applying Bloom's taxonomy to

| Table 17.8 |
| --- |

## *Patient Teaching/Learning Recommendations*[3,5,26]

Select a physical environment conducive to teaching and learning. (Check for temperature, noise, smell, cleanliness, and safety.)

Teach one or two units at one session (if necessary) instead of the entire program.

Use clear and concise verbal instructions.

Provide written instructions and pictures of the desired movement.

Demonstrate the correct movement.

Ask the patient to reproduce the correct movement by guiding the patient (if necessary) to reproduce the correct movement.

Provide specific and movement-related feedback by demonstrating the incorrect and correct movement.

motor learning, the cognitive domain commences in the cognitive or "what to do" stage and continues throughout the associative and autonomous performance stages. Cognitive learning in the "what to do" stage involves teaching from the simplest behavior to the most complex. Similarities to other already known or learned tasks should be described. The patient needs to verbalize the task components and the requirements for completion. Also, the use of mental practice (rehearsal) can improve the patient's learning of the task.

At the beginning of motor learning, the patient may need to be cognitively prompted to the critical aspects of the task. The patient is very dependent on visual and auditory feedback, listening to the therapist, and watching the therapist performing the skill. The therapist has to establish clear references for measuring the patient's accuracy of task performance. The environment must be controlled to allow the patient to concentrate on the task. Any extraneous distractors (such as noise) should be eliminated. After the task is performed for the first time, the patient should be asked to evaluate his or her performance and identify problems and solutions. During this early cognitive motor learning stage, the patient may need feedback after each trial of the task.

In the associative stage, from the cognitive perspective, the patient may require variable feedback (such as summed). This can increase the depth of cognitive processes and improve retention. In the associative or "how to do" stage of motor learning, cognitive monitoring is decreased. The patient is becoming more dependent on the psychomotor part of learning. To increase the patient's knowledge and retention, the therapist can focus on variable practice order (such as random) and also variable feedback (such as summed). Encouraging consistency of performance is also important cognitively for better organization of the motor task.

In the last phase of motor learning ("how to succeed"), the patient receives a minimal level of cognitive monitoring. The therapist's feedback is offered occasionally and only when errors are clear and obvious. The learner's role is to demonstrate strong decision-making skills and be able to correctly self-evaluate.

The affective domain of Bloom's taxonomy is characterized by the manner in which the learner deals with the new information emotionally, such as feelings, values, appreciation, enthusiasms, motivations, and attitudes.[27] When applying the affective domain to motor learning, the therapist's role is essential to encourage and motivate the patient to learn and become independent when performing the skill. During the affective stage of learning, if the patient is motivated, he or she will be able to complete the task and become autonomous. From the affective perspective, the therapist may need to check the patient's level of excitement and try to calm the patient. Stress and anxiety can impair the learning process. To enhance the patient's enthusiasm for learning, the therapist must provide encouragement for practice and feedback.

In the cognitive stage of the motor task, the therapist must praise the patient for being able to cognitively learn the task and demonstrate the task, even if the performance had errors. Recognizing the patient's willingness to learn and act on the learned information increases the patient's motivation and self-efficacy. Asking the patient to mentally think about the skill (mental rehearsal) can decrease the patient's anxiety when performing the skill.

In the associative phase of motor learning, the patient needs to be able to increase his or her ability to make decisions and also perform self-assessments. The therapist should continue to provide feedback for enhancing the patient's motivation and encourage the patient to self-assess their achievements. The teaching should avoid excessive augmented feedback. In the autonomous stage of motor learning, the patient needs to be challenged to make decisions and focus on the competitive aspect of their task performance.

Bloom's psychomotor domain of learning includes using new information and trying to execute a simple skill or part of a more complex skill.[27] The therapist should use sensory cues to guide the patient's motor activity. In the early part of the psychomotor stage, the patient may learn a complex skill by imitation or trial and error. The therapist may need to emphasize closed skills initially in a closed environment and gradually progress to open skills in an open, unpredictable environment. Adequacy of performance is achieved by practicing and using intrinsic and augmented feedback. When applying the psychomotor domain to early motor learning, the therapist can focus on errors that are consistent during movement. The patient's motor performance should be controlled to minimize errors. Complex tasks need to be broken down into parts. Each part must be practiced separately before integrating the whole skill. Repeated practice of the same task is important to improve the patient's performance.

In the associative part of motor learning, the patient is able to practice the task and refine the performance. In this stage, the patient needs adequate rest periods, especially if a task is complex or long. From the psychomotor domain, the patient, as the learner, needs manual guidance to assist in production of movement. The patient's dependence on visual feedback decreases and use of proprioceptive feedback increases. Helping the patient to "feel" the movement can decrease errors and improve accuracy. The task must be related to functional skills and the patient's goals for function. In the associative motor stage, the psychomotor domain of learning encourages organized and consistent motor practice. The therapist should not use facilitation and guided movements. The environment should progress toward open, changeable surroundings similar to the ones found at home, at work, and in the community.

In the final autonomous motor learning stage, from the psychomotor perspective, the patient's learned responses have become habitual and the movements are performed with confidence and proficiency. The patient is independently performing the task. This last motor stage should stress consistency of performance, especially in relation to variable environments, open skills, and variations of the task. High levels of practice of the task are appropriate. Also, competitive aspects of the task must be encouraged during practice.

When applying Bloom's taxonomy for movement performances, the therapist should first set goals with the patient, encourage the patient to practice, give feedback, and provide motivation. The patient should be involved in decision making using a patient-centered examination, evaluation, and plan of care. The patient's (and family's) needs, preferences, lifestyle, socioeconomic status, and culture should be included in the plan. The therapist must encourage the patient's progression of motor skills from the cognitive to affective and physical performance.

For example, the cognitive stage may be marked by awkward, slow movements that the patient is consciously trying to control. The therapist can assess the patient's learning by asking open-ended questions or by having the patient explain the material. Initially, the patient has to think before doing the movement. Performance may be reduced and there will be inaccuracies in the movements. Some patients may be frustrated. The therapist's accurate feedback and support are necessary. Identifying and enhancing the learner's attitude toward accurate performance can increase the patient's adherence to learning. The patient's motivation could be increased by designing an activity program that is simple and clear; for example, oral teaching can be reinforced with demonstrations and a plain handout containing pictures of the task. Also, when using the patient's prior learning, especially with older adults, the learner can spend less time thinking about every detail and start to associate the new skill with another skill already known.[26] As a progression of the psychomotor stage, the movements begin to look smoother and the patient feels less awkward. The patient is confident with the performance and becomes independent. Finally, the patient also no longer needs to rely on the therapist for feedback.

# Patient Education for Older Adults Related to Exercises/Activities and Internet Utilization

## Objectives

After completing Chapter 18, the reader will be able to:

- Describe teaching and learning considerations for home exercise programs for older adults.

- Determine learning goals and special considerations for written home exercise material for older adults.

- Discuss the importance of using the Internet to supplement patient education for older adults.

- Explain special recommendations related to content and navigational features of health Web sites for older adults.

## Teaching Physical Activities and Exercises to Older Adults

The most significant demographic trend in the United States is the aging of its population. In 2011, the baby boomer population will begin to turn 65.[29] By 2030, the number of older Americans will double to approximately 70 million.[29] This means that one person in every five will be an older adult.[29] The growing number and proportion of older adults will increase demands on the American health care system, including physical and occupational rehabilitation. Rehabilitation health care providers need to consider and try to prevent the major disablement factors of older adults: (1) physiologic aging, (2) chronic diseases and disorders, and (3) levels of activity.[30] Although exercise and physical activity are the most important elements to maintaining physical and mental health, many older adults favor being sedentary and, as a result, are physically unfit.

## THE IMPORTANCE OF PHYSICAL ACTIVITIES FOR OLDER ADULTS

Older adults' physical activity generally decreases with advancing age. Physical and occupational therapists and assistants should provide patient education about the importance of physical activity in the treatment of the most common chronic medical conditions associated with old age. Being physically active can reduce the risk of high blood pressure, diabetes, stroke, and osteoporosis.[29,30] Nevertheless, approximately 60% of older adults in the United States are still physically inactive, refusing to participate in physical activities.[29] Older adults need first-hand education to understand that strengthening exercises done in moderation that are specially designed for them can actually improve strength, balance, and endurance regardless of age or disability. In general, exercise and physical activity can even enhance the health of individuals who are 90 years old or older, and patients who are frail or have various disabilities and disorders.[29,30] During the regular aging process, physical activity can help to prevent or delay disabilities. The five types of exercises and activities that are beneficial for older adults are strength, endurance, flexibility, balance, and aerobic programs (**Table 18.1**).[29]

Teaching and learning in physical and occupational rehabilitation must emphasize to older adults the benefits of strengthening exercises for functionality and prevention of obesity, diabetes, and osteoporosis. Balance and flexibility exercises help the older adult patient avoid falls. Falling is a widely recognized cause of hip fractures for elderly individuals, leading to disability and loss of independence.[2,29] Endurance training using aerobic programs also can delay or prevent many disorders associated with aging such as diabetes, heart disease, or stroke. Aerobic exercises can reduce many health risks of chronic disorders such as obesity, heart disease, high blood pressure, stroke, type 2 diabetes, and certain types of cancer. Weight-bearing aerobic programs can also help to decrease risks for osteoporosis and relieve chronic muscular pain. In the long run, aerobic conditioning maintains older adults' mobility and reduces cognitive decline.[2]

## GENERAL CONSIDERATIONS WHEN TEACHING HOME EXERCISE PROGRAMS TO OLDER ADULTS

In physical and occupational rehabilitation, motivating the older adult patient to perform exercises is a recognized challenge. Appropriate teaching and learning techniques can help older patients and clients increase their physical activity and slow the progression of their disabilities. The most important behavioral factors during the teaching and learning process are the patient's motivation and self-efficacy. As previously mentioned in this text, to improve motivation, a significant concept in the beginning of the teaching and learning process is

| Table 18.1 | **General Types of Exercises Recommended for Older Adults[29]** | |
|---|---|
| Strengthening exercises | Toe stands, squats, wall push-ups, finger marching, T-Band resistance exercises, or moderate intensity weight lifting (for major muscle groups). |
| Endurance exercises | Aerobic exercises that increase cardiovascular endurance such as bicycling, walking, swimming, or jogging. |
| Flexibility program | Stretching exercises. |
| Balance activities | Backward walking, toe walking, heel walking, sideways walking, or martial arts activities such as Tai Chi. |

to establish a therapeutic relationship with the patient. This association based on empathy, compassion, and caring allows the therapist to create, together with the patient, efficient and effective rehabilitation goals and outcomes. Additionally, this therapeutic alliance constitutes the foundation of the shared teaching and learning process. Patients and therapists teach and learn from each other.

The teaching and learning process may not always be smooth and sometimes may even fail. Nevertheless, only through cooperation with the patient in a patient-centered care plan can the therapist create the most effective teaching and learning framework for the patient. The patient education structure must always be based on and supported by the therapist's personal experiences and relationships with his or her patients and patients' families.

Teaching and learning for older adults in general must include the following basic requirements: (1) a clear understanding of health status and choices for interventions; (2) an active participation in the decision-making process; (3) an ability to cope with the health status, the prognosis, and the outcomes; (4) the potential to follow the rehabilitation plan of care including the home exercise program (HEP); and (5) the responsibility for continuation of care and promotion of a healthy lifestyle (**Table 18.2**).[2,30]

Teaching and learning recommendations may also include the following:[2,31]

■ Assessing of the learner's interest, past experiences, and level of motivation

■ Organizing the teaching and learning environment (such as using a quiet, clean, and comfortable room at the patient's preferred temperature; having enough light without glare; sitting near the patient so the patient can see the teacher; speaking clearly and slowly; inviting the patient's family, caregiver, or a friend to the session; or teaching brief sessions)

| Table 18.2 | *Basic Teaching and Learning Goals for Older Adults*[2,30] |
|---|---|
| | Must provide a clear understanding of health status and choices for interventions. |
| | Must be based on the patient's active participation in the decision-making process (using a patient-centered teaching and learning plan). |
| | Must increase the patient's ability to cope with the health status, the prognosis, and outcomes. |
| | Must enhance the patient's potential to follow the plan of care (including the HEP as a continuum of care). |
| | Must increase the patient's (or caregiver's) responsibility for continuation of care and health promotion. |

- Breaking up large pieces of information into small units
- Teaching one step at a time
- Using demonstrations
- Encouraging the patient to practice each step
- Finding out the patient's learning preference (such as reading, listening, watching, or doing)
- Adjusting the teaching method to the patient's learning style and special needs (for example, for a visual learner the teacher may give the patient a picture of the skill to be taught at the beginning of the learning process)
- Using large print (at least 16 points and not italics) for patients with vision problems
- Reinforcing and clarifying the information, such as having the family, caregiver, or friend participate in the teaching and learning session; giving the patient written material for home; or reviewing the material with the patient when the patient returns to therapy

Teaching and learning must be adapted to each patient's age, developmental needs, culture, and language. The teaching and learning process must be an interdisciplinary effort. At the beginning of the 21st century, the Institute of Medicine developed strategies for health care professionals' education to enhance patient care quality and safety.[32] All clinicians, including physical and occupational therapists, must ensure they are working as part of an interdisciplinary team, practicing evidence-based medicine, delivering patient-centered care, focusing on quality improvement, and using information technology.[32] Patient teaching skills must be integrated into all learning experiences of health care professionals. The therapists should be expert clinicians while delivering patient education characterized by clear and simple messages using layman's terminology.[32] Also, explaining new words and asking the patient to repeat the terms as necessary can help therapists deliver effective patient teaching and learning.

The therapist as the teacher must be able to obtain the patient's attention, motivation, and participation. An overview of the learning process, including objectives and outcomes and the type of information to be communicated, should be provided to the patient from the beginning of the teaching and learning process.[31] The therapist as the teacher should stimulate the learner's recall of previous learning and also relate the learner's prior known information to new topics or concepts.[31] The learning process must be monitored by the therapist in conjunction with the patient's goals, outcomes, and learning styles.[31] Learning units, objectives, and outcomes should be organized over a period of time by breaking down the topics or concepts into smaller steps or units. The therapist also should determine with the patient the best sequence for learning. Some patients may prefer to learn from simple to complex and others from concrete to abstract or familiar to unfamiliar.[31] Teaching and learning should progress at a comfortable pace to accommodate the patient's learning style and preferences.

Feedback is required on a regular basis or as needed by the learner. The feedback must include accurate information about results. The patient as the learner needs opportunities to practice and repeat the information or skill as necessary. Successful learning of a new behavior should be rewarded to increase the patient's motivation, locus of control, and efficacy.

The learning environment must be monitored for extraneous variables that influence the teaching and learning process.[31] These variables can be conditions that have a negative impact on the patient's learning such as pain or discomfort, anxiety, fear, frustration, feelings of failure, shame, embarrassment, boredom, or time pressures.

When teaching exercises to the physically active older adult, the therapist must know that an active, generally healthy patient has different goals than an older sedentary adult in poor health.[2] The active older patient, who may have been exercising for many years, may wish to preserve his or her function and independence.[2] As a result, the physically active individual may need to be challenged to increase the intensity of exercises, especially when performing resistance training. Contrarily, the sedentary older adult patient may have a negative attitude toward exercise and no intention of becoming physically active. For this patient, a behavioral modification program (as previously described in Chapter 8) should be applied to increase the patient's motivation to perform an exercise or activity.[2]

Another consideration in regard to exercises is related to the fact that the frail older adult patient with disabilities (especially cardiac disorders) may need to receive a monitored, graded exercise stress test prior to starting any exercise program including an HEP.[2,31] In some situations, cardiac testing may not be feasible for an older adult in poor health, because a stress test may present a physical and emotional challenge to the patient. For such patients, the exercise activity should be functionally based and closely monitored by the therapist (mostly for blood pressure and heart rate).

As a general directive for teaching and learning exercises, the HEP should be specific to the patient's needs and presented in an understandable format. For the healthy older adult, the ideal home exercise program should be tailored to the patient's requirements using a combination of aerobic, resistance, stretching, and balance training. An effective exercise will target large muscle groups (such as legs, arms, shoulders, calves, and back).[29] Older individuals who are generally healthy should train aerobically at moderate intensity 3 to 5 days per week for a duration of 5 to 60 minutes per session.[2,29] For both types of patients (healthy and frail older adults), the teaching and learning process of exercises including the HEP must be assessed, analyzed, and reevaluated periodically to assure it is still meeting the patient's needs. Additionally, both groups need creative, varied (customized as necessary), and functional HEPs that lead to continuous involvement to preserve and improve function as necessary.

The HEP represents an extension of the interventions. The exercise program starts on the first day of interventions and continues through the day of discontinuation of physical therapy.[26,31] However, the patient may not always be ready for exercises. Consequently, the therapist has to identify signs regarding the patient's state of readiness and motivation for action. As described in Chapter 8 of this book, patient motivation and readiness to change are fundamental to behavioral modifications, including the beginning of an HEP. Using the transtheoretical model of change (TMC) can enhance an individual's self-control and willingness to change. Many times, the patient needs help to identify barriers to their participation in an exercise program. When the patient is in the precontemplation stage of change, the therapist has to help the patient identify personal goals that can contribute to exercise performance. In the contemplation stage, the patient needs encouragement by evaluating the pros and cons of an exercise program. A patient in the action phase of change typically is better motivated to adhere to the program.

Additionally, it is very important to link the HEP with the patient's problems, goals, and outcomes.[2,26] The HEP should be presented as part of the total process of patient education and rehabilitation. Teaching exercises to a group of patients with similar goals can also increase motivation. Furthermore, the HEP must be tailored to the patient's usual activities and lifestyle. For example, a patient who likes to play golf will become motivated by performing exercises to improve his or her golf swing. The exercise has to reflect the activity (or activities) to which the patient will be returning after the rehabilitation is completed. Changes in the patient's lifestyle, such as asking the patient to start an exercise program that can interfere with his or her daily schedule, can harmfully affect the patient's motivation and adherence with the program.

## SPECIAL CONSIDERATIONS WHEN TEACHING HOME EXERCISE PROGRAMS TO OLDER ADULTS

Special considerations for older patients with hearing impairments require the therapist to speak slowly, clearly, distinctly, and in a normal tone of voice (not loudly).[31] Shouting or speaking in a raised voice distorts language sounds and also gives the impression of anger.

Speaking in a high-pitched voice makes it difficult to hear. The therapist must look directly at the patient and be at the same eye level with the patient.[31] Pronunciation should not be exaggerated so that the patient can lip read (speech read) or pick up visual signs (such as expressions, gestures, or pantomime).[31] Hands must be away from the therapist's face and adequate lighting in the room is necessary for the patient's lip reading.

When the patient wears a hearing aid, it should be checked for proper functioning and whether the hearing aid battery is working.[26] The external auditory canal can be checked for excessive earwax. Interfering sounds must be reduced. Background noises such as exercise machines, whirring computers, or office equipment can mask what the therapist is saying.[26] The therapist can keep a notepad nearby to write down information in case the patient has difficulty understanding it verbally. The therapist should be careful with pronunciations of letters such as *m, n, b, c, d, e, t,* and *v.* Presbycusis (hearing loss associated with aging) is most often accompanied by a significant loss of high-frequency speech sounds affecting reception of consonants (*sh, ka, fa, ba, ta, za,* etc.).[26] Numbers need to be stated separately, such as 6 and 5, and not 65. When the topic is changed, the patient should be informed by pausing briefly or gesturing toward or gently touching the patient (or asking a question).

Special considerations for older patients who have vision impairments require the therapist to introduce him- or herself and other people in the room.[26] The patient should be asked if he or she wants assistance to move around and to provide directions. The rehabilitation area should be adequately lighted and the therapist needs sufficient light on his or her face.[26] Glare must be minimized. The patient needs to be asked if he or she wants assistance to sit down and directions must be provided. The therapist should make sure the patient has brought and is wearing eyeglasses. When using printed information, such as the HEP, it must be written in a large print size (such as 16 points), with simple fonts and typeface that is easy to read.[26] If the patient has difficulty reading, the therapist can tape record the instructions, or use large diagrams and pictures. Print information can also be presented to the patient in Braille.[26]

## GENERAL CONSIDERATIONS WHEN WRITING HOME EXERCISE PROGRAMS FOR OLDER ADULTS

The HEP should be written at a fifth- or sixth-grade reading level[26] and should include no more than two or three main ideas. The patient has to know only what they need. Any extraneous information or details will be confusing. Words must be chosen carefully. It is recommended to use words with only one or two syllables. Complex words (such as inflammation) must be replaced with simple ones (such as redness).[26] A conversational style is best to allow the patient to feel they are talking with a friend. The HEP may include diagrams, drawings, or pictures of exercises or activities. These should be uncomplicated.

The HEP should be written in the patient's primary language.[26] Cultural differences must be considered. Preferred terms may vary even within an ethnic or racial group. The messages must be tailored to each cultural or ethnic group and subgroup. Groups may have different needs, values, and beliefs that will affect how they interpret the message. Talking with patients and understanding their cultural values before writing an HEP is recommended.

Technical terms must be avoided and short sentences must be used as much as possible. Each sentence in the HEP must present only one idea and contain no more than one three-syllable word.[26] The HEP should be written in clear layman's terms and be concise. The words must make sense to the patient and be consistent with the therapist's verbal information, written illustrations, and demonstrations. When a family member or a caregiver is involved in rehabilitation, he or she should be familiarized with the home program early in rehabilitation (usually at the beginning of therapy) to allow an easier transition at the discontinuation of therapy.[26] The exercises or activities presented in the HEP must be simple and clear. The program can include approximately two to four exercises or activities. These must incorporate the following: the number of repetitions of activities or exercises, the number of sets, how long to hold, the amount of exercise resistance, positions for performing the exercises or activities, the duration of exercises or activities, the frequency, and the method of progression.[26] The exercises and activities must be sorted in a logical manner so the patient does not have to change positions too much when performing them.

Written patient material must be personalized, demonstrating that the material is customized for the patient. Personalizing patient material is very effective for all older adult patients, and especially for patients with limited literacy because the information focuses on important data that is relevant just for them. Written or printed materials need to have the patient's name on the cover.[26] The written or printed information must first be read together with the patient. If it is necessary, the patient can highlight the key aspects. Illustrations may need to have the patient circle or draw an arrow pointing to the key feature of a movement in the exercise program.[2] The information can be reinforced by videotaping the patient and the therapist while performing the exercises (activities).[2] In physical therapy, teaching and learning strategies using live and videotaped modeling are more effective for retention than a handout alone.[33,34] The videotaped session can provide feedback to the patient for better performance.[33] Additionally, it is recommended that the patient demonstrates the HEP at each visit.[33]

Formatting also can make a difference in readability (**Table 18.3**). Printed materials for older adults must use serif typeface such as **Times New Roman** or **Georgia**.[35,36] Because these serif typeface fonts have tails on the ends, they can create an illusionary line to guide the reader's eye across the print. Sans serif typefaces (such as **Arial**) do not have this capability and are harder to read on printed pages.[36] The type sizes should be 12 points (at least), 13 points, or 14 points. Times New Roman should use 14 points.[35] For patients who have visual impairments, 16-point or 18-point types are the best choices.[35] Headings must be larger to stand out; however, other than headings, fonts larger than 14 points must not be used for patients who do not have vision problems.[35] Printed materials need white space to provide relaxation from reading for the eyes and to help older adults focus their attention. It is best to use both uppercase and lowercase letters because readers in general are more familiar with reading that way.[36] Uppercase letters can be used for headlines or when emphasizing an idea. Letters that are all uppercase are difficult to read and should not be used.[36] When the text is double spaced it is easier to read; otherwise, the lines seem to be blurry and may need to be read over and over again.[36] Italics, bold, and underlining

| Table 18.3 | *Basic Recommendations for Printed Materials for Older Adults*[35,36] |
|---|---|

Use easy to read serif typeface fonts (such as Times New Roman or Georgia).

For patients without vision problems, use 12-, 13-, or 14-point type sizes. Times New Roman should be 14-point type. For patients with vision impairments, use 14- or 16-point type.

Headings must stand out.

Use a mix of uppercase (good for headlines) and lowercase letters. Do not use all capital letters.

Double space the text.

Align the text to the left (called left justified).

Write short lines (approximately 50 to 65 characters).

Be careful when using italics, bold, and underlining.

Do not use sentences divided by illustrations.

Be careful when using colors such as yellow, blue, or green.

Use contrast between the letters (or illustrations) and the background of the paper.

Do not use glossy or thin paper.

should not be overused because it will make the text less readable; for example, italicized letters can appear squeezed together.[36] Aligning the text to the left margin also makes it easier to read.[36]

When using an illustration of an exercise, the sentences describing the exercise should not be wrapped around the illustration.[36] Typically sentences divided by illustrations are hard to read. When using colors, it is often difficult to identify yellow, blue, or green, especially if they are close to each other.[36] Also, using blue or green text on a yellow background (or vice versa) may cause the words to blend into the background.[36] Printed material for older patients needs to have contrast, such as using a black type against a white background.[2,36] Patterned backgrounds or text appearing across an illustration are not easy to read.[36]

Each written line should be short, containing approximately 50 to 65 characters;[36] otherwise, the patient may inadvertently skip to another line. To reduce the line length, it is suggested to use two columns (but without making the lines too short).

Paper selection is also important; for example, it is hard to read material printed on a glossy paper because it creates a shine.[35] Also, paper that is very thin should not be used because the reader can see through it to the other side of the page.

# Patient Education and Older Adults' Use of the Internet

Physical and occupational therapists can use the Internet to provide information to their patients. Many rehabilitation facilities successfully use Web sites to make usable rehabilitation-based health information available to prospective and current patients (clients).

## INTERNET AND WEB SITES AS A SUPPLEMENT TO PATIENT EDUCATION

Health information delivered through the Internet can be a major influence in patients' decisions in regard to management of their care. Patients as health care consumers make use of clinical guidelines and Web sites that disseminate evidence-based information on treatments and their effectiveness.[37] Patients and clients can learn about the risk of disease or injury, how to detect problems, and ways to get their health back when sick or injured. Using the Internet, patients can take a more proactive role toward their own health.[37] Patients who ask questions, express opinions, and state their preferences regarding treatment have measurably better health outcomes than those who do not communicate with their health care providers.[37] As a result, this form of cooperation between the patient and the provider promotes a patient-centered care approach. In regard to older adults, the majority use the Internet to locate health information,[37] although not all older adults have computer accessibility. However, as a tool, the Internet allows the older patient population, similar to their younger counterparts, to take a more active role in their health care and work collaboratively with their health care provider.

In physical and occupational therapy, the Internet can be a helpful supplement to patient education. Having a Web site can assist therapists to communicate to their patients (clients) teaching and learning material appropriate for the patient population and related to their educational goals. Although personal interaction with patients is extremely important, being able to provide specific information on a Web site can augment the in-office patient education.

Web sites created for older adult patients (clients) should include specific considerations regarding the content of the material and the navigational features. In general, the Web site should be extremely user friendly and simple to navigate. The ability to perform complex actions decreases with age.[38,39] These actions may include the ability to simultaneously remember and process new information, to perform complex cognitive tasks, and to comprehend text. Although these decreased abilities are not usually dramatic, their presence can interfere with the performance of some relatively simple tasks such as using a computer.[39] Older adults process information more slowly than younger adults; however, there are effective ways to present text on a Web site to mediate these age-related changes.

## Designing a Web Site for the Older Adult

The general considerations for Web site content include the following:[38,39]

- Presenting information in a clear and familiar way (to reduce the number of presumptions)

- Using positive statements and an active voice

- Using simple language (perhaps providing a separate glossary of technical terms)

- Communicating the material in a logical way

- Dividing lengthy documents into short sections

- Using text-relevant images

- Providing open captioning (or access to a static version) as text alternatives to animation, video, or audio

The information presented in the Web site must be accurate and complete. Additionally, the Web site should include a disclosure related to notifying the user about the purpose of the site.[39] The site has to clarify whether its primary function is to market products and services or provide rehabilitation information to its patients and clients. If the Web site's functions include both types, the users need to be appropriately informed. The users also need to know about any profiling or collection of information associated with the use of the Web site.[38]

The recommendations for writing Web site content are generally similar to the ones for printed materials. A good background can enhance the content of the page and attract the user's attention to particular segments or graphics.[38] The contrast between the background and the content is also significant because any lightening of the contrast can diminish readability. The contrast colors should be carefully selected. Typically, analogous colors (colors next to each other on the color wheel such as blue and green) offer the least amount of contrast whereas complimentary colors (colors opposite to each other on the color wheel such as purple and yellow) offer the most.[38] The traditional design of a Web page is dark text on a white or light background. However, some older individuals may prefer to have light text on a dark background, especially on a Web site. Both are acceptable as long as the contrast between the text and the background is strong. Also, patterned wallpaper-type backgrounds must never be used because they are disruptive and may give the illusion of text-twisting.[38] The font of the text should preferably be between 12- and 14-point, depending on the typeface.[38] Headings always need to be larger than the body text. Stylized or novelty typefaces should not be used for blocks of text. The same recommendation applies to italics and underlined text. Content written in italics can appear shaky and unstable, whereas underlining may look blurry.[38] The content needs to be written with enough space between the letters and use a left justification by aligning the text along the left margin of the page.

## WEB SITE NAVIGATIONAL FEATURES FOR THE OLDER ADULT

The general considerations for the navigational features when designing a Web site for older adults may include the following:[38,39]

- Having a simple and uncomplicated organization of the Web site.
- Using explicit step-by-step navigation procedures (whenever possible).
- Reducing the navigational clicks to a minimum (to decrease prompts that need to be memorized).
- Placing a consistent toolbar near the top of the screen where it is highly visible (can help with usage and navigation).
- Using single mouse clicks instead of double (considering individuals who may have arthritis of the hands).
- Labeling the links.
- Using a standard page design and the same symbols and icons throughout the Web site.
- Having the same set of navigation buttons in the same place on each page (allowing the reader to move easier from one Web page or section of the Web site to another).
- Labeling each page in the same location (using the name of the Web site).
- Including text with any icons and using large buttons (that do not require precise mouse movements for activation). An icon is a small pictogram. Computer icons may represent a file, folder, application, or device on a computer operating system.[38,39] In today's modern usage, the icon can represent any indicator the users want it to be. User friendliness demands that computer icons are distinct from each other, self-explanatory, and easily visible under all possible user setups.

Additional navigational considerations for a Web site for older adults may include using pull-down menus sparingly and avoiding automatic scrolling.[38] If manual scrolling is required, it should incorporate specific scrolling icons on each page. Buttons such as Previous Page and Next Page must be provided to allow the reader to review or move forward. Any icons must also have text hyperlinks.[38] Each Web site should include a help menu with several means for obtaining assistance. The support could be in the form of a tutorial (how to use the site), toll-free telephone number (for people who prefer to talk to a person), an email address option, and/or a frequently asked questions (FAQ) page (that includes technical and site content questions).[39] The FAQ page must be current, reflecting the visitors' questions. Additionally, the Web site must be continuously evaluated for its friendliness and accessibility features.

# TEACHING AND LEARNING CONSIDERATIONS FOR WELLNESS, HEALTH PROMOTION, AND DISEASE PREVENTION

## Objectives

After completing Chapter 19, the reader will be able to:

- Discuss the importance of teaching and learning concepts for wellness, health promotion, and disease prevention.

- Determine patients' values and readiness related to health promotion and disease prevention.

- List physical and occupational therapy teaching goals and major areas of emphasis for 21st-century health promotion and disease prevention.

- Apply prevention measures for prediabetes/diabetes and falls.

## The Importance of Wellness, Health Promotion, and Disease Prevention in Physical and Occupational Therapy

Concepts of wellness, health promotion, and disease prevention are all part of occupational and physical therapy teaching and learning. The American Occupational Therapy Association's (AOTA's) Centennial Vision toward the year 2017 includes health and wellness as an overarching area of practice.[40,41] The year 2020 Vision Statement for physical therapy also includes prevention and wellness services.[42] For physical and occupational therapy, wellness and health promotion are societal needs that relate to people's emotional and physical well-being. Factors that increase the need for health and wellness in American society include the growing aging population that has increasing longevity, health effects from the rising rates of obesity, the increased health care disparities affecting treatment and services, and other outside factors such as technological advances and imbalances in life roles. Disease prevention, health promotion, and wellness programs are expanding for both professions in areas of senior wellness, prediabetes and diabetes prevention, avoidance of falls, home and business modifications to enhance wellness, managing patients and clients with obesity, and other specific community-based health promotion activities.[40,42]

In Western society, people believe that health is the most favorable state for a person and that illness and disease should be avoided. The medical model in Western society promotes disease cures as the ultimate goal. Sometimes, society may not focus on wellness, disease prevention, and health promotion. Some individuals try to change their lifestyles only after receiving a diagnosis of an illness. Ideally, people should not require illness to evolve and change. Unfortunately, some individuals need to make changes but cannot unless forced by circumstances. Health care providers are aware that many people need changes in their self-concept to be able to make informed choices for their health. Using the patient-centered care approach, health care providers have been able to gradually increase their patients' active participation in health care decisions. By participating in their self-care, many patients attain self-respect and self-worth and, at the same time, a greater feeling of independence and control. Usually, changes in an individual's self-concept can facilitate fundamental transformations in their belief system. Patient teaching and learning helps to make these changes possible. Physical and occupational therapists and assistants play an important role in helping individuals of all ages make the decision to change and improve their health. They encourage people to examine their lifestyles and consider moving toward wellness and good health.

## 21st-Century Goals for Health Promotion and Disease Prevention in Physical and Occupational Therapy

Physical and occupational therapists and assistants play an important role in disease prevention and promotion of physical activity and exercises to enhance health and avoid diseases or disorders. The 21st-century goals of physical and occupational rehabilitation include prevention of stroke, arthritis, diabetes/prediabetes, and falls in older individuals (**Table 19.1**). Encouraging people to adopt healthy lifestyle choices constitutes a large aspect of physical and occupational therapy teaching and learning. Prevention and health promotion activities include the therapist's clinical teaching and learning as well as other proactive activities in the community such as health screenings, health education, and risk assessment programs.[40,42] For example, therapists perform screenings for scoliosis, develop exercise programs in the community to prevent obesity among teenagers and adults, and educate older adults about fall prevention.

Teaching and learning health promotion and disease prevention requires physical and occupational therapists to increase their focus on evidence-based research related not only to their profession, but also to medicine and public health.[40,42] Currently, near the implementation of the Healthy People 2020 program, the American health care community needs population-based strategies that focus on primary prevention of chronic diseases. The resources for public health programs are limited. All health care providers, including those in physical and occupational therapy, have the responsibility to apply their ideas and find innovative prevention initiatives that work. Students in medical and allied health schools must be encouraged to learn how to advance their future practices in order to increasingly become engaged in preventive and proactive strategies for their patients and clients. Proactive strategies, especially in health promotion, can include not only the latest therapeutic techniques, but also any intervention that is meaningful to patients and clients. For example, if a person has difficulty walking because of being overweight and uses a wheelchair to ambulate in the community, the therapist may need to consider strategies other than only exercise. The best health promotion teaching and learning for this individual may be a combination of several options and patient-specific physical activities (such as weight lifting while sitting in the wheelchair). These will enable patients to adhere to patient education strategies and also safely participate in society.

The American Physical Therapy Association (APTA) and the AOTA have expanded their efforts toward improving patient safety, performance, and function.[41,42] Both national organizations support interventional and preventative plans to help individuals who have had a stroke or who have arthritis and also to prevent the consequences of falls for people older than 65 years of age. Specifically, the APTA has been trying to convince the U.S. Congress to enact legislation regarding public health issues where physical therapy can have a significant role in the prevention of disease and disorders.[41] Physical and occupational therapists and assistants are in the forefront of stroke and arthritis prevention and initiation of health promotion programs related to physical activity and nutrition. The U.S. Congress hopefully will authorize education campaigns for stroke prevention and establish a clearinghouse to support communities whose goals are to improve stroke care. As of

| Table 19.1 | *Major Areas of Health Promotion/Disease Prevention in Physical and Occupational Rehabilitation in the 21st Century[41,42]* |
|---|---|
| Stroke prevention. | |
| Arthritis prevention. | |
| Diabetes and prediabetes prevention. | |
| Prevention of falls in older adults. | |
| Obesity prevention. | |
| Promotion of regular physical activity/exercise. | |

January 2009, several health-related organizations (in addition to APTA and AOTA), including the American Heart Association and American Stroke Association, were still waiting for the Stroke Treatment and Ongoing Prevention Act (the STOP Stroke Act) to be approved by the full Senate.[43]

The APTA also is trying to convince Congress to pass legislation that will use the knowledge and expertise of physical therapists to promote physical activity and prevent and reduce obesity in the United States.[42] Obesity is a growing epidemic and a severe public health problem.[44] It is projected that by the year 2030, more than 86% of American adults will be overweight.[45] This estimates an appreciable financial burden for American health care. It is expected that one in every six dollars spent on health care will go towards overweight and obesity-related health problems.[45] Some legislators have been trying to intervene and find solutions to the problem. On July 23, 2008, Senators Chris Dodd (D-CT), Tom Harkin (D-IA), and Jeff Bingaman (D-NM) introduced the Federal Obesity Prevention Act of 2008.[46] Currently, the goals of the Obesity Prevention Act seem to be concentrating primarily on the nutritional aspects of health, promoting dietary changes in children's meals. Hopefully, in its final form the Obesity Prevention Act will also integrate physical activity for people of all ages. Important aspects of improving and maintaining good health include both choosing nutritious foods and engaging in regular physical activity. Regular physical activity can enhance health and prevent disease.[44]

Encouraging children and adults to adopt a healthy lifestyle through nutrition and activities/exercises can make a big difference in health promotion. Physical and occupational therapists have the capability to provide individualized assessments, prevent exercise-related injuries, and consider health factors that influence the type, duration, and intensity of physical activity. Many individuals who are overweight and trying to lose weight experience injury when starting an unsupervised exercise program. Physical and occupational therapists are particularly qualified to be of help. For example, individuals who are healthy can start an aerobic activity of minimum to moderate intensity for 5 days per week, coupled with flexibility and relaxation exercises.[42] However, if they lack conditioning, they need to learn how to avoid injuries from high resistance and high impact activities.[42] The best conditioning program for an individual who is overweight (just beginning a diet coupled with exercise) would be a customized plan designed especially for individual. Such a program has to be enjoyable and also support the person's maintenance of healthy weight reduction.

# Concepts of Wellness, Health Promotion, and Disease Prevention in Physical and Occupational Therapy

The concept of wellness is the condition of being in good health.[41] Wellness is described as a person's being in good physical and emotional health and appreciating and enjoying his or her good health.

## CONCEPTS OF WELLNESS AND HEALTH PROMOTION

Wellness is typically a result of a lifestyle geared toward well-being. The individual chooses to reach his or her optimum potential of health regardless of the presence or absence of a disabling condition. Health promotion is the science and art of helping individuals change their lifestyle to move toward a state of optimal health.[47] Health promotion can improve the state of an individual's overall health. In occupational and physical therapy, wellness and health promotion are the necessary steps that guide a person toward a healthy lifestyle. These steps may include exercise, nutrition, stress reduction, fitness, good mental and spiritual health, proper rest, or a combination of these. An individual must have health awareness to be able to choose a lifestyle for health and happiness.[47] Health promotion that includes teaching and learning can increase a person's health awareness and ability to integrate all senses to balance their state of health.

Teaching and learning for wellness and health promotion is a regular part of physical and occupational therapy patient education interventions. Physical and occupational therapists and assistants have always been teaching their patients and clients about wellness and health promotion topics. Furthermore, they have been incorporating these topics into their patient management programs. The national strategy for improving American health includes supporting health care providers to initiate new subspecialties in their area of practice that will fully concentrate on lifestyle management and prevention of chronic disease and disability.[42] Physical and occupational therapy practices of the 21st century may change health care environments to entirely focus on wellness, health promotion, and disease prevention. Many physical and occupational therapists already offer fitness, wellness, and other health promotion programs as a continuum of their rehabilitative care. Expanding physical and occupational therapists' roles in health promotion could help nationally educate people on how to redesign their lifestyles. Because health promotion enables people to increase their control over and improve their health, the focus of teaching and learning is health awareness and choosing a lifestyle for health and happiness.

Wellness is a dynamic state of health functioning through harmonious interactions between a person's internal and external environments.[47] As a complex mechanism, wellness consists of many different variables such as physical, social, environmental, emotional, intellectual, and spiritual.[47] People's individual values and their interpretations of health also play an important role when teaching and learning wellness and health promotion (**Table 19.2**).[47,48]

Promoting health and wellness has to increase a person's own awareness about health. There are four major health models that relate to a person's own concept about health and wellness: clinical, role performance, adaptive, and eudaemonistic.[47,48] The clinical model is defined as an individual, narrow interpretation of health.[47] In this model, the person wrongly believes that the absence of signs and symptoms of disease or injury actually means a healthy lifestyle. The clinical model is a passive state of freedom from illness. In the clinical model, the person's own health beliefs and lifestyle places him or her at high risk for disease. By being free of observable signs and symptoms, the individual does not address larger life issues that harmfully affects his or her health.[47] For example, a person who regularly

| Table 19.2 | *Interpretations of Health*[47,48] |
|---|---|
| Clinical model | Health is the absence of signs and symptoms (most narrow interpretation). |
| Role performance model | Health is the ability to perform roles and tasks in society. |
| Adaptive model | Health is the ability to adapt and survive environmental changes. |
| Eudaemonistic model | Health is well-being and self-realization (best interpretation). |

uses tobacco and lives a sedentary lifestyle is likely, sooner or later, to experience signs and symptoms that relates to his or her lifestyle pattern. This will happen regardless of the fact that the signs and symptoms are not apparent at this time. Individuals who believe in the clinical model have a very limited view about health. They just expect to be treated for signs and symptoms of illness and return to the same way of life as before.[48] The individuals who believe in the clinical model are not concerned with changing lifestyles for wellness and health promotion.

The role performance model considers health as the state of optimum capacity of the individual as long as the person is able to perform his or her roles and tasks in society.[47] If people can perform these roles and tasks, they are considered healthy. For example, even if an individual is overweight, inactive, and has diabetes, the individual considers him- or herself healthy as long as he or she is able to perform his or her daily responsibilities in the social environment.[47] This individual will not want to change his or her lifestyle as long as he or she is able to assume a role and work. Illness, and perhaps change, may occur only if the individual is unable to work or perform societal roles. The role performance model incorporates psychological and social standards of health.[48] Also, if an individual cannot work it means illness, even if the individual appears clinically healthy.

The adaptive model considers the environment as a central factor in which the individual can engage in effective interaction with both the physical and social environment.[47] The model links the clinical and the role performance models. In the adaptive model, health may be a process instead of a state of being.[48] Illness, as an opposite of health, is failure in the adaptation system and the inability to cope with changes in the environment.[48] As a result, adaptive behavior requires an individual to remain healthy, considering his or her ability to grow, change, and survive environmental transformations.[48] When an individual has a disorder, the interventions will help him or her adapt and cope with it. In this model, the individual believes staying healthy is based on his or her own ability to cope or adapt to the illness and his or her successful interaction with the environment.[47] Good health is flexible adaptation to the environment and interaction with it for maximal benefit. In this model, an individual will receive the necessary interventions to eliminate signs and symptoms and interact again with his or her physical and social environment.[47] However, the individual will not consider the reasons for the signs and symptoms causing the disorder as long as he or she is able to adapt to it.

The eudaemonistic model is the best model of health.[47] This concept extends the definition of health to include an individual's well-being and self-realization. In the eudaemonistic model, health is not a biological or physical measure, but an ability of an individual to do what he or she wants.[47] Health represents the fulfillment of an individual's full potential in regard to happiness and aspirations. In the eudaemonistic model, health is characterized by a high level of wellness and satisfaction with life.

In addition to the above models, which consider the person's values about health, two other models can help determine whether an individual is likely to participate in wellness and health promotion activities: the health belief model and the health locus of control model. The health belief model (HBM) predicts which individuals would participate in health promotion activities.[48] The model states that a relation exists between an individual's beliefs about health and his or her actions.[48] Factors that influence a person's health concepts include personal expectations in regard to health and illness, earlier experiences with health and illness, sociocultural context, and age and developmental state.[48] For example, relative to age, many older adults believe they should tolerate a particular illness or disability because normally they have greater susceptibility to poor health than younger people. The health belief model is also based on a person's individual perceptions about health, the necessary modifying factors, and the likelihood of action. Some individuals may perceive the threat to their health to be serious. As an example, if a person who uses tobacco believes there is a severe threat to his or her health, he or she may be able to become motivated and try to change. The health belief model is important in teaching wellness and health promotion because it provides an insight into the relationship between the way a person sees their state of health and their response to health, illness, or health promotion.[48]

The health locus of control model is characterized by people's belief in themselves or others in regard to health.[48] Some individuals will believe they are able to change their health for the better whereas others may think that outside forces are largely in control of their well-being.

## CONCEPTS OF DISEASE PREVENTION

In health care, disease prevention is defined as any activity that can reduce an individual's mortality and morbidity from disease.[47] Disease prevention focuses on maintaining an individual's health by avoiding possible risk factors that decrease their health such as disease, disorder, or injury.[47] For patient teaching, prevention or preventive measure is a method of educating an individual or a group of individuals to be able to avoid an injury, disorder, or disease. Teaching and learning disease prevention can identify the risk factors that may cause health problems and also provide protective measures to avoid such threats.[47] These risks for a person's health may have a behavioral, genetic, environmental, or sociocultural characteristic or could be a combination of these. For example, genetic risk factors occur in individuals whose close relatives have heart disease, diabetes, cancer, or osteoporosis. These individuals have a greater risk and are more likely to develop the diseases themselves. To exemplify this even more, the Centers for Disease Control and Prevention (CDC) found that women age 35 years or older with a family history of osteoporosis are 2.3 times more likely to have the disease.[49] Genetically, the association grew stronger, to 8.4 times, when two or more close relatives had a family history of osteoporosis.[49] Consequently, individuals identified in these groups should learn how to implement preventive services (such as screenings) prior to being diagnosed with osteoporosis.

The prevention of risk factors can be implemented at three levels, primary, secondary, and tertiary prevention.[47] Primary prevention is the most cost-effective form of health care because it occurs prior to the onset of the disease.[47] The focus of primary prevention is to identify and reduce the risk factors for the development of the disease. Teaching and learning for primary prevention can help avoid the suffering, the cost, and the emotional burden related to the disease. Secondary prevention is not as cost-effective as primary.[47] The main benefit of secondary prevention is its concentration on early detection of health problems, and trying to stop or slow down the progression of the disease.[47] Measures of secondary prevention can include identification and treatment of asymptomatic individuals who have already developed risk factors or preclinical disease;[47] however, these individuals do not clinically exhibit the disease. Teaching and learning for secondary prevention concentrates mostly on convincing the individuals to have screening tests done, such as for hyperlipidemia, hypertension, or breast and prostate cancer. Consequently, the course of an illness can be altered with medications or other early interventions to maximize the person's well-being and minimize suffering. Tertiary prevention is perhaps the least cost-effective because its main goal is attempting to minimize the negative effects of the disease.[47] Although the illness already has occurred and caused damages to an individual, the tertiary prevention measures try to restore the individual's function and prevent complications of the disease. At this point, tertiary prevention activities are already late because the disease is established. Nevertheless, teaching and learning can minimize the impact of the disease. Physical and occupational therapists have a big role in tertiary prevention because they work with patients and clients who have chronic diseases and disabilities. Both forms of rehabilitation are helping individuals minimize disabilities through involvement in lifelong fitness programs.

## PATIENT READINESS TO LEARN ABOUT HEALTH PROMOTION AND DISEASE PREVENTION

Teaching and learning disease prevention and health promotion requires therapists to evaluate each patient's readiness and motivation to follow programs and change behavior. Many individuals may believe they are at risk for various disorders but are not ready to drastically modify their lifestyles. As a result, they will not cooperate with preventative measures. As a general rule, to cooperate with prevention strategies, the individual must understand that his or her current behavior is a serious threat to his or her health.[50,51] Then, the individual should be convinced that the therapist's or other health care provider's recommendations are highly beneficial for him or her.[51] The last step for starting the prevention measures is increasing the individual's certainty that the benefits to change overcome the barriers.[51] The health belief model (HBM) mentioned earlier in this chapter can be applied for health promotion and prevention strategies.[50] As a hypothetical example, a 37-year-old man is more than 100 pounds overweight and also has diabetes and high blood pressure. His perceived susceptibility is that he knows his vulnerability to serious health problems such as a stroke or a heart attack. Although his physician told him that losing weight will probably eliminate his diabetes and hypertension, he was not sure about the perceived severity of the problem. This individual needed to understand the risks associated with being overweight and having high blood pressure and diabetes. The 37-year-old man realized the risks when he had his right big toe amputated due to diabetes. At that time, he recognized the perceived threat from being overweight (having his foot amputated) and the perceived benefits for losing weight. Only then did this individual become convinced that going through a weight loss program (eating less) and buying a membership in a gym (starting a regular exercise program) would be more beneficial than suffering and possibly having another amputation. The financial barriers of paying for the weight loss program and the gym membership did not compare to his pain and suffering and perceived future health risks.

The other model of behavioral change, called the transtheoretical model (TTM), includes five stages of change that can assist the therapist in planning teaching and learning for prevention.[51] For the previous hypothetical example, the 37-year-old man who is overweight and has diabetes and hypertension, the therapist may need to provide preventative teaching and learning considering the individual's motivation in the TTM process of change. In the precontemplation stage, the man is not thinking about making a change and losing weight. He may be resistant to change and may need more information relative to the risk factors for obesity, diabetes, and hypertension. In the precontemplation stage, teaching and learning may need to be customized to the person's specific health risks. The therapist should not criticize or coerce the person but try to build a rapport and explore his health concerns. If the 37-year-old man is in the contemplation phase, he may want to make changes to his condition in the late future (say 6 or 7 months). He may be unsure of how to go about the change. Some days he may want to lose weight and other days he may not. Even if his right toe was amputated, in the contemplation phase, this individual is still unsure about the change. In the contemplation stage, the therapist may need, in a gentle and gradual way, to find a discrepancy between where the person is and where the person wants to be. The therapist may be able to inform the individual that his current behavior is not leading toward significant goals for his future health. This can increase the person's motivation to make changes and lose the weight. In the preparation stage of change, the 37-year-old man may be thinking of taking steps in the near future (in approximately 1 month or sooner). In this phase, teaching and learning has to help the individual consider all options for change (including risks and benefits). In this hypothetical example, the individual may feel that the reason to lose weight is more important than other health risks. In the action stage of change, the man is ready to start the weight loss and the exercise program. He is looking for support from others to implement the behavioral change. Teaching and learning must increase his self-efficacy[51] and enhance his belief about his capability to produce the change. In the maintenance stage of change, this patient needs teaching and learning to sustain his behavioral change and prevent him from going back to his previous, harmful health behavior.

## Delivering Disease Prevention Services in Physical and Occupational Therapy

When delivering disease prevention services, physical and occupational therapists should first assess their current disease prevention practice and identify a specific need for their patient population. For example, practices that involve older adults whose risk factors are falls at home may need to target fall prevention as a topic. Others, who treat adults with impairments secondary to type 2 diabetes, may focus on prediabetes and diabetes prevention education. Also, regardless of the patient population, therapists may have to think about the disease prevention topic based on the needs of their community. The target audience can be older adults, adults, children, school systems, industry and businesses, and other specific populations such as people with type 2 diabetes, hypertension, multiple sclerosis, or other disorders and diseases in need of health education.

The second step in delivering organized prevention services is to develop a preventive care protocol that includes goals and objectives for the program.[52] The purpose of the prevention program should be considered and the general goals identified. Examples of goals could be patient health education, screenings or assessments, or teaching exercise/fitness programs.

The third step of a prevention program is to develop the program.[52] The therapist must identify all the characteristics of the activity[52] in order to make the necessary preparations for its implementation. For example, for a scoliosis screening program, the physical therapist needs to know his or her state's standards in regard to the program. These standards may include screening objectives, the reimbursement policy, and other state regulations. The goals of the screening program have to be related to the physical criteria, health and community resources for referrals, and implementation of educational and informational programs and materials for students, parents (or guardians), children's services personnel, and members of the school district. The educational material for scoliosis screening may need to include (dependent on each state) the legal basis for screening (regulations and/or guidelines), types of scoliosis, treatment and effects of nontreatment, psychological considerations for positive findings, screening techniques (including use of the scoliometer), criteria for referral, reporting, recording and follow-up procedures, organization of the screening program, and current research. The educational material may need written handouts and a Powerpoint/video presentation.[52] The logistics for delivery of the program include the location, parking access, time and length of the screening, the number of people attending, and the necessary cost.[52]

The last stage of the prevention program is to evaluate the results of the educational services that were provided.[52] The audience can evaluate the program. The therapist also can ask for feedback, depending on the number of participants and the length of the session. Additional considerations for a disease prevention program may include development of the written material and determining the optimal pace of the program. As an example, children's screening programs should be less structured and be shorter than those for adults. Older adults involved in an exercise program may have to start slowly and incorporate activities that are important for their everyday routine.

## DISEASE PREVENTION TOPICS FOR PREDIABETES AND DIABETES

Prediabetes is a condition in which blood glucose levels are higher than normal but not high enough to be considered diabetes. In the United States, approximately 56 million Americans currently have this condition, which leaves people at risk not only for developing type 2 diabetes, but also for cardiovascular complications.[53] Furthermore, approximately one of every three persons born in 2000 will develop diabetes in their lifetime.[53] The lifetime risk of developing diabetes is even greater for Native Americans, Asian Americans, Pacific Islanders, African Americans, and Hispanic Americans.[53] Many people with prediabetes are asymptomatic. Prevention for prediabetes is very important because typically, type 2 diabetes cannot be cured but only treated once an individual acquires the disorder. The chance for individuals to have prediabetes is related to two major risk factors, obesity and a sedentary lifestyle.[53] Both of these factors increase the risk of insulin resistance in which tissue, muscle, fat, and liver cells fail to use insulin effectively. With the onset of insulin resistance, the pancreas compensates by producing more insulin. Gradually, the pancreas's capacity to secrete insulin in response to meals weakens and the timing of insulin secretion also becomes abnormal.

Physical and occupational therapists can use teaching and learning strategies promoting lifestyle modifications to prevent prediabetes. People with prediabetes who lose at least 7% of their body weight by engaging in a moderate physical activity for at least 150 minutes weekly can prevent or delay diabetes (returning their blood glucose to normal levels).[53] Changing sedentary lifestyles is one of the most important aspects of preventing prediabetes and delaying type 2 diabetes.[53] In addition to reducing caloric intake (especially fats), increasing physical activity is a must in prediabetes prevention. In physical and occupational therapy, patient or client education should concentrate on teaching the following simple activities:

- Taking the stairs instead of the elevator
- Parking at the far end of the parking lot
- Taking a brisk walk daily

- Doing strengthening exercises with weights three to four times per week
- Creating a patient-specific activity plan with the patient

The patient-specific activity plan can include aerobic conditioning for at least three times per week with no more than two consecutive days without activity; moderate to vigorous intensity aerobics starting at 50% of the maximum heart rate (MHR) and going up to 70% of the MHR; and duration should be at least 150 minutes per week of the moderate (at 50% of the MHR) aerobic activity or 90 minutes per week of vigorous (70% of the MHR) activity.[53] For muscle strengthening activities, the patient or client needs to learn to exercise all major muscle groups three times per week by lifting weights (starting with a weight that cannot be lifted more than 8 to 10 times per set) and progressing accordingly.

New research shows that interval training produces greater changes in exercise capacity than traditional aerobic training.[54,55] From the physiological perspective to improving insulin sensitivity in prediabetes, interval training provides a more powerful stimulus than traditional low-to-moderate intensity aerobic conditioning.[54] Interval training also can help patients with obesity and cardiovascular risk factors such as diastolic hypertension.[55] Interval training involves bouts of high exercise intensity (between 15 seconds and 4 minutes at 90% of the MHR) followed by a recovery period of equal or longer duration than the associated work interval. For example, on a treadmill machine that includes an incline, an individual can walk at a comfortable pace of 3.5 mph for 7 minutes. After that, he or she needs to set the incline at level 2 and also increase the speed to 4.5 mph for only 2 minutes. The individual can alternate a few times the comfortable pace with a high intensity walk. Care must be taken that the person does not experience dizziness or lightheadedness.

For patients who already have diabetes, physical and occupational therapy teaching and learning should focus on the following topics: control of blood pressure (to prevent diabetes complications such as heart disease and stroke, and also eye, kidney, and nerve disorders); control of blood lipids (to reduce cardiovascular complications); early detection of eye disease (to prevent development of vision loss); early detection of kidney disease by lowering blood pressure (to prevent decline in kidney function); and a comprehensive foot care program (to prevent the possibility of peripheral vascular disease and amputation).[26] In regard to the foot care program, the following recommendations should be included in the patient education program:[26]

- Washing feet daily without soaking (in warm, not hot, water)
- Drying feet properly, especially between the toes (to prevent fungal infections)
- Inspecting feet daily for sores, cuts, blisters, redness, or calluses
- Applying lotion (not between the toes) after washing and drying
- Cutting (not too short) toenails weekly or having a foot doctor (podiatrist) cut them
- Asking the podiatrist to check for corns and calluses
- Wearing comfortable-fitting socks (or slippers at home) to protect feet and avoid blisters

- Wearing comfortable-fitting shoes (breaking in shoes slowly)

- Visiting a podiatrist as necessary (to check for circulation and nerve function)

Moreover, patients with diabetes need specific teaching and learning related to their skin care to keep skin hydrated and to avoid fungal infections.[26] Drinking fluids is also very important to keep skin moist and healthy.

## DISEASE PREVENTION TOPICS FOR OLDER ADULTS

Physical and occupational therapists as health care providers need to concentrate their practice efforts in particular areas of concern to older individuals. As discussed in Chapter 18, increasing physical activity for older adults is an important part of physical and occupational therapy. Promotion of physical activity in older adults should avoid ageism that discourages them from reaching their potential. At the same time, physical therapists should recognize that many older patients may not be able to attain high levels of activity. The most important consideration should be helping older adults decrease sedentary behavior and start an exercise program. Some older individuals may be able to perform vigorous activity and high levels of exercise if they already have sufficient strength and experience with exercises; however, the majority of older adults may need to take a gradual approach to activities to minimize risk of injury. It is also important to consider that adults who are deconditioned need activities that require little effort and short duration (5 to 10 minutes at the most) performed a few times during the day. The American College of Sports Medicine (ACSM) includes several recommendations for physical activity of older adults.[56] Generally, the ACSM advises older adults to use a combination of physical activities including aerobic, endurance, strength, balance, and flexibility.[56] This blend of exercises allows healthier benefits than just a single form of movement. Moderate intensity aerobics should be performed 3 to 5 days per week for at least 30 minutes; flexibility, including balance exercises, are needed daily; and strength training is best done 2 to 3 days per week.[56] Additionally, older adults who have one or more medical conditions need to perform activities that also treat their health-related situation. Physical and occupational therapists must plan all the therapeutic activities with the individuals, integrating prevention into the regular physical and occupational rehabilitation interventions.

Another critical area of disease prevention and promotion of physical and occupational therapy is fall prevention for older adults and patients (clients) with disabilities. Falls are the leading cause of injury and accidental death in adults over the age of 65 years.[29] Every year, approximately one in three older adults will suffer a fall.[29] Falls have many causes, which vary from unfamiliar surroundings and improper footwear, to cumbersome furniture arrangements, distractions, or adverse effects of medications combined with age-related physical changes, and various medical conditions.[26] The World Health Organization classified the risk factors for falls in four large categories: biological, behavioral, environmental, and socioeconomic.[57] The biological risk factors may be any or a combination of aging; decline in physical, cognitive, and affective capabilities; and comorbidities associated with chronic illnesses.[57] The behavioral risks may include sedentary lifestyle, side effects of medications, inappropriate footwear, or alcohol use/abuse.[57] The environmental factors could be an interaction of behavioral or biological and environmental hazards.[57] These can be found at home or in public surroundings due to slippery surfaces, narrow steps, uneven sidewalks, or insufficient lighting. The last large group of risk factors, the socioeconomic ones, may include low income and inadequate housing, limited access to medical care, or lack of community resources including patient education.[57]

The majority of falls and fall-related injuries are preventable using fall prevention measures. The proposal from the World Health Organization for fall prevention includes three large strategies: (1) increasing awareness of the importance of fall prevention and interventions, (2) developing research-based assessment tools for determining the risk factors for falls, and (3) facilitating specific research-based fall interventions that are culturally appropriate.[57] In regard to the teaching and learning aspect of fall prevention, it is internationally recognized that patient education is an essential strategy for effective fall interventions. Teaching and learning should be directed at not only older individuals who are at risk for falling, but also health care providers and people responsible for the design and construction of housing and public places used by older adults.[57]

Although health care providers are aware of the importance of preventing falls, it is their responsibility to continuously evaluate their patients' risks for falling and provide the necessary individualized patient and health education as well as support services for prevention and intervention. Physical and occupational therapists have the opportunity to work closely with older adults and are able to assess and improve the biological, behavioral, environmental, and socioeconomic risk factors for falls. For example, physical and occupational therapists and assistants can provide a detailed environmental assessment for each patient and make recommendations to maximize independence and reduce hazards (**Table 19.3**).[2,26]

In a patient's home, the assessment evaluates for clear and unobstructed entryways and hallways (especially if using a wheelchair); accessible furniture arrangement in the living room and bedrooms; installation of handheld shower heads, grab bars, and bath controls in the bathroom; and/or lowering the sink and countertops to accommodate wheelchairs in the kitchen.[26] In many situations, therapists may work with contractors and builders to gradually introduce the necessary changes and train patients to work with the environmental additions for better accommodation.[26] Home environments that are modified for greater accessibility can also promote energy conservation and help with fall prevention.

In addition to environmental modifications, physical therapists can use teaching and learning for older adults to help engage them in a broad range of physical activities that are performed on a regular basis. The physical therapist will need to perform a comprehensive assessment prior to starting an activity program to evaluate range of motion, muscle strength, and sensory integrity.[26] Physical therapists can use various tests and measures to determine the patient's risk of falling. Different tools are available to assess a variety of factors that may contribute to a patient's fall risk. Environmental factors, medications, physical impairments, and/or cardiopulmonary problems should be identified to create a customized plan of activities and exercises. Generally, tailored exercise programs for older adults need to include balance, flexibility, and strengthening programs that can reduce the risk of injuries

| Table 19.3 | **Examples of Recommendations to Prevent Falls at Home**[2,26] |
|---|---|
| Stairways, hallways, and pathways need good lighting (with light switches at the top and bottom of stairs). |
| Walking areas must be uncluttered. |
| All carpets must be fixed firmly to the floor. Nonslip strips should be placed on tile and wooden floors. |
| Stairs must have handrails on both sides (from top to bottom). The handrails should be tightly fastened. |

and falls.[2,26] Dynamic balance activities such as using Tai Chi techniques may be appropriate.[58] Although using Tai Chi to prevent falls is still controversial, this Chinese form of martial arts may help reduce the risk of falls in elderly, frail adults.[58] Institutionalized older adults who were prone to falls that used a Tai Chi exercise program increased their knee and ankle strength as well as their balance, flexibility, and mobility.[58] In addition to physical strength, Tai Chi also enhanced the individuals' confidence in fall avoidance.

Physical and occupational therapists and assistants can actively involve their patients in the fall prevention process so they better understand their personal fall risk factors and intervention priorities. Teaching patients how to identify and solve problems is an important part of physical and occupational therapy interventions. Therapists can use evidence-based research to prioritize and target areas involved in falls. Fall prevention programs should address multiple risk factors. Among these factors, variables such as the patient's medications, vision, assistive devices, and the types of shoes used in ambulation are also important for a comprehensive assessment of falls.[26] The patient must learn that multiple medications can cause dizziness, drowsiness, and balance problems. Consequently, the patient should review his or her medications with the physician and/or pharmacist.[26] Dizziness can also occur with hearing loss. The patient can visit his or her regular physician or an audiologist to check his or her hearing. Poor vision can also reduce postural stability, increasing the risk of falls in older adults. Poor visual acuity, contrast sensitivity, and depth perception can reduce the ability of older adults to detect environmental hazards.[26] Regular (at least yearly) eye examinations are required to check for appropriate prescription glasses. Fall prevention education for older adults must also include the type of shoes they wear at home or outside the home. Well-fitting slippers with nonskid soles are important for avoiding falls at home, especially at night.[26] Good lighting (especially at night) can reduce the chance of falling. Also, adding bright tape strips on stairs and nightlights in bathrooms may increase the individual's safety when visiting the bathroom at night.

Section

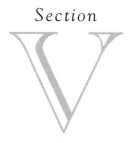

# CONCLUSIONS

## Section V Summary

Section V of this book introduced topics in the area of teaching and learning for motor performance including the significance of motor practice and feedback. Bloom's taxonomy of educational objectives was applied to physical and occupational therapy's teaching of motor tasks. Instructional techniques for home exercise programs for older adults, taking into consideration impairments and functional limitations when designing written materials and Web sites, also were included. Section V concluded with applications of teaching and learning approaches to wellness, health promotion, and disease prevention.

## Section V Case Study

### PATIENT EDUCATION FOR MOTOR LEARNING

Per the APTA's *Guide to Physical Therapist Practice*,[59] the patient physical therapy diagnostic classification pattern is:

Impaired motor function and sensory integrity associated with progressive disorders of the central nervous system

ICD-9-CM Codes: 332 Parkinson's disease

The APTA's *Guide to Physical Therapist Practice*[59] recommendations for patient-related instruction:

Instruction, education, and training of patient and caregivers regarding:

- Current condition (pathology/pathophysiology, impairments, functional limitations, or disabilities)
- Enhancement of performance
- Health, wellness, and fitness programs
- Plan of care
- Risk factors (pathology/pathophysiology, impairments, functional limitations, or disabilities)
- Transitions across settings
- Transitions to new roles

### Patient Description

The patient, Mrs. D., is a 67-year-old woman with a medical diagnosis of idiopathic Parkinson's disease (PD). She was diagnosed with PD 1 year ago. She lives at home with her husband of 35 years. Mrs. D. is a retired pediatrician. The patient's husband is a 75-year-old retired accountant. They have one child who is married and lives in Europe. They like to travel and spend summers in Europe.

Immediately after her diagnosis, Mrs. D. used a new type of medication called Neupro. This medication consisted of a patch that contains rotigotine, a form of dopamine neurotransmitter. Nine months ago, while driving her golf cart, she fell asleep due to side effects of the medication. Rotigotine causes sudden somnolence. The golf cart hit a tree and injured Mrs. D., fracturing her right hip. She required surgery with an open reduction and internal fixation. Postsurgery she received physical therapy. After her accident she refused anti-Parkinsonian medications. This withdrawal of medication caused a reoccurrence of Parkinson symptoms. She decided to commence physical therapy for her Parkinson symptoms.

Currently, Mrs. D. describes her symptoms as slowness and difficulty of movement, especially when getting out of a chair. She also has a slight tremor in both hands while at rest.

Mrs. D.'s primary impairments include shuffling gait, slow speed, and diminished arm swing. Mrs. D. requires gait training. Her physical therapy motor learning will include goals to improve stepping, lengthen stride, broaden base of support, and increase arm swing.

### Guiding Ideas to Prepare a Motor Learning Program Using Fitts and Posner's Stages

- Indicate the motor learning strategies necessary for the cognitive stage (visual practice, feedback, and a controlled environment).

- Indicate the motor learning strategies necessary for the associative phase (proprioceptive cues, self-modifications of skill, using prior learning experience, and using motivation).

- Indicate the motor learning strategies necessary for the autonomous stage (highly organized tasks, simultaneous tasks, and changeable environments).

## General Teaching and Learning Points:

- Evaluate patient's learning style.

- Evaluate patient's motivation for learning.

- Understand patient's medical history, educational level, and personal interests.

- Use patient-centered care.

- Structure the learning environment.

## Specific Points for Cognitive ("What To Do") Stage of Learning:

- The patient tries to form a general understanding of the motor skill.

- The patient gathers the information through observation (visual learning), verbal feedback, and kinesthetically (proprioceptively) through the muscle spindles.

- The patient attempts to define her goal and the general methods for achievement of the goal.

- The patient's performance may be slow and may include errors (uses trial and error).

- The patient may need to practice the motor skill many times.

- The therapist must offer feedback and supervision (especially for patient's safety).

- The environment must be controlled for noise or distractions.

## Specific Points for Associative ("How to Do") Stage of Learning:

- The patient starts to understand how parts of the motor skill relate to each other.

- The patient will make few errors during practice of the skill.

- The patient recognizes and corrects her performance errors.

- The patient uses mostly kinesthetic (proprioceptive) feedback to perfect the skill.

- The patient can modify the skill in relation to the environment.

- The patient may want to integrate the skill in her golf practice.

- The therapist's involvement (including feedback) decreases.

Specific Points for Autonomous ("How To Succeed") Stage of Learning:

- The patient may be able to automatically perform the motor skill.
- The patient may want to practice the skill on the golf course.
- The patient may want to succeed at playing golf again.
- The patient concentrates on environmental details and makes corrections.

# Section V References

1. Shumway-Cook A, Woollacott MH. *Motor Control: Translating Research into Clinical Practice.* 3rd ed. Philadelphia: Lippincott Williams & Wilkins; 2007.
2. Jones JC, Rose DJ. *Physical Activity Instruction of Older Adults.* Champaign, IL: Human Kinetics; 2005.
3. Kisner C, Colby LA. *Therapeutic Exercise: Foundations and Techniques.* 5th ed. Philadelphia: F.A. Davis; 2007.
4. Rothstein JM, Wolf SL, Roy SH. *The Rehabilitation Specialist's Handbook.* Philadelphia: F.A. Davis; 2005.
5. Shepard KF, Jensen GM, eds. *Handbook of Teaching for Physical Therapists.* 2nd ed. Woburn, MA: Butterworth-Heinemann; 2002.
6. O'Sullivan SB, Schmitz TJ. *Physical Rehabilitation.* 5th ed. Philadelphia: F.A. Davis; 2007.
7. Allen Preissler M. Associative learning of pictures and words by low-functioning children with autism. *Autism.* 2008;12(3):231–248.
8. Gentile AM. Implicit and explicit processes during acquisition of functional skills. *Scand J Occup Ther.* 1998;5:7–16.
9. Brown AS. A review of the tip-of-the-tongue experience. *Psychol Bull.* 1991;109(2):204–223.
10. Eldridge LL, Masterman D, Knowlton BJ. Intact implicit learning in Alzheimer's disease. *Behav Neurosci.* 2002;116:722–726.
11. Muslimovic D, Post B, Speelman JD, et al. Motor procedural learning in Parkinson's disease. *Brain.* 2007;130:2887–2897.
12. Osman M, Wilkinson L, Beigi M, et al. Patients with Parkinson's disease learn to control complex systems via procedural as well as non-procedural learning. *Neuropsychol.* 2008;46(9): 2355–2363.
13. Wong TS, Schwartz JL, Karimipour DJ, et al. An education theory-based method to teach a procedural skill. *Arch Dermatol.* 2004;140(11):1357–1361.
14. Gentile AM. A working model of skill acquisition with application to teaching. *Quest.* 1972;17:3–23.
15. Dickstein R, Deutsch JE. Motor imagery in physical therapist practice. *Phys Ther.* 2007; 87(7):942–953.
16. Randal KE, McEwen IR. Writing patient-centered functional goals. *Phys Ther.* 2000;80(12): 1197–1203.
17. Lin CHJ, Sullivan KJ, Wu AD, et al. Effect of task practice order on motor skill learning in adults with Parkinson disease: a pilot study. *Phys Ther.* 2007;87(9):1120–1131.
18. Beekhuizen KS, Field-Fote EC. Sensory stimulation augments the effects of massed practice training in persons with tetraplegia. *Arch Phys Med Rehabil.* 2008;89(4):602–608.

19. Maslovat D, Chua R, Lee TD, et al. Contextual interference: single task versus multi-task learning. *Motor Control.* 2004;8:213–233.

20. Brady F. The contextual interference effect and sport skills. *Percept Motor Skill.* 2008;106(2): 461–472.

21. Jarus T, Gutman T. Effects of cognitive processes and task complexity on acquisition, retention, and transfer of motor skills. *Can J Occup Ther.* 2001;68(5):280–289.

22. Allami N, Paulignan Y, Brovelli A, et al. Visuo-motor learning combination of different rates of motor imagery and physical practice. *Exp Brain Res.* 2008;184(1):105–113.

23. Huang VS, Shadmehr R, Diedrichsen J. Active learning: learning a motor skill without a coach. *J Neurophysiol.* 2008;100(2):879–887.

24. Sullivan KJ, Kantak SS, Burtner PA. Motor learning in children: feedback effects on skill acquisition. *Phys Ther.* 2008;88(6):720–732.

25. Voelcker-Rehage C. Motor-skill learning in older adults—a review of studies on age-related differences. *Eur Rev Aging Phys Activity.* 2008;5(1):5–16.

26. Dreeben O. *Physical Therapy Clinical Handbook for PTAs.* Sudbury, MA: Jones and Bartlett; 2008.

27. Bloom BS. *Taxonomy of Educational Objectives, Handbook I: The Cognitive Domain.* New York: David McKay; 1956.

28. Hagstrom F. Formative learning and assessment. *Commun Disord Q.* 2006;28(1):24–36.

29. Centers for Disease Control and Prevention, Department of Health and Human Services. Healthy aging for older adults. Available at: http://www.cdc.gov. Accessed July 2008.

30. Frontera WR, Slovik DM, Dawson DM, eds. *Exercise in Rehabilitation Medicine.* 2nd ed. Champaign, IL: Human Kinetics; 2006.

31. Dreeben O. *Introduction to Physical Therapy for PTAs.* Sudbury, MA: Jones and Bartlett; 2007.

32. Greiner AC, Knebel E, eds. *Health Professions Education: A Bridge to Quality.* Washington, DC: National Academies Press; 2003.

33. Reo JA, Mercer VS. Effects of live, videotaped, or written instruction on learning an upper-extremity exercise program. *Phys Ther.* 2004;84(7):622–635.

34. Friedrich S, Cermak T, Maderbacher P. The effect of brochure use versus therapist teaching on patients performing therapeutic exercise and changes in impairment status. *Phys Ther.* 1996;76(10):1082–1089.

35. National Institutes of Health. National Institute on Aging. Making your printed health materials senior friendly. Available at: http://www.nia.nih.gov/HealthInformation/Publications/srfriendly.htm. Accessed July 2008.

36. Hazzard W, Blass J, Halter J, Ouslander J, Tinetti M, eds. *Principles of Geriatric Medicine and Gerontology.* 4th ed. New York: McGraw-Hill, Health Professions Division; 1999.

37. Campbell RJ, Nolfi DA. Teaching elderly adults to use the Internet to access health care information: before-after study. *J Med Internet Res.* 2005;7(2):1–19.

38. National Institutes of Health. Senior health: Helping older adults search for health information online: a toolkit for trainers from the National Institute on Aging. Welcome to module 9: evaluating health websites. Available at: http://nihseniorhealth.gov/toolkit/toolkit.html. Accessed July 2008.

39. Charness N, Holley P. The new media and older adults. *Am Behav Sci.* 2004;48(4):416–433.

40. American Occupational Therapy Association. Occupational therapy practice areas for the 21st century. Available at: http://www.aota.org. Accessed August 2008.

41. American Occupational Therapy Association. Occupational therapy's role in prevention and wellness. Available at: http://www.aota.org. Accessed August 2008.

42. American Physical Therapy Association. Public health initiatives resource center. Available at: http://www.apta.org. Accessed August 2008.

43. American Heart Association. STOP Stroke Act. Available at: http://www.americanheart.org/presenter.jhtml?identifier=3010937. Accessed January 2009.

44. The Obesity Society. Obesity statistics: U.S. obesity trends. Available at: http://www.obesity.org/statistics/obesity_trends.asp. Accessed January 2009.

45. Wang Y, Beydoun MA, Liang L, et al. Will all Americans become overweight or obese? Estimating the progression and cost of the U.S. obesity epidemic. *Obesity.* 2008;16(10): 2323–2330.

46. Dodd C. Dodd, Harkin, Bingaman call for new obesity taskforce. Introduce bill to fight obesity epidemic nationwide. July 23, 2008. Available at: http://www.dodd.senate.gov. Accessed July 2008.

47. Craven RF, Hirnle CJ. *Fundamental of Nursing: Human Health and Function.* Philadelphia: Lippincott Williams & Wilkins; 2006.

48. Hemphill-Pearson BJ, ed. *Assessments in Occupational Therapy Mental Health: An Integrative Approach.* 2nd ed. Thorofare, NJ: SLACK; 2008.

49. Centers for Disease Control and Prevention, Department of Health and Human Services. The importance of genomics. Available at: http://www.cdc.gov. Accessed August 2008.

50. Miller W, Heather, N, eds. *Treating Addictive Behaviors.* 2nd ed. New York: Plenum Press; 1999.

51. Glanz K, Rimer BK, Lewis FM, eds. *Health Behavior and Health Education. Theory, Research and Practice.* San Francisco, CA: Wiley & Sons; 2002.

52. British Columbia Ministry of Health Services. GPAC (Guidelines and Protocols Advisory Committee): Guidelines eligible for the condition based incentives. Available at: http://www.bcguidelines.ca/gpac/eligible.html. Accessed August 2008.

53. Centers for Disease Control and Prevention, National Center for Chronic Disease Prevention and Health Promotion. What is prediabetes? Available at: http://www.cdc.gov. Accessed August 2008.

54. Earnest C. Exercise interval training: an improved stimulus for improving the physiology of pre-diabetes. *Med Hypotheses.* 2008;71(5):752–761.

55. Schjerve IE, Tyldum GA, Tjønna AE, et al. Both aerobic endurance and strength training programmes improve cardiovascular health in obese adults. *Clin Sci.* 2008; 115(9):283–293.

56. Nelson ME, Rejeski WJ, Blair SN, et al. Physical activity and public health in older adults: recommendation from the American College of Sports Medicine and the American Heart Association. *J Am Coll Sports Med.* 2007;1–11. Available at: http://www.acsm-msse.org. Accessed August 2008.

57. World Health Organization. Ageing and life course. Family and community health. *WHO Global Report on Fall Prevention in Older Age.* 2007;1–53. Available at: http://www.who.int. Accessed August 2008.

58. Choi JH, Moon JS, Song R. Effects of Sun-style Tai Chi exercise on physical fitness and fall prevention in fall-prone older adults. *J Adv Nurs.* 2005;51(2):150–157.

59. American Physical Therapy Association. *Guide to Physical Therapist Practice.* 2nd ed. Alexandria, VA: APTA; 2001.

# GLOSSARY

**ACSM**   The American College of Sports Medicine is an international organization that promotes scientific research, education, and practical applications of sports medicine; its goal is to preserve and improve individuals' physical performance, health, fitness, and quality of life. Physical and occupational therapists can be members of the ACSM.

**adherence behavioral strategies**   Adjusting interventions to patients' routines and lifestyles to increase patients' adherence; using reminders or cues for interventions (such as emails, phone calls, or cards); creating written/verbal contracts.

**affective domain**   Learning domain that is part of Bloom's taxonomy of learning. In the affective domain of learning, the learner deals with new information emotionally. This domain may include feelings, values, appreciation, enthusiasms, motivations, and attitudes.

**AMA**   The American Medical Association is the national organization of physicians, residents, and medical students. It promotes the art and science of medicine including public health; establishes and supports ethical, educational, and clinical standards for the medical profession; and advocates for the integrity of the physician–patient relationship.

**ambivalence**   A state of having emotions (positive and negative) or of having thoughts or actions in contradiction with each other when they are related to the same object, idea, or person. The term is also commonly used when a person experiences uncertainty or indecisiveness concerning something.

**andragogy**   The process of engaging adult learners in the learning experience; in the 21st century, the term defines an alternative to pedagogy and refers to learner-focused education for people of all ages.

**AOTA**    The American Occupational Therapy Association is the national professional association of occupational therapy practitioners and students. Its goal is to improve the quality of occupational therapy services. Its centennial (by 2017) vision for the occupational therapy profession is to become a powerful, science-driven and evidence-based, widely recognized, and globally connected (including a diverse workforce) organization.

**APTA**    The American Physical Therapy Association is the national professional association representing and promoting the profession of physical therapy. Its goal is to advance physical therapy practice, research, and education. Its mission is to further the role of physical therapy in diagnosis and treatment of movement dysfunctions, prevention, and enhancement of the physical health and functional abilities of members of the public.

**associative learning**    A form of learning in which the response becomes associated with a particular stimulus; learning is based on the relationship between two stimuli or between a stimulus and a behavior. Examples of associative learning are classical and operant conditioning.

**Bandura principle**    A principle stating that most human behavior is learned observationally through modeling. It promotes an individual's learning by observing others' behavior and attitudes, and the outcomes of those behaviors. It is used in schools and in clinical situations. Effective modeling requires attention, retention, reproduction, and motivation. Modeling is also the basis for explaining a variety of behaviors in children.

**basic patient communication objectives**    Informing the patient about his or her condition and methods of intervention; educating patients by using proper teaching and learning techniques; addressing patient understanding; and ensuring that the patient has future access to the information.

**behaviorism**    Learning theories based on behavioral psychology stating that behaviors are acquired through conditioning. In behaviorism, there are only two ways to change behavior and encourage learning: classical (Pavlovian) conditioning and operational conditioning.

**beneficence**    A moral obligation to promote good and prevent or remove harm; to promote the welfare, health, and safety of society and individuals in accordance with their beliefs, values, preferences, and life goals.

**bioethics**    The philosophical study of the ethical controversies brought about by advances in biology and medicine; an applied form of ethics incorporated into allied health professional ethics.

**Bloom's taxonomy of learning**    A design and evaluation tool for training and learning. The taxonomy is a system of categories of learning behaviors to assist in the design and assessment of American education. Bloom's taxonomy classifies instructional activities as they progress in difficulty. It includes six learning levels: knowledge, comprehension, application, analysis, synthesis, and evaluation.

**brain-dominance learning theory**    A learning theory explaining that individuals use different sides of their brain to process different kinds of information.

**CAPTE**   The Commission on Accreditation in Physical Therapy Education is the only accreditation agency recognized by the U.S. Department of Education and the Council for Higher Education Accreditation to accredit entry-level physical therapist and physical therapist assistant education programs. The CAPTE's mission is to serve the public by establishing and applying standards that assure quality and continuous improvement in the entry-level preparation of physical therapists and physical therapist assistants, and that reflect the evolving nature of education, research, and practice.

**care ethics**   Also called ethics of care; it is a normative ethical theory about what makes actions right or wrong. Care ethics draws from the traditional female experiences of care-giving and being partial toward persons who have needs and vulnerability. The funda-mental moral commitments of care ethics expand the aims of medical practice to include caring and trying to cure patients, and the willingness to maintain a continual relationship with these patients. Care ethics contrasts with deontological and teleological ethics, which stress the importance of universal standards and impartiality.

**CARF**   The Commission on Accreditation of Rehabilitation Facilities is an interna-tional, nonprofit organization that provides rigorous accreditation standards and surveyors for organizations working in the human services field worldwide. Among the many areas of practice represented in the CARF standards are aging services; behavioral health, which includes psychosocial rehabilitation and assertive community treatment; child and youth services; employment and community services; medical rehabilitation (including physical and occupational); and opioid treatment programs.

**CDC**   The Centers for Disease Control and Prevention is an American agency charged with tracking and investigating public health trends. The CDC's mission is to promote health and quality of life by preventing and controlling disease, injury, and disability.

**classical conditioning**   A form of associative learning (also called Pavlovian); has to do with conditioning of behaviors that were elicited from an association between two stim-uli. Classical conditioning involves involuntary, reflexive behaviors.

**cognitive domain**   Learning domain that is part of Bloom's taxonomy of learning. In this domain, the learner deals with new information by increasing his or her knowledge and developing theoretical skills.

**cognitivism**   Learning theories based on cognitive psychology; learning cannot be described in terms of a change in behavior because behavior is not a factor of learning. Cognitivism uses the learner's internal mental processes to help him or her increase cognitive structur-ing. The learner is viewed as an information processor, similar to a computer. Information comes in, is processed, and leads to certain outcomes. Any previous experience and knowl-edge may augment the process of learning.

**communication skills for increased adherence**   Communication skills used by the health care provider to understand the patient's perspective on a disease, its causes, and its possi-ble interventions, and as a result, to increase the patient's adherence with interventions. These may include carefully listening to the patient's replies and trying to pick up clues to the patient's understanding as well as his or her ability to adhere to a recommended intervention.

**communication strategies**    Strategies suggested to be used in physical and occupational therapy to improve communication with the patient or client. Communication strategies may include expressing empathy, avoiding argumentation, developing discrepancy between the patient's behavior and important personal goals, involving family members, referring the patient to a support group, using motivational interviewing (to increase self-efficacy and confidence), recognizing small positive steps the patient is taking, using supportive statements, helping the patient set reasonable and reachable goals, and expressing the belief that the patient can achieve the goals.

**concept words**    Describe a general idea or an abstract framework. Patients can often misunderstand concept words in written material.

**confidentiality**    Relates to the concept of privacy and protection of privileged information; refers to an ethical and legal principle associated with several professions including the ones in physical and occupational therapy. In regard to medical information, confidentiality is the right of the patient to have personal, identifiable medical information kept private.

**consequentialism**    Also known as utilitarianism; an ethical theory stating that the consequences of a particular action form the basis for any valid moral judgment about that action; that the moral worth of an action is solely determined by its contribution to its overall utility in maximizing happiness among all persons. Thus, from a consequentialist standpoint, a morally right action is one that produces a good outcome, or consequence.

**constructivism**    Learning theories stating that knowledge is uniquely constructed by each individual. Constructivism is based on a combination of cognitive psychology and operant conditioning theory within behavioral psychology. The basic premise is that learning (cognition) is the result of mental construction. Learners learn by fitting new information together with what they already know. As a result, learners must actively build knowledge and skills.

**COTA**    A Certified Occupational Therapist Assistant (also known as an occupational therapy assistant) works under the direction of the occupational therapist; provides rehabilitative services to individuals with physical, mental, or developmental impairments.

**cultural competence** An awareness of, sensitivity to, and knowledge of the meaning of culture. It includes openness and willingness to learn about cultural issues and the ability to understand one's own biases, values, attitudes, beliefs, and behaviors.

**debriefing**    Used in learning theories to facilitate the cognitive process of learning by promoting discussion and reflection of the information that was learned.

**declarative learning**    Also called explicit learning; an active process in which people seek out the structure of any information presented to them. Declarative learning requires attention, awareness, and reflection. Declarative learning is an analytical, language-based, and memory-dependent approach to acquiring and retaining knowledge.

**deontological ethics**   Focuses on the rightness or wrongness of an action as opposed to the rightness or wrongness of the consequences of those actions. It is a form of ethics based on the duty or obligation of the action.

**divine command theory**   States that ethical standards depend solely on God. Any act that conforms to the law of God is right whereas acts that break God's law are wrong.

**effective listening skills**   Listening with undivided attention to the other person. Effective listening skills may involve using verbal and nonverbal expressions when listening, acknowledging the other person's whole message, checking with the other person about the meaning of the message, and asking the other person questions to clarify their meaning.

**ethical relativism**   Promotes the idea that all moral principles are equally valid relative to cultural preferences.

**experiential learning theory**   A form of education that occurs as a direct participation in life events. This form of learning involves a direct encounter with the phenomena being studied. It may include the following steps: setting a positive climate for learning, clarifying the learner's purposes, organizing and making available learning resources, sharing feelings and thoughts with learners (but not dominating them), and balancing intellectual and emotional components of learning.

**Flesch-Kincaid formula**   A readability formula; translates the formula's 0–100 score to a U.S. grade level, making it easier for teachers, parents, librarians, and others to judge the readability level of various books and texts.

**fundamental literacy skills**   Skills concerning understanding the meaning of information found in applications, forms, graphs, or schedules. Fundamental literacy skills can be categorized as prose literacy (understanding the meaning of information found in newspapers, books, magazines, or online) and quantitative literacy (understanding the meaning and being able to use basic and advanced mathematical operations).

**generalizability**   A statistical theory regarding generalizing about the findings of a research study. In research, generalizability is a framework for conceptualizing, investigating, and designing reliable observations for studies.

**generalizability in motor learning**   The transfer of learned information from one environment to another. It is used to examine the application of a learned skill to other similar tasks without practice.

**Gunning Fog Formula**   Determines the readability level of materials between fourth grade and college. It is considered one of the easier methods for calculating material readability.

**habituation**   Causes a decrease in a response due to a harmful or noxious stimulus. In physical therapy, habituation training can be used as an intervention for certain cases of dizziness and balance impairments caused by benign paroxysmal positional vertigo (BPPV).

**health education**   Planned, systematic, sequential (if necessary), and logical process of teaching and learning provided to individuals, groups, and/or communities for wellness, prevention, and health promotion. The focus of health education in physical and occupational rehabilitation is based on societal needs to change and improve health behaviors.

**health literacy**    The degree to which individuals have the capacity to obtain, process, and understand basic health information and services necessary to make appropriate health decisions.

**health promotion**    The science and art of helping individuals change their lifestyle to move toward a state of optimal health.

**HEP**    The home exercise program is a combination of specific exercises and activities planned by therapists for their patients. HEP reinforces clinical interventions and also contributes to patient's continuum of care (after discharge from therapy). HEP consists of exercise booklets, customized written instructions/drawings, or/and computer-generated information and drawings.

**humanistic learning theory**    Promotes the learner's feelings, choice, freedom, and motivation. The theory states that feeling positive about oneself facilitates the learning process. As a teaching trend, the humanistic theory was created as a reaction against scientific reductionism, which explained everything on the basis of science.

**information processing theory**    Studies cognition and cognitive development in relation to the reasoning processes of the mind. These processes are considered similar to a computer. To learn something new, learners must focus on new information, compare the new information with the old, and create new mental groupings for the new information. The theory includes four major learning stages: attention, processing, memory storage, and action.

**informed consent**    Requires the health care professional and provider to describe all relevant treatment options to the patient, noting the benefits and risks.

**Joint Commission**    An independent, not-for-profit organization that accredits and certifies more than 15,000 health care organizations and programs in the United States. The Joint Commission accreditation and certification is recognized nationwide as a symbol of quality that reflects an organization's commitment to meeting certain performance standards. Its mission is to continuously improve the safety and quality of care provided to the public through the provision of health care accreditation and related services that support performance improvement in health care organizations. (Formerly the Joint Commission on Accreditation of Healthcare Organizations, JCAHO.)

**justice**    In health care, a bioethical principle that a health care provider distributes equal and fair interventions.

**knowledge of performance**    Refers to feedback that gives the patient specific information on how a movement is performed or gives a correction to the specific movement.

**knowledge of results**    Refers to feedback regarding how well the overall task attempt was performed.

**Kolb's cycle of learning**    David Kolb's experiential learning theory stating that learning is a continuous process. The theory includes four distinct learning styles or preferences, which are based on four dynamic learning cycles: concrete experience, reflective observation, abstract conceptualization, and active experimentation.

**learning environment**   Physical and psychological variables contributing to teaching and learning. Physical variables are represented by a classroom or a room where teaching and learning takes place. Psychological variables are represented by surrounding environment such as light, temperature, sound, and student's own variables (such as hunger, thirst, boredom, or illness). In health care, the learning environment must be physically and psychologically comfortable for learners, especially for adult learners.

**LEP**   Limited English proficiency; language difficulties found in some individuals learning English as a second language. These difficulties do not in themselves constitute language impairments.

**locus of control**   Defined by psychologists as an individual's generalized expectations concerning control over future events. It refers to a person's belief about what causes the good or bad results in his or her life. It can be either internal (meaning the person believes he or she controls his or her own life) or external (meaning the person believes the environment, a higher power, or other people controls his or her life).

**Maslow's Hierarchy of Needs**   A humanistic form of learning proposed by Abraham Maslow. He believed that learning is not an end in itself; it is the means to progress towards self-development, which he called self-actualization. In order to learn and develop, an individual must meet all his or her levels of needs to progress to self-actualization. These needs start with physiological ones and end with competency, confidence, independence, prestige, and full use of talents and capacities. Learning can contribute to a person's psychological health.

**motivation**   A psychological force that moves a person to take action in the direction of meeting a need or goal.

**motivational interviewing in patient education**   A directive, patient-centered counseling style to elicit behavioral change by helping patients to explore and resolve their ambivalence.

**motor control**   A person's ability to regulate or direct the mechanisms needed for movement to occur. Brain structures and complex processes of cognition, perception, and environment must work harmoniously together to produce smooth movements and actions for a particular task.

**motor learning**   A system of internal processes working together to obtain relatively permanent changes in an individual's ability to perform a skillful task. It includes acquisition and retention of a skilled movement. Motor learning is also the interval process or state reflecting a person's current capability for producing a particular movement

**motor learning (stages of)**   Created by Fitts and Posner as a three-stage model; includes cognitive, associative, and autonomous stages. The three stages are considered the classical representation of motor learning.

**motor performance**   Includes only acquisition of a skilled movement; it is the most frequent measure of learning that assesses temporary acquisition of a skill.

**motor skills**    Tasks individuals demonstrate when performing movements. The basic characteristics of motor skills are: (1) there must be an achievable goal; (2) the skill must be voluntarily performed; and (3) body movements must take place to achieve the goal.

**multiple intelligences**    An educational theory developed by psychologist Howard Gardner. It describes an array of different kinds of intelligences exhibited by human beings. Gardner originally identified seven main intelligences: linguistic, logical-mathematical, spatial, bodily-kinesthetic, musical, interpersonal, and intrapersonal; he later added the naturalistic intelligence. The theory suggests that schools should offer student-centered education to help students develop the intelligences in which they may be weaker.

**negligence**    Conduct that is culpable because it falls short of what a reasonable person would do to protect another individual from possible risks of harm; a health care provider's conduct that falls below the standard established by the law for the protection of others.

**neuroethics**    The subcategory of bioethics concerned with neuroscience and neurotechnology; combines neuroscience with ethical and social issues of the 21st century.

**nonassociative learning**    Also called single event learning; the most basic form of learning. It requires a single stimulus (repeated frequently) for the learning to take place. There are two simple forms of nonassociative learning, habituation and sensitization.

**nonmaleficence**    Involves refraining from action that might harm others.

**numeracy**    To be able to read and interpret numbers. Persons having limited literacy skills also have limited numeracy abilities.

**older adults**    Those 65 years of age or older. They are the most rapidly growing U.S. demographic. By 2030, the number of older Americans will double to approximately 70 million.

**operant conditioning**    An associative and trial and error type of learning. It requires a voluntary behavior. In operant conditioning, a behavior produces events. The events can be rewarding experiences or negative experiences. The behavior changes as a result of such events. If the consequences of a behavior are pleasant, the preceding behavior becomes more frequent. If the consequences are unpleasant, the behavior will diminish and in some cases will become extinct.

**OT**    An occupational therapist is a health care provider who helps patients improve their ability to perform tasks in living and working environments. The OT works with individuals who suffer from a physically, mentally, developmentally, or emotionally disabling condition. Occupational therapists use treatments to recover, develop, or maintain the daily living and work skills of their patients.

**patient autonomy**    The capability and right of patients to control the course of their own medical treatment and participate in the treatment decision-making process. Autonomy gives the patient the right to refuse or choose their treatment.

**patient-centered care**    A form of health care management that considers patients (and their loved ones) an integral part of the care team who collaborate with health care professionals in making clinical decisions. As partners in care, patients are involved in the planning process and encouraged to take responsibility for their own health. Patient-centered care also considers patients' cultural traditions, their personal preferences and values, their family situations, and their lifestyles.

**patient education**   Planned, systematic, sequential, and logical process of teaching and learning provided to patients and clients in all clinical settings. The focus of patient education in physical and occupational rehabilitation is based on the patient's examination, evaluation, and plan of care.

**patient empowerment**   Involves educating and encouraging patients to expand their role in their decision-making health-related behaviors and self-management of care.

**patient satisfaction**   A general concept that reflects the overall experience of an individual receiving examination and treatment in a specific environment in a particular period of time.

**pedagogy**   A teacher-centered style of teaching that places the student in a submissive role requiring obedience to the teacher's instructions.

**predictors of adherence in patient education**   Psychological factors such as motivation, self-efficacy, and locus of control.

**presbycusis**   Loss of auditory acuity and sensitivity as a result of aging.

**presbyopia**   Loss of visual acuity and sensitivity as a result of aging.

**procedural learning**   Also called implicit learning; learning tasks that can be performed automatically (without conscious thinking). It can be acquired gradually through repetition of motor tasks. This form of learning does not require awareness, attention, and higher order cognitive processes. Procedural learning of motor tasks can last longer than declarative (or explicit) learning, to the point where the individual can lose the ability to explain how to perform the task. It can be used to learn motor activities such as riding a bike, swimming, touch-typing, or playing a musical instrument.

**psychomotor domain for motor tasks**   Learning domain that is part of Bloom's taxonomy of learning. The learner uses new information to try to execute a simple skill or part of a skill.

**PT**   A physical therapist is a health care provider who helps to restore function, improve mobility, relieve pain, and prevent or limit permanent physical disabilities of patients suffering from injuries or disease. The physical therapist restores, maintains, and promotes overall fitness and health.

**PTA**   The physical therapist assistant helps the physical therapist to provide treatment that improves patient mobility, relieves pain, and prevents or lessens physical disabilities of patients. The physical therapist assistant performs a variety of physical therapy tasks under the direction and supervision of a physical therapist.

**reinforcement**   To be able to cause the same response again or the strengthening of a response. In learning, reinforcement can be an event that increases the likelihood that a given response will recur again. For reinforcement to occur in learning, the learner always needs specific knowledge of learning results (feedback) and reward for learning.

**retention**    In learning, it is the act of retaining information. Retention is affected by the degree of first-time learning process. If the student did not learn the material well initially, he or she will not retain it well either. Participants' retention is directly affected by their amount of practice during the learning process.

**retention test in motor learning**    Test used during motor practice; can evaluate an individual's motor performance in the same environment in which the individual originally learned the motor skill. Retention test in motor learning can assess acquisition of a motor skill.

**self-efficacy**    A person's belief or confidence in his or her ability to succeed at making a change.

**sensitization**    A form of training totally opposite to habituation. Sensitization causes an increased response due to a harmful or noxious stimulus. In physical therapy, sensitization may be used to increase a patient's sensitivity to a threatening stimulus in order to enhance his or her awareness of the stimulus. This form of training may be necessary to reduce the possibility of accidental falls in older individuals.

**SMOG readability formula**    Can be used by comparing the total number of words containing three or more syllables with the SMOG conversion table. This is one of the most common and easy-to-use readability formulas.

**Social Learning Theory**    Explains human behavior in terms of continuous reciprocal interaction among cognitive, behavioral, and environmental influences.

**Stages of Change Model (SCM)**    Originally developed in the late 1970s and early 1980s by James Prochaska and Carlo DiClemente when they were studying how smokers were able to give up their addiction. The idea is that behavior change does not happen in one step, but progresses through different stages of change. Individuals must decide by themselves when a stage is completed and when it is time to move on to the next stage. Their decision must come from the inside. The stages of change are precontemplation, contemplation, preparation, action, maintenance, and relapse.

**syllogism**    A form of deductive reasoning that explains a notion from the general to the specific.

**teleological ethics**    Also called consequentialism or utilitarianism (see *consequentialism*); states that the moral worth of an action is solely determined by its contribution to its overall utility in maximizing happiness among all persons.

**transfer test in motor learning**    Evaluation of motor performance in a different environment than where practice occurred.

**transference**    The learner's ability to use the information taught in a new setting. Transference can be positive and negative. Positive transference occurs when the learner is able to apply a taught behavior to another task. Negative transference occurs when the learner is not able to apply a taught behavior to another task.

**value judgment words**    Words describing the amount or threshold for action. Value judgment words are difficult to comprehend and should not be used in written patient education materials. Examples in rehabilitation: asking a patient to exercise "regularly" or not to lift anything "heavy" without explaining the meaning of these two value judgment words.

**variables affecting patient satisfaction**   Establishment of a sense of trust between the patient and the health care provider, perceptive listening and careful observation of small details that give a glimpse into the life of the patient, and determining the patient's needs.

**veracity**   Also called truthfulness; an ethical principle that promotes honesty and telling the truth. Veracity binds both the health care provider and the patient in an association of truth. The patient must tell the truth to receive the appropriate health care. The health care provider must disclose factual information so the patient can exercise his or her personal autonomy.

**virtue ethics**   Focuses on helping people develop good character traits, such as kindness and generosity. These character traits will, in turn, allow a person to make correct decisions later in life.

**wellness**   A person being in good physical and emotional health and appreciating and enjoying their good health.

**written interaction**   Written material that encourages individuals to better learn the material. Examples of written interaction: writing a short question and asking the individual to write the answer; asking the person a few questions and requesting answers.

# INDEX